FLASH REVIWE

FOR THE CLINICAL BOARD EXAM
OF ANESTHESIA AND INTENSIVE
CARE

Dr. AYMAN H. SULTAN
Consultant Anesthesia

Co-Authored by:

Dr. ATIF M. SAIT
Consultant anesthesia

Dr. TAREEF N. ASHOUR
Consultant anesthesia

Dr. AHMAD F. BOGARI
Consultant anesthesia

Dr. FAYEZ A. MAHMOUD
Consultant anesthesia

Dr. ABDULKHALEK A. ABDULJALEEL
Consultant anesthesia

Dr. MOHAMMAD A. NYAZ
Consultant anesthesia

Reviewed and Edited By:

Dr. FAYEZ A. MAHMOUD

Contents:

Preface

During my preparation for the final exam of Anesthesia and Critical Care board I had a lot of long cases as a mock exam with the senior regional pioneer consultants in the field and I collected information about these cases as much as I could in a simple way to be reviewed easily and effectively in short time before the exam.

After the exam, I noticed that these notes were of a great help to achieve the success, so I decided to make them available in a professional way for me as quick refreshment source and for other's those planning to have clinical exam in this specialty as concise review material.

As I am now an anesthesia and critical care consultant and the residents training program director, I reviewed this information again from other prospects and involved some of well-known colleagues to review as well to have theiropinions and input in the materials.

I hope this book will help you in your preparation and I hope by that to help the future colleagues in many other clinical viva exams.

Best regards for all.

Dr. Ayman H. Sultan

Abdominal Aortic Aneurism

High risk surgery with the potential for perioperative complications including cardiac and renal effects

1. Potential for large fluid shifts, temperature fluctuations, blood loss and hemodynamic instability requiring invasive monitoring and vasoactive medications.
2. Hemodynamic, metabolic, and end-organ effects of aortic clamping/unclamping with potential for ischemic insults to the heart, brain, kidneys, and spinal cord
3. Comorbid disease (Coronary Artery Disease, Diabetes, Chronic Kidney Disease, HTN, Smoking, Advanced age…etc.)
4. Post-operative pain management

Anesthetic Goals/Conflicts:

- Optimize perioperative myocardial O_2 supply-demand relationship by
    - minimizing hemodynamic changes associated with aortic clamping and unclamping
    - minimizing stress response to induction. emergence, and post-operative pain
- Minimize distal ischemic complications specifically:
  - renal dysfunction - visceral ischemia - spinal cord ischemia
- Adequate post-operative pain control

History: Determine comorbidities, assess end organ perfusion status, identify clinical risk factors, and functional capacity

PE: Assess peripheral pulses, BP, U/O. Focussed cardiopulmonary exam, document neuro-deficits

Investigations: CBC, Coagulation, electrolytes, ECG/Echo as per AHA guidelines/CT for aneurysm anatomy/X-clamp location

Optimization:

For ruptured: optimize volume, HGb, cross match, coagulation.
Elective: cardiology consultation for risk stratification, consider Beta blockers for intermediate or high-riskpatients, hold ACEi. Discontinue ASA/Plavix/Coumadin and bridge as necessary. Consider Endo-Vascular Aneurism Repair for high-risk patients not tolerating open procedure. Consider autologous blood donation or ANH

Anesthetic Options: GA for elective cases, Avoid epidural in unstable hemodynamics (nomorbidity/ mortality benefit). GA / Regional for EVAR.

Room Setup: 5-lead, temperature monitoring, foley, 4U PRBCs, fluid warmers, cell-saver, invasive lines, vasopressors, antihypertensives, forced air warmers. PAC/TEE if severe Left Ventricular dysfunction or supra-celiac X-clamp.

Intraoperative Management: Stable induction, have patient prepared and surgeon available if ruptured. Prior to X-clamp, minimize fluids, give heparin 100U/kg. Mannitol .25g/kg prior to cross clamp for renal protection. May need afterload reduction (BB/NTG/↑anesthetic) if high X-clamp, distal perfusion techniques. Anticipate hypotension with clamp release, volume resuscitation, ↓anesthetic, pressors, reverse heparin.

Post-operative: Ventilate if ruptured/large fluid shifts, pulmonary comorbidities, obese esp. with supra-celiac clamp. Otherwise extubate, HDU.

Timing of procedure: Between 5.5-6.0 cm, risk of surgery = 1 year risk of rupture, clear benefit > 6.0 cm. 1 year risk of rupture = 9.4%, 10.2%, 32.5% for aneurysms bw 5.5-5.9 cm, 6.0-6.9cm and > 7.0cm respectively.

Achondroplasia

1. Potential difficult airway
    a. difficult BMV, subglottic stenosis, facial anomalies, cervical spine instability (odontoid hypoplasia)
2. Neurologic complications:
    a. Spinal stenosis, hydrocephalus (cervical kyphoscoliosis)
3. Cardiopulmonary complications
    a. Kyphoscoliosis, OSA and central sleep apnea, RLD with Cor-pulmonale
4. Difficult neuraxial anesthesia: kyphoscoliosis, narrow epidural space, prolapsed discs, deformed vertebral bodies
5. Difficult IV access, monitoring and positioning

Anesthetic Goals/Conflicts:

- Safe establishment of airway
- Identification and optimization of cardiorespiratory complications
- Goals for pHTN if applicable

1. Potential difficult intubation and ventilation
    - Large tongue, mandibular hypertrophy, thickened vocal cords, glottic stenosis
2. Potential for increased ICP, brain mass, pituitary tumor
3. Coexisting Disease
    - Cardiac dysfunction: HTN, LVH, diastolic dysfunction, acromegalic cardiomyopathy; Conduction defects; CAD
    - Respiratory: OSA in 70% of males with potential for RV failure (Cor pulmonale)
    - CNS: Susceptible to peripheral neuropathies → ensure correct positioning
    - Miscellaneous.: Glucose intolerance; vascular ischemia (hand) Osteoporosis; Osteoarthritis
4. Postoperative: Post-extubation subglottic edema

Anesthetic Goals/Conflicts:

- Optimize perioperative endocrine function (stress dose steroids), consult endocrinology
- Assess and manage any increase in ICP, avoid aggravating factors
- Provide still field for microscopic surgery
- Controlled emergence (minimizing bucking / coughing / vomiting to decrease risk of bleeding and CSF leakage)
- Monitor for postoperative complications e.g.: DI, SIADH

Addison's Disease (Adrenal Insufficiency)

1. Potential life-threatening Addisonian crisis
   - Shock, dehydration, hypotension, anorexia, acute abdomen, hypoglycemia, fever
   - Highest risk postoperatively
2. Cardiovascular abnormalities
   - Hypotension with decrease SVR and LV stroke index
   - Cardiac conduction abnormalities d/t hyperkalemia
   - Hypovolemia (2-3L)
3. Electrolyte imbalance
   - Hyponatremia, Hyperkalemia, Hypoglycemia
4. Pharmacologic considerations
   - Risk of hyperkalemic arrest with succinylcholine
   - Decreased respiratory response to circulating catecholamines
5. Perioperative steroid replacement

Anesthetic Goals/Conflicts:

- Anticipate and prevent cardiovascular collapse secondary to Addisonian crisis with appropriate supplemental steroid dosing
- Pre-operative correction of fluid and electrolyte abnormalities

History and examination: Assess disease severity (dental caries, reduced exercise tolerance, postural hypotension, arrhythmia, hypovolemia, muscle weakness, fatigue, abdominal pain, N/V, anorexia, confusion, seizures, weight loss, azotemia, hyperpigmentation, hypoglycemia, infections)
Assess the adequacy of steroid replacement – 20mg/d prednisone x 5 days atrisk for HPA suppression (5-20/d x 4 weeks)

Investigations: CBC, Electrolytes, BUN / Cr, ACTH stimulation test

Optimization: -Correct electrolytes abnormalities,
-Steroids – hydrocortisone 300mg/d (adequate mineralocorticoid activity) – add fludrocortisones 0.05-0.1 mg/d PO once hydrocortisone is tapered to 15-20 mg PO q am and 5-10 mg PO q pm
- IV fluids (NS or D5/NS) 2-3 L or more. - Identify and correct precipitating factor

Anesthetic Options: Local, regional, general

Anesthetic Setup: Standard emergency drugs, Hydrocortisone, consider arterial and PAC catheterization if cardiac filling pressures indicated or in major surgery

Management of Anesthesia: No specific anesthesia regimen superior, avoid etomidate (adrenal suppression), Myocardial sensitivity to drugs (narcotics / barbiturates), Muscle weakness / weight loss may require a reduction in muscle relaxant dose, may not seechanges in Heart Rate despite decreased SVR, Check electrolytes, glucose intraoperatively; emergence may be prolonged.

Post-operative: CXR for pneumothorax if adrenalectomy (up to 20%), Pancreatitis risk with left adrenalectomy, Consider ICU d/t risk of Addisonian crisis postoperatively, monitor for respiratory weakness post-operatively.

Anaphylaxis

1- Considerations for the pediatric patient (physiology, pharmacokinetics, cooperation)

2- **Potential difficult intubation and/or ventilation**

a. dynamic airway status as patient grows or disease progresses

3- Possible co-existing Pathology

a. Potential aspiration risk
b. Potential for unstable or immobile cervical spine
c. Developmental Delay
d. Obstructive sleep apnea
    i. pHTN and cor-pulmonale
e. hydrocephalus with increase. ICP
f. Multiple congenital anomalies
    i. Congenital Heart Disease
    ii. Metabolic D/O – hypoglycemia

Anesthetic Goals/Conflicts:

iii.

1. Identify co-existing Pathology:
    - Difficult intubation / ventilation; Aspiration risk; Cervical spine stability; Presence of OSA; Associated anomalies
2. Plan airway management
    - Appropriate equipment & personnel
    - Minimize anesthetic related post-operative respiratory depression

Goal of Pre-operative assessment is to identify pre-existing pathology

Hx: Determine airway anomaly and Associated syndromes, assess for aspiration risk, OSA, unstable c-spine, Associated conditions (developmental delay, hydrocephalus, congenital cardiac disease)

PE: Careful airway exam. Predictors of difficult BMV (midface hypoplasia, macroglossia), predictors ofdifficult intubation. Cardiac examination – CHD, pHTN. Check for ease of IV access.

Investigations: Dictated by procedure. Glucose of neonate. Consider c-spine x-rays for stability, ECHO to rule out congenital cardiac disease. Sleep study/oximetry if suspected OSA.

Optimization: Aspiration prophylaxis if appropriate (ranitidine 0.5 mg/kg IV; metoclopramide 0.1 mg/kg) no pre-operative sedation if risk of airway obstruction, anti-sialagogue (glycopyrrolate 5-10mcg/kg or atropine 10-20 mcg/kg).

Room Setup: Standard monitors and IV placed prior to induction or airway management. Preoxygenate if possible. Difficult airway cart. Consider ENT specialist in the room, neck prepped and draped, rigid bronchoscopy.

Induction: Awake vs. SV induction (Inhalational vs. TIVA), consider lidocaine neb pre-operative

Intraoperative Management: Minimize long-acting respiratory depressants.

Post-operative: Often more difficult airway after the surgery – similar preparation as pre-operative; Consider post-operative ventilation, HDU/ICU.

Complications: Loss of airway, aspiration.

Special: Syndromes associated with potential difficult ventilation/intubation: Teacher Collins, Pierre

Robin, Apert, Down s., Crouzon, Goldenhar, Klippel Feil, Beckwith-Wiedemann, Hurler syndrome, laryngeal webs, cystic hygroma, choanal atresia.

Airway Syndromes

1. Multisystem infiltrative disease with potential for:
    a. **Difficult Airway:** Macroglossia, laryngo-tracheo-bronchial tree involvement.
    b. **CVS:** Restrictive cardiomyopathy, complete heart block, risk of sudden death, autonomic neuropathy
    c. **Respiratory:** Rare pulmonary interstitial disease
    d. **Renal:** Nephrotic syndrome and renal failure
    e. **Gastro Intestinal**: Increased risk of aspiration secondary to autonomic/peripheral neuropathy

2. Amyloid associated illnesses
    a. Multiple myeloma, RA, hypothyroidism, chronic infection or inflammation
3. Considerations for medical therapy:
    a. Steroids/Chemotherapy

Amyloidosis

Degenerative disease of motor ganglia in anterior horn of the spinal cord and spinal pyramidal tracts (upper and lower motor neuron death), and muscle atrophy

1. Risk of **Aspiration** - Bulbar weakness
2. **Respiratory dysfunction** - weakness +/- chronic aspiration
3. **Autonomic instability** – orthostatic hypotension and resting tachycardia
4. **Altered respiratory response to NMB** - Hyperkalemic respiratory response to succinylcholine - NdMB sensitivity
5. Medications: Pyridostigmine, riluzole (liver dysfunction)

Anesthetic Goals/Conflicts:

- Anticipate need for postoperative ventilation
- Maximize respiratory function with muscle strength, secretion management, pain management
- Prevent aspiration
- Avoid hyperthermia
- Conflicts: RSI vs. avoidance of NMB, regional vs. neurological deficits

Hx: *Evidence of respiratory embarrassments*, pneumonia, ability to cough, functional capacity.

Bulbar dysfunction, swallowing difficulty, dysphagia, dysarthria, gag reflex
Autonomic symptoms: orthostatic hypotension, syncope, resting tachycardia.
Medications: Riluzole – reduce damage to motor neurons by decreasing release of glutamate, can be hepatotoxic, pyridostigmine

PE: neurologic, respiratory, and cardiac examination (orthostatic BP)

Investigations: Usual bloodwork, consider PFTs/ABGs/CXR/ECG

Optimization: Neurology consult, physiotherapy, aspiration prophylaxis
Anesthetic Options: All options ok, regional/neuraxial preferred, RSI, judicious use of NMBs

Room Setup: Assistant for RSI, consider arterial line.

Post-operative: Fully reversed, may require respiratory support

Special:

- Usual age 40-60, men: women 1.5:1
- Association with lung carcinoma
- Upper and lower motor neuron dysfunction
- Fasciculations, asymmetric muscle weakness, autonomic dysfunction, leg cramps
- Sparing of sensory apparatus, coordination, intellect, extraocular muscles, sacral PNS innervating bowel/ bladder sphincreaseters

Acromegaly

Anesthetic emergency characterized by Hypotension, Hypoxemia, and increase. Airway pressures

DDx - Tension Pneumothorax, Dynamic hyperinflation, PE, Bronchospasm, Aspiration, Pulmonary embolism, Transfusion reaction, Mediastinal mass, Carcinoid

Emergency Management

- Stop administration of antigen and inform surgeon – prepare to terminate procedure
- Scan monitors: rate, rhythm, BP, $EtCO_2$, SaO_2, PIP, Temperature
- Hand ventilates with 100% O_2, discontinue anesthetic agents
- Secure the Temporize with vasopressors and fluids
- Examine patient for flushing, urticaria, wheezing, and adequacy of CO
- Move quickly to administration of **Epinephrine**, 10-20ug boluses (1-3ug/kg) titrated up to 500ug
  - 0.3 – 0.5 mls SC of 1:1000 (300 – 500 mcg)
  - 10ug/kg (0.1ml/kg 1:10000) in PALS

Secondary Management

- **Catecholamines**: Epinephrine infusion 5-10ug/min (1ug/kg/min in PALS),
- **Bronchodilators** for bronchospasm
- **Antihistamines**: Ranitidine 50 mg IV q8h reg
- **Corticosteroids**: Hydrocortisone 100 mg IV q6h reg, methylprednisolone 1mg/kg IV
- Serum tryptase (within 1-2 hrs), monitor in HDU x 24hrs

Presentation: CV (74%), cutaneous (70%), bronchospasm (44%)

Hx: After anaphylaxis episode: a detailed history is important to determine what agents were administeredand what was the temporal sequence

PE: Cardiovascular collapse: persistent hypotension, pulmonary hypertension, RV dysfunction, tachycardia. Respiratory: lower respiratory obstruction, laryngeal edema/obstruction (may persist 5-32 hours despite vigorous therapy). Derma: flushing, pruritus, urticaria, angioedema; GI – cramps, diarrhea;

Investigations: After resuscitation: red-top tube for mast cell tryptase (preferably within 1-2 hrs of reaction) Repeat 24 History later. Consider blood and urine for histamine concentrations.

Optimization: pre-treatment with steroids and anti-histamines is NOT effective in preventing anaphylaxis; test dose Abx and other potential allergens; latex free environment

Options: Neuraxial - Patients under neuraxial anesthesia may be partially sympathectomized, requiring even larger doses of epinephrine.

Post-operative: ICU setting. These patients can relapse – don 't send them home for at least 24 hrs. Consultation with immunology re: biochemical testing

Special: Muscle relaxants, latex, antibiotics.

Amyotrophic Lateral Sclerosis

FOOT SURGERY, NOT ANKLE! NEVER USE EPI!

No Specific Contraindications, disadvantages include high failure rate, slow onset 10-25mins and calf tourniquet pain not covered (ankle tourniquet ok).

Anatomy: 5 nerves, 3 superficial, 2 deep

Complications: Nerve injection (19% transient), 0.4% permanent, local pain 40%, hematoma, infection, LA toxicity or cardiac arrest < 0.01%

Technique: CAS monitors, leg on pillow to elevate foot, 3 x 10cc LA (25G needle)
Posterior Tibial N: Lies posterior to posterior tibial artery, gives off lateral and medial plantar. Insert needle in grove behind medial malleolus and advance until bone contacted. Withdraw 1-2mmand inject 2-3mls local. Withdraw again to skin, fan lateral and medial with 2mls each time.

Deep Peroneal: Lateral to EHL tendon and medial to anterior tibial tendon. Needle perp. to skin until it contacts bone, withdraw 1-2 mm, inject 2-3 cc

Superficial Peroneal: From same site as DP block, skin wheal to sup aspect of lateral malleolus ~ 10mls

Saphenous Nerve: From same site as DP block, skin weal to sup aspect of med malleolus ~ 10mls

Sural Nerve: Located midway between lateral asp. ofthe Achilles tendon and the sup asp of the lateral malleolus,

Point the needle anteriorly towards
fan like pattern fibular, inject 5-7mls

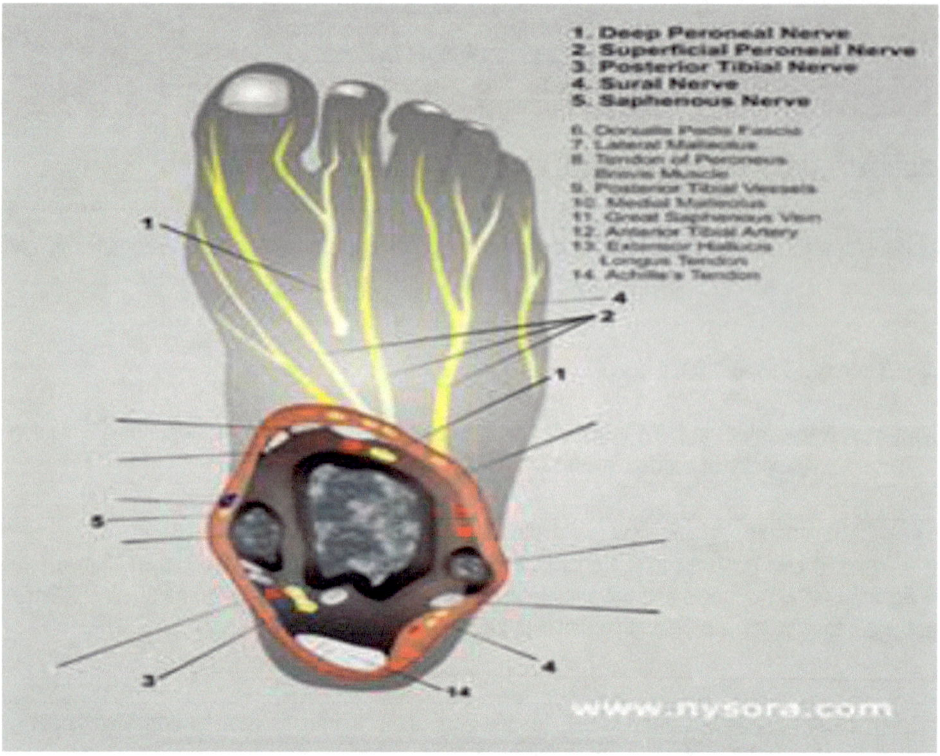

1. Deep Peroneal Nerve
2. Superficial Peroneal Nerve
3. Posterior Tibial Nerve
4. Sural Nerve
5. Saphenous Nerve
www.nysora.com

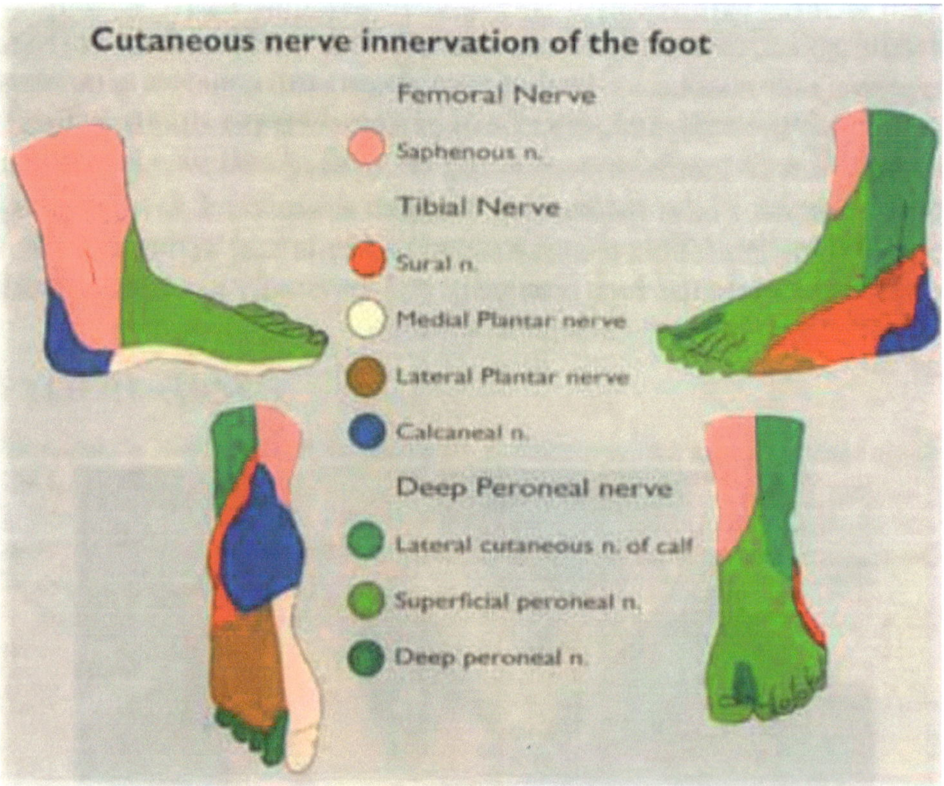

Cutaneous nerve innervation of the foot
Femoral Nerve
Saphenous n.
Tibial Nerve
Sural n.
Medial Plantar nerve
Lateral Plantar nerve
Calcaneal n.
Deep Peroneal nerve
Lateral cutaneous n. of calf
Superficial peroneal n.
Deep peroneal n.

Ankylosing Spondylitis

1. Potential for difficult airway
   - o Decreased C-spine mobility
   - o Possible Temporomandibular joint (TMJ) disease
2. Potential for cervical spine instability with Atlanto-Axial subluxation
3. Axial spine fusion
   - o Neuraxial anaesthesia may be technically difficult
   - o Care with patient positioning
4. Multisystem disease with extra-articular features:
   - o Cardiac: Ischemia, cardiomyopathy, conduction defects, pericardial effusion
   - o Respiratory: restrictive respiratory disease with Pulmonary fibrosis, pHTN, apical fibro-bullous disease (1.5-15%)
   - o Neuro: Spondylolisthesis (cord compression), uveitis
   - o Renal dysfunction – NSAID nephropathy
5. Medications - NSAIDS, Steroids, MTX, TNF-alpha
   a. Marrow suppression, platelet dysfunction, renal impairment, steroid coverage

Anesthetic Goals/Conflicts:

· Anticipate difficult airway

Trauma/Neuro: Need to rapidly secure difficult airway in an unstable patient

Hx/Px: Airway for ease of intubation; Atlanto-Axial Instability; assess axial mobility – positioning, neuraxial; identify comorbid disease
cardiac: functional capacity, Ischemia/failure, cor pulmonale, palpitations, evidence of pHTN; Meds

Investigations: CBC, electrolytes, BUN, Cr, ECG (conduction Dz, pHTN), CXR, +/-PFTs / ABG, ECHO

Optimization: Aspiration prophylaxis, Laparoscopic procedure preferred for RLD, aggressive multimodal analgesia; There is no clear consensus regarding the management of anti-TNF-a blockers in the peri- operative period

Anesthetic Options: Neuraxial techniques may still be used but likely to be difficult. Brachial plexus blocks are relatively contraindicated given RLD; GA with ETT (AFOI, awake DL, light wand), LMA

- given restrictive disease but AI and apical bullae may complicate**Room Setup:** Difficult airway cart, CAS + 5, consider A line. Transcutaneous pacer if conduction Dz; further invasive lines may be indicated depending on extra-articular features; SSEPs forspine surgery

Intraoperative Management: Consider comorbidities (AI, pHTN…) Careful positioning/padding; Rapid desaturation withRLD; Caution with increase. vent pressures with bulla (pneumothorax).

Post-operative: Low threshold for post-operative ventilation if significant restrictive lung (RF – poor pre-operative respiratory function, upper Abd/thoracic surgery, long procedure)

Complications: failed intubation (LMA); respiratory failure; failed regional (may need to control difficult airway), tension pneumothorax

Parturient: no improvement in symptoms with pregnancy; most have vaginal delivery; difficult regional; conflict = difficult regional vs. Difficult airway & aspiration risk

Anorexia, BMI <17.5

1- Delayed gastric emptying and risk of aspiration
2- Fluid and electrolyte abnormalities
    a. Hypovolemia (dehydration)
    b. Hyponatremia, hypokalemia
3- Cardiac Dysfunction
    a. Low-output cardiac failure - decreased cardiac muscle and contractility
    b. Potential cardiac arrhythmias - electrolyte abnormalities, prolonged QT
    c. Autonomic disturbances
4- Malnutrition: Anemia, thrombocytopenia
5- Medications: Antidepressants

Anesthetic Goals/Conflicts:

- Prevent aspiration – prophylaxis
- Conflict RSI vs. hemodynamic instability
- Identify underlying cardiac

dysfunctionRestore electrolytes and volume pre-operatively

Aortic Stenosis

1. Increased risk of **perioperative cardiac complications**: Ischemia/MI/arrhythmias/CHF
2. Identify severity of disease and **high-risk markers** (angina, syncope, CHF)
3. Cardiac physiologic changes
    a. **fixed left ventricular output:** obstruction with limited ability to increase. CO
    b. hypertrophied ventricle with **diastolic dysfunction** (reduced ventricular compliance)
        i. Sensitive to volume depletion, Dependent on atrial kick, subendocardial ischemia (↑ muscle mass, ↓ coronary perfusionpressure)
    c. **altered myocardial oxygen supply / demand**
    d. **systolic dysfunction** (impaired contractility) occurs late in disease
4. **Co-existing disease**
    a. CAD / other valve disease / pHTN / Advanced Age
5. **Ineffective CPR**

Anesthetic Goals/Conflicts:

- Hemodynamic goals of Ao Stenosis: HR 60-90 (avoid tachycardia; avoid bradycardia), maintain or augment preload, maintain contractility, **avoid decreases in afterload**
- Monitor for ischemia, and optimize favorable myocardial oxygen supply/demand relationships
- Pregnancy
- Increase risk of CHF with increased volume, and the risk of ischemia with decreased afterload and tachycardia
- early slow epidural to limits tachycardia, avoid spinals and decreased afterload

Hx: Determine signs of angina, syncope or CHF (50% mortality <5, 3, 2 years). Determine valve area (Normal AVA 2.6-3.5cm^2, Mild >1.5cm^2, gradient <25mmHg, Mod AS 1.0-1.5cm^2, gradient 25- 40mmHg, Severe <1.0cm^2, Critical <0.7cm^2). Functional capacity. Associated CAD/pHTN/arrhythmias

PE: Narrow pulse pressure, pulsus parvis (reduced pulse volume) et tardus (slow) usually with AVA<0.7cm. Displaced apical impulse, murmur of Ao stenosis (SEM late peaking crescendo-decrescendo, radiating to the neck) Reduced or silent S2. Evidence CHF. S4 (atrial kick into non-compliant ventricle). S3 (filling into non- compliant ventricle). Rales, wheezes, elevated JVP, hepatosplenomegaly.

Investigations: CBC, LFTs, Coags, BUN, Cr, CXR, ECG: LVH +/- strain, LBBB, Echo. Cardiac Cath: Assess coronaries and AV gradient.

Optimization: Cardiology Consult. Consider AVR repair/replacement prior to elective sx. Volume resuscitates vs diuresis for CHF. Rate Control.

Anesthetic Options: Any that maintain hemodynamics (avoid SAB), slow titrated epidural. Severe AS maybe a relative contraindication to neuraxial anesthesia.

Room Setup: 5 lead ECG/invasive lines, PAC relative contraindication dt risk of arrhythmias, TEE. Short acting BB 's, phenyl, lido/amiodarone for ectopy, defibrillator pads.

Intraoperative Management: Opioid based induction, judicious etom/keta/benzo, avoid excessive drop in SVR or contractility (volatiles assoc. with junx rhythm. Avoid tachycardia on emergence.

Post-operative: Monitor for ischemia, adequate analgesia.

Aortic Regurgitation

AR can be acute or chronic resulting in pressure and volume overload of the LV and reduced forward CO

1. Increased Risk of perioperative cardiac complications (CHF/MI)
2. Hemodynamic alterations associated with AR and associated hemodynamic goals
    a. Acute – volume/pressure overload, sympathetic stimulation, increased LVEDP / ischemia and arrhythmias, **cardiogenic shock**
    b. Chonic – ventricular dilation and hypertrophy, pulmonary hypertension, LV/RV failure
3. Associated co-morbidities:
    a. Other valvular pathology (MS of rheumatic heart disease)
    b. Ischemic heart disease
    c. Endocarditis
    d. Aortic dilation / dissection
    e. Connective tissue diseases (rheumatoid arthritis, ankylosing spondylitis.)
    f. Marfan 's syndrome
4. Management of medical therapy

Anesthetic Goals/Conflicts:

Fast, full, and forward

- Maintain forward flow: High N HR (~90bpm), NSR, maintain, adequate preload (may require augmentation), decrease afterload (maintain adequate CPP), maintain contractility

Hx: Evaluate underlying etiology, onset, severity, symptoms (**CHF**/orthopnea/PND), arrhythmias. Assess for comorbidities: **Aortic stenosis**, **CAD**, MCTD, **pulmonary hypertension**.

PE: Assess volume status, JVP, edema, rales. Displaced LV impulse = cardiac enlargement. Wide pulse pressure, decreased diastolic blood pressure, bounding perph. pulse. De Musset 's sign – head bobbing with systole, Corrigan 's sign – water hammer / collapsing.

Auscultate for murmur: Diastolic -blowingll murmur at LSB. Abdominal distention and pain – splanchnic ischemia. PE findings pHTN.

Investigations: usual BW, ECG – LVH, conduction disorders, CXR – cardiomegaly **ECHO**-EF/severity of AR, PAP.

Optimization: Cardiology consult, Consider valve replacement or valvuloplasty prior to elective surgery

Class 1 indications for repair/replacement: 1) NYHA III-IV HF History / N syst fnx, 2) NYHA IIHistory / N syst fnx but progressive dilatation 3. Patients with angina 4. Patients with mild-mod LV dysfunction 5.

Patients undergoing cardiac surgery for other reason
consider light anxiolysis to avoid increase in SVR. Ensure adequate afterload reduction. Hold diuretics and ACEi. Manage anticoagulation for a. fib. Arrange post-operative monitored care

Anesthetic Options: GA / Neuraxial (anticipate and avoid significant drops in preload) Pregnancy – early epidural to avoid adrenergic increase. in SVR during labour

Room Setup: Inotropes (milrinone, dobutamine, epinephrine), nitride/NTG, 5lead, +- PAC/TEE

Intraoperative management: Induction, preserve preload & contractility / NSR / HR~90bpm / slight afterload reduction.

Post-operative: CSICU or ICU for post-operative cardiac monitoring. Observe for: hypotension,ischemia/ infarct, LV failure, cardiogenic shock, pHTN +/- RV failure.
Avoid myocardial depressants or increased SVR. Post AVR may require inotropes

- Preventable perioperative event with no definitive treatment and significant mortality

- Conflict between aspiration risk and:
    - Airway quality
    - Cardiopulmonary reserve
    - Feasibility and tolerance for regional techniques

- Consider aspiration in differential diagnosis of bronchospasm with hypoxemia

Anesthetic Goals/Conflicts:

- RSI and HD instability
- Maintain oxygenation
- Prevent complications: Pneumonia, ARDS, sepsis, barotrauma secondary to high PIP

Hx & Px: RF for aspiration: Hx of difficult airway, HISTORY &N surgery/radiation, DM, NM D/O, reflux, dysphagia, peptic ulcer disease, Cardiopulmonary – exercise tolerance, edema, angina

Manifestations: gastric contents in oropharynx, hypoxemia, increase PIP, bronchospasm, copious tracheal secretions, coughing, laryngospasm, rales, chest retraction, dyspnea, CXR changes

Optimization: avoid GA, antacids, H2 antagonist, metoclopramide, ng suctioning prior to induction and extubation, cricoid pressure, consider awake intubation, extubate awake

Anesthetic Options: GA, local, regional (avoid depression of laryngeal reflexes by excess sedation)

Intraoperative Management:

- Perform immediate tracheal suctioning prior to positive pressure ventilation
- If ETT is in the trachea, place the patient head down, with right lateral tilt (protect left long)
- Pass a suction catheter down the ETT
- Maintain oxygenation: PPV with 100% FiO2, PEEP

- Perform bronchoscopy if particulate aspiration
- Cancel elective surgery. Emergency surgery should be restricted to theminimum procedure consistent with patient safety

Post-operative: If patient remains stable throughout event without significant desaturation/hypotension ...etc. could consider discharge from Post Anesthesia Care Unit after 2 hours of observation

- Provide supportive care: fluid management, H2 blockers, intermittent pulmonary toilet
- Empiric antibiotics if compromised patient, fulminant course, high bacterial load

o Prophylaxis is indicated for known aspiration of feculent material
  - Bronchodilators to relieve large airway closure in less damaged areas of the lung
  - Consider Extra Corporeal Membrane Oxygenation (ECMO) support if oxygenation cannot be maintained

Asthma

reversible expiratory obstruction due to hyperactive bronchi with inflammation, mucous hypersecretion and bronchoconstriction

1. High risk for perioperative respiratory complications including **respiratory failure**
   - FEV1 < 40% indicates severe obstruction,
   - Normal or high $PaCO_2$ suggestive of fatigue and impending failure
2. **Perioperative Bronchospasm**
3. **Barotrauma and Pneumothorax**
4. Potential for Status Asthmaticus & Pulmonary Tamponade
   - Identify patients at risk: previous attacks, frequency of hospitalizations, steroids, can 't speak, increase. WOB, silent chest, confusion, increased or Normal CO_2.
   - Ddx Wheezing: FB, aspiration, anaphylaxis, cardiogenic edema, tracheal stenosis
   - Medical Management Salbutamol, Ipratropium, Epinephrine,Corticosteroids, Aminophylline, MgSo4, SEVO, Heliox, glycopyrrolate, atropine
   - Ventilatory strategies and consideration for ECMO

Anesthetic Goals/Conflicts:

Aspiration

- Indication of intubation: pH <7.2, unremitting hypoxia SaO2 <90%, progressive exhaustion, decreased level of consciousness. Hypercarbia although a marker of severe disease is not anindication for intubation.

Medications:

Salbutamol: MDI 4-20 puffs/hour, Neb 5-10mg q 15mins prn, IV 4mcg/kg load then 0.1-0.2mcg/kg/min
Epinephrine (1:1000) 4-8mcg/min
Ipratropium: MDI 4-20 puffs/hour, Neb 0.5mg q 30-60mins prn
Corticosteroids: Methylprednisolone 40-125mg/ q6h or Hydrocortisone
500 mg IV Aminophylline: 3-6 mg/kg load and 0.2-0.9 mg/kg/hr infusion
MgSo4: 2-4 grams over 20 mins, then 1gram/hour infusion

- Thiopental/Histamine releasing narcotics/NdMR. Watch for tachydysrhythmias due to Rx

Intubation: Ketamine/Lidocaine/Benzo 's/Narcotics, avoid STP/Histamine release/NDMBs such as mivacurium/cis-atracurium. Avoid Cholinesterase inhibitors.

Ventilator: FiO_2 = 1, TV 6-8ml/kg, RATE 6-8/min, PEEP <5, Keep PIP < 50 cm/h20, square wave flow (increase VI). May need to disconnect patient for dynamic hyperinflation and chest compression. If severe bronchospasm on intubation and can 't ventilates, confirm tube placement, r/o pneumothorax and then give IV adrenaline. Maintain with Volatile, consider ECMO!

Bronchospasm:

1. Optimize pre-operative with bronchodilators
2. Avoid histamine release
   - Morphine, Atracurium
3. Deep plane of anaesthesia prior to airway manipulation
   - Consider broncho dilating anaesthetic agents: ketamine, sevoflurane
4. Extubation plan
   - Deep extubation +- LMA
   - Opioids prior to emergence – remifentanil

American Society of Regional Anesthesia and Pain Medicine (ASRA) ***Consensus (2002)***

General: Use extreme caution in neuraxial blocks on patients taking more than one anticoagulant

Thrombolytics:

- Don 't do neuraxial technique. If administered inadvertently, fibrinogen level may be helpful

Unfractionated Heparin

- Low dose SC prophylactic dosing not a contraindication but hold until afteradministration of block
- Check platelets after > 4 days of UFH (HIT)
- Intraoperative IV dosing (e.g., vascular surgery) acceptable 1 hour after needle
- Remove catheter with 2 conditions: 1) 2-4 hours after last heparin dose; 2)Patient 's coagulation status documented. Restart anticoagulation 1 hour after catheter removal
- Bloody/difficult insertion + UFH may increase risk but not contraindication to proceeding

LMWH

- Don 't monitor *Xa*; peak effects 2 hours after administration.
- If bloody tap – inform surgeon, avoid LMWH for 24 hours
- Low dose (prophylactic) LMWH: delay needle for > 10-12h
    - Enoxaparin 0.5 mg/kg every 12 hours
    - Dalteparin 5000 units every 12 hours
- High dose (treatment) LMWH: delay needle for > 24h
    - Enoxaparin 1 mg/kg every 12 hours
    - Enoxaparin 1.5 mg/kg daily
    - Dalteparin 120 U/kg every 12 hours
    - Dalteparin 200 U/kg daily, or
    - Tinzaparin 175 U/kg daily

- Post-operative BID LMWH (high dose): delay at least 24h after needle; notcompatible with catheters left in situ and may start 2h after catheter removal
- Post-operative daily LMWH (low dose): delay at least 6-8h after needle; compatible with catheters left in situ but must be removed >10-12 Historyafter last dose and restarted > 2h after removal

Oral Anticoagulants (Warfarin)

- Discontinue therapy 4-5 days pre-operatively, document normal INR (<1.5)
- If warfarin initiated > 24h pre-operative, check INR prior to block
- Document INR < 1.5 prior to catheter removal, monitor daily if on therapy
- Monitor neurological status minimum 24h after catheter removal, longer if INR > 1.5

Antiplatelet Agents

- NSAIDs (including ASA) do not increase the risk of spinal hematoma
- Discontinue clopidogrel > 7 days; Ticlopidine > 14 days before needle
- Glycoprotein IIb/IIIa inhibitors – Eptifibatide (integrillin) and Tirofiban (Aggrastat) delay > 4-8h after administration; Abciximab (ReoPro) delay > 24-48h after administration
- Avoid neuraxial technique in patients on more than one antiplatelet agent

Herbal Drugs

- No data and no contraindication to block (do not increase the risk of hematoma ontheir own)

Thrombin Inhibitors (Desirudin, lepirudin, bivalirudin, argatroban)

- Increased risk of bleeding, but nospecific recommendations

Fondaparinux (Arixtra)

- Minimal data, but increased risk of hematoma
- Recommend single atraumatic pass, no indwelling catheters

Interscalene: *for shoulder surgery, ulnar sparing*

Specific Contraindications: Unable to tolerate reduced FEV1 by 25% (interscalene) i.e., FEV1 < 1L; Contralateral vocal cord paralysis

Complications: 100% Phrenic, Pneumo 0.2%, Horner's, Intravascular injection, 13-24% hypotension/ brady,inadvertent SAB, Epidural block.

Anatomy: Roots/Trunks

Approach: Palpate interscalene groove with head supine and rotated 30 deg away. EJ crosses the groove at the level at the cricoid cartilage. Skin wheel at the level of the CC, 22g 1.5ll needle inserted perpendicularly in slightly medial and caudal direction. Stimulating Phrenic = Too anterior, Trapezius = posterior. Look for motor activity of the arm, wrist or hand, but deltoid OK. 30-40mL local.

Supraclavicular: *for any upper extremity surgery that does not req the shoulder*

Specific Contraindications: avoid bilateral due to risk of bilateral pneumothorax or phrenic nerve block.

Complications: Phrenic Nerve (50-60%), Horner's, Nerve Injury 0.02-0.4%), Cardiac arrest 0.01%, Hematoma, local pain (40%). Highest incidence of pneumothorax, however should be less than 5%

Anatomy: Trunks at the lateral border of Ant. Scalene, most reliable U/E block

Approach: Palpate interscalene groove at its most inf point, just post to subclavian pulse (SP); the latter can be felt in a plane just medial to the midpoint of the clavicle. After a skin wheal, a 22g 1.5ll needle is directed just ↑ and post to the SP and directed caudally at a very flat angle against the skin. Obs for muscle contraction. of the forearm. 25-40mL. If U hit rib, the needle is withdrawn and reval path. The plumb-bob 'techn is another SC approach. The needle entry site is immediately. sup to the clavicle, just lateral to the point where the SCM is attached to the clavicle. The angle of needle entry is 90° to the table. If you contact rib, try manipulating in an ant to post direction or walk along rib.

Infraclavicular: *Misses skin of axillae and proximal medial arm (intercostobrachial, Medial brachii cut nerves)*

Anatomy: *Cords, beyond the first rib*

Specific contraindications: ***None****, safer than supraclavicular*

Complications: Pneumo(rare), hemo, and chylothorax (with a left-sided block) are possible and occur at a higher rate than with the supraclavicular approach. Phrenic = rare.

Approach: When performing, the patient lies supine with the head slightly turned away from the side of the procedure. The operative limb is abducted to 90° and the axillary pulse is identified. The midpoint of the clavicle is identified and 2 cm caudal to this point a needle is inserted at a 45° angle and directed toward the axillary art pulsation. With a 4-in, 21-gauge insulated nerve stimulator needle, motor activity inthe hand is sought. Or you may use the coracoid approach which is 2cm medial and inf. to the coracoid process. Needle insertion is perp. to floor. If no twitch aims cephalad then caudad. Do not accept.
Musculocutaneous N as it may leave the sheath at this point in 50% of pts.

Axillary: *Musculocutaneous nerve has already left the sheath at this point and is in coracobrachialis, good for procedures distal to elbow. Can block with 5-10ml in CB abv artery, fanning technique or at elbow.*

Complications: Hematoma, IV injection, Nerve injuries

Approach: The pulse of the axillary artery is identified as high (proximal) in the axilla as possible. Using an "immobile needle" technique, a 22-gauge, 1.5-in needle is inserted until bright red blood is aspirated. The needle is then slightly advanced or withdrawn until blood aspiration ceases. Injection can be performed posteriorly, anteriorly, or in both locations in relation to the artery. A total of 40 mL of local anesthetic is usually injected; distal pressure on the sheath during the injection may promote better cephalad spread of the solution within the sheath.

Intercostobrachial Nerve Block (T2): *for anesthesia to medial arm/tourniquet pain*

Approach: The intercostobrachial nerve derives from the T2 somatic intercostal nerve, whereas the medial brachial cutaneous nerve derives from C8 and T1. Both become superficial and cutaneous at the pectoral ridge over the humeral head. They are easily blocked, with the arm abducted, by means of a linear injection (field block) from the deltoid prominence superiorly to the most inferior aspect of the medial upper arm (Figure 17–3). A total of 5 mL of local anesthesia is used.

Nerve Blocks at the Elbow:

Ulnar Nerve: Flex elbow 30degrees, 2 cm proximal to groove bw medial epicond and olec. Process. 5ml of LA.

Median Nerve: Intercondylar Line, Medial to Biceps Tendon and 1 cm medial to brachial artery at this IC line. Elicit paras. or motor respiratory. or hit periosteum and withdraw 0.5-1cm.
Inject 3-5 ml.

Radial Nerve: Same Intercondylar line, 2 cm lateral to BT.
Nerve is deep, can elicit paresthesia move in a fan shape

or hit bone and withdraw 0.5cm. Inject 5ml. Aim towards lateral epicondyle on insertion

Lateral Cutaneous Nerve of the Forearm: Branch of MSC N. Inject just below fascia lateral to BT and medial toradial nerve. 2-3ml LA.

Medial Cutaneous Nerve of the Forearm: Branch of medial cord. SC infiltration from biceps tendon to medial epicondyle.

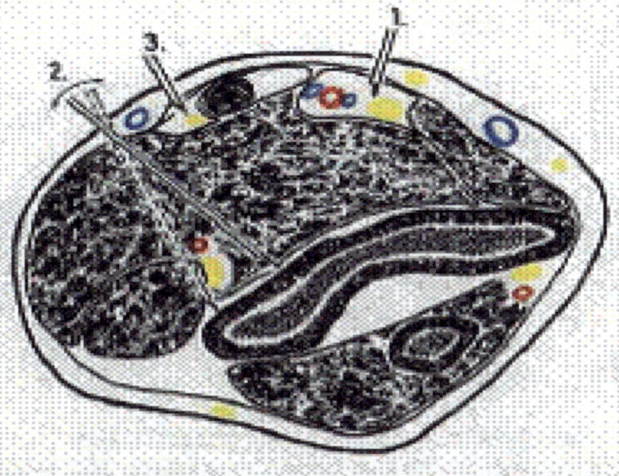

10-12. Cross-section of arm at elbow. *(1)* Median nerve . *(2)* Radial nerve block. *(3)* Lateral cutaneous nerve of m block. (Note nerve under deep fascia and close to bi- tendon.)

Brachial Plexus Blocks ½

1. Confirm the diagnosis of brain death and confirm wishes of patient and family
   - NDD by 2 physicians not involved with transplant (see below)
2. Physiologic Consequences of Brain death
   - Hemodynamic instability (myocardial dysfunction, vasomotor tone, hypovolemia -)
   - Pulmonary dysfunction - ARDS and Hypoxemia (pulmonary edema - Neuro vs. cardiac, VAP)
   - Neuro-endocrine dysfunction
     - DI (70%), hypokalemia, Hypothyroid, hypocortisolemia, Hyperglycemia
   - Coagulopathy / DIC (brain release of thromboplastin)
   - Poliokothermia secondary to hypothalamic dysfunction
3. Etiology of Brain Death and secondary injuries
   - Trauma (potential for multi-organ involvement, pulmonary / cardiac contusions)

Anesthetic Goals

- maintain end-organ perfusion (monitoring, fluids, vasopressors & ventilatory support)
  - SBP > 100 mmHg, PO_2 >100 mmHg, U/O 100 mL/History (1-1.5 ml/kg/History), Hb > 100g/L, CVP 5-10 mmHg, FiO_2 < 40% for lung retrieval
- Strategies for organ preservation using free radical scavengers including mannitol, superoxide dismutase, and the free radical synthesis blocker allopurinol
- Consider hormone replacement therapy (improve solid organ retrieval)
  - Methylprednisolone 15 mg/kg q24h
  - Tetra-iodothyronine (T4) IV: 20 mcg bolus followed by 10 mcg infusion

Minimal clinical criteria for NDD: etiology of NDD in absence of conditions mimicking NDD, Deep unresponsive coma & bilat absence of motor response (excludes spinal reflex), No corneal/pupil responses (pupils' mid-size or greater) with no brain stem reflexes (gag/cough, vestibulo-ocular, facial motor response), Positive apnea test ($PaCO_2$≥60 or ≥20mmHg increase.) Absent confounding factors. Minimal T=34 °C. Ancillary test if Unable to determine min criteria: 4 vessel Angio of common/internal/vertebral arteries.

Brain death hemodynamics - initial ischemia results in unopposed vagal stimulation (brady, blocks, hypotension, low CO), progression to midbrain results in vagal stimulation with marked sympathetic activation (tachy, arrhythmias, HTN), finally complete brainstem ischemia - loss of vagal tone with unopposed sympathetic activation, Herniation of brainstem - loss of sympathetic activation with profound hypotension **Hx/Px:** Review history preceding NDD (etiology, e.g. trauma), secondary injuries, current meds/ventilation to maintain organ perfusion, Vitals/Temperature, U/O

- followed by 2.4 units/ infusion

Investigations: CBC, Lytes, BUN, Cr, Group & Screen, ABG (looking for anemia, electrolyte abnormalities (DI), renal insufficiency, acidosis). Imaging: CXR (lines & tubes, pulmonary edema, aspiration etc.), ECG (rhythm, ischemia), ECHO (EF, wall motion abnormalities, contusions)

Optimization: Lung protection ventilatory strategy, (Vt 6-8, plat < 30 mmHg, PEEP to minimize FiO2, SaO_2 > 95%, colloids > crystalloid), triple hormone therapy, glycemic control, euthermia

Anesthetic Options: volatile & narcotic with inotrope/vasopressors for hemodynamic ctrl only (no Awareness)

Room Setup: CAS, 5 lead, A-line, CVC, Foley, temperature probe

Intraoperative Management: Vasopressors (epinephrine, vasopressin) to support blood pressure, DA and phenylephrine suggested to improve splanchnic perfusion. Vasodilators (phentolamine, alprostadil [lung retrieval]) to improve perfusion during cross-clamping, heparin prior to x-clamp, Active warming Direct chromotropes (**isoproterenol, DA**) to treat brady as brain dead patient unresponsive to vagolytics

Post-operative: appropriate disposition of remains

Bradycardia

Does the patient have a **pulse**? → if not, immediate ACLS
Most important Question is **sinus bradycardia** or not?

Brachial Plexus Blocks 2/2

- Anesthetic drugs → suxamethonium, anticholinesterases, opioids, Neuraxial blockade
- Cardiac drugs → β-blockers, CCB, Clonidine, Digoxin, phenylephrine

3. Cardiac: * ischemia * conduction system disease → SSS, heart block
4. Nerves
    - Vagal mediated → pain, oculo-cardiac, peritoneal stretch, ECT
    - Baroreceptor mediated → ICP, HTN, carotid sinus manipulation
5. Endocrine: *hypothyroidism *hypothermia

Emergency Management

1. Inform surgeon, Scan monitors: rate, rhythm, BP, EtCO2, SaO_2, temperature
2. Hand ventilates with 100% O_2
3. Examine patient for pulse or signs of adequate perfusion

Develop DDx and treat as per ACLS protocol

Bronchiectasis

1. Risk for severe Respiratory Complications
    a. Auto-PEEP & pulmonary tamponade
    b. Mucus plugging d/t impaired mucociliary activity
    c. Recurrent lung infections / abscess
    d. Massive hemoptysis

2. Chronic Hypoxemia & Hypercarbia
    a. pHTN & RVF
3. Associated therapy: Postural Drainage, Abx 's, Chest Physio.
4. Underlying etiology: Cystic Fibrosis, congenital cartilage defunction, HIV, TB, infection, inflammation, Rheumatoid arthritis

Anesthetic Goals/Conflicts:

- Optimize pre-operative lung function with postural drainage and Abx therapy
- Prevent contamination of good lung with purulent sputum (consider lung isolation)
- Avoid instrumentation of the airway or nasal intubations (chronic sinusitis)

Bronchopleural Fistula

1. Possible life-threatening emergency from ineffective PPV, tension pneumothorax or lung flooding
    a. Requirement for lung isolation
        i. Minimizes air leak and facilitates ventilation

2. Prevent soiling of contralateral lung if abscess/ empyemapresent

3. Comorbid disease / etiology forBPF
    a. Lung abscess/ empyema
        - Systemic Inflammatory Response (SIRS), Multi-organ failure, EtOH abuse, IVDU, steroids, DM
    b. Post lung resection
        - COPD, arrhythmia, malignancy, CAD
    c. Trauma
    d. Spontaneous pneumo/ bullous disease

Anesthetic Goals / Conflicts

- isolation of affected side to support ventilation and prevent cross-contamination
- prepare for and be ready to resuscitate from cardio or respiratory collapse
- facilitate early extubation post-thoracotomy

Hx: acute or chronic; stable or unstable; post-operative resection vs. infective vs. trauma; air leak, dyspnea, fever, pleuritic pain, purulent sputum or drainage, Comorbidities - 4Ms, COPD (severity, meds, exacerbations, smoking), RHF (SOB, syncope, jaundice, fatigue, edema), functional capacity

PX: signs of SIRS, ease of intubation/lung isolation, Tracheal deviation, subcu emphysema; Comorbid disease - COPD (increase AP diameter, prolonged expiration, wheeze); Estimate the loss of VT through the fistula (bubbling through the chest tube), Quantify the difference between inhaled and exhaled tidal volumes (spirometry); CVS - pHTN/RHF: loud P2, RV heaves, TR murmur, elevated JVP, hepatic congestion, peripheral edema; Trauma: other injuries

Invistigations: CBC (sepsis), Lytes, Bun, Cr (paraneoplastic syndromes), INR/PTT (epidural), ABG, x-match; CXR/CT (pneumothorax, chest tube, bullae, empyema, chronic lung disease), ECHO (RHF), ECG(RVH - R > S in V1, p-pulmonal

Optimization: chest tube, drain empyema, aspiration prophylaxis, anti-sialagogue (FOB), Resuscitate

Anesthetic Setup: 5 lead, +/- TEA, Artline, +/-CVC, FOB, multiple ETT (DLT, SLT, blockers), CPAP, HFJV, Chest tube tray and thoracic surgeon in room

Management: D/C chest tube suction (dec. leak), SV lung isolation with DLT ideal (AFOI vs. asleep SV induction vs. RSI with DLT / bronchial SLT, if PPV - low Vt, low pressures, watch for contralateral lung contamination; HFJV allows ventilation with lower Pk pressures; surgeon can pack the lung once the chest is open; early extubation, good analgesia (TEA, Paravertebral, intercostals, PCA)

Complications: ·Tension pneumothorax, Inability to ventilate with hypoxemia and hypercarbia (Consider briefly clamping chest tube), Outpouring of pus and lung flooding, Complications from OLV: hypoxemia, Sepsis, Pain, Persistent air leak
, atrial arrhythmia, demand ischemia if septic), PFTs (baseline)

Burns (>10% BSA 3$^{rd.}$ degree or 25% 1-2Nd degree)

1. Trauma Pt / Emergency
2. Potential Difficult airway with inhalational injury (ALI)
    a. Coexisting CN & CO Toxicity necessitating 100% O2 and early potentially hyperbaric chamber
3. Hypovolemia: Volume Resuscitate with Parkland formula – 4cc/kg/%BSA
4. Multi-organ dysfunction:
    a. Cardiogenic shock (circulating mediators, increase SVR, dec. CBF)
    b. ALI/ARDS, aireway sluffing, ARF, Rhabdomyolysis, Sepsis, hypothermia
5. Altered Pharmacology
    a. Suxamethonium hyperkalemia > 24 hrs, resistance to NdMRs
    b. Susceptibility to myocardial depressants
6. Recurrent Procedures: Difficult IV Access & monitoring; blood loss; pain; remote location

Anesthetic Goals Conflicts:

- Early and safe airway management: Avoid Suxamethonium > 24 hrs – 2 years after injury
    - o Assume inhalational injury and provide 100% O2, investigate for cyanide and CO toxicity
- Volume resuscitation
- Avoid End-organ damage, U/O 1ml/kg, ARDS ventilation strategy

ATLS: Assess for inhalational burn, early intubation, 1.0 FiO2, stop burning process (brush chemicals off, copious water), large bore IV access in non-burned area (groin), volume resuscitate. Provide adequate analgesia – multimodal approach

Transfer: >10%, extremes of age, sensitive areas (face, hands, perineum), comorbidities\

Hx: AMPLE history, tetanus status, Type & location burn – chemical (alk worse than acid), thermal, electrical (deep muscle necrosis, rhabdom, ARF); Associated trauma (covert injury). Inhalational injury - dyspnea, hoarseness, carbonaceous sputum, singed facial hair. CN toxicity (HISTORY /A, dizzy, tachycardia, tachypnea, lethargy, Sz, coma); CO Toxicity (HISTORY /A, dizziness, confusion, N/V, visual changes, CNS dysfunction).

PE: Vitals +temperature, ABCDE, airway for ease of intubation U/O, C-spine. CNS exam for CO toxicity vs head trauma. CVS: Volume status, cap refill Respiratory: focused airway exam for inhalational injury. Burn area (%BSA - Rule of 9's; palm = 1%TBSA); burn severity

Investigations: CBC, Lytes, Coag Profile, urine myoglobin, ABG (lactic acidosis with CN toxicity), Co- oximetry, Serum Cyanide (tox >0.2mg/L, lethal >1mg/L), ECG, CXR, Diagnostic FOB

Optimization: 100% O2, volume resuscitation as per Parkland formula (4 cc/kg/%BSA – 50% in 1st 8hrs, 50% in next 16 hrs). Consider HBO for CO (>30%); CN- toxicity – HBO, e
(150mg/kg), hydroxocobalamin. Maintain U/O 1cc/kg/hr – Consider
to increase. solubility (correct met acidosis). Consider inotropes for
strategy. Early enteral feeding.

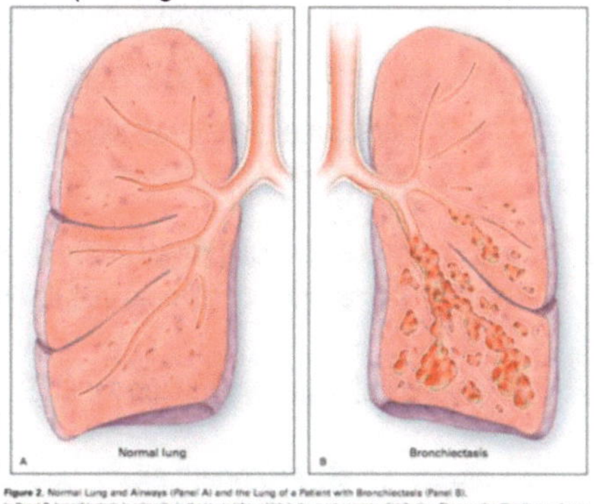

Figure 2. Normal Lung and Airways (Panel A) and the Lung of a Patient with Bronchiectasis (Panel B).
In Panel B, bronchiectasis is primarily in the lower lobe, which is the most common distribution. The saccular dilatations and grape-like clusters with pools of mucus are signs of severe bronchiectasis.

Room Setup: CAS +5lead, temperature, Hot OR, Art line (samplin
foley, vasopressors, PRBC. Large bore IV 's, difficult airway cart. A
outcomes.

Intraoperative Management: Regional vs GA. Avoid Suxamethon
ofNdMRs (peak resistance 2-6 wks., starts 48hrs) Difficult airway –
vs.SV induction if uncooperative; RSI if OK; Avoid ++ propofol due
Ketamine. ++ analgesia; lung protection; volume resuscitate.

Post-operative: Burn unit; HDU; ICU; multi-modal analgesia

1- Potential airway emergency with complete airway obstruction
2- Disease of acute airway edema
   a. refractory to conventional treatment of airway edema (**corticosteroids, epinephrine, antihistamines)**
   b. precipitated by emotional stress, trauma, oral surgery, or direct laryngoscopy

Anesthetic Goals/Conflicts:

- Prevent recurrent episodes with long-term prophylaxis
  - **anabolic steroids, anti-fibrinolytics**
- Prevent acute perioperative episode
  - Avoidance of airway instrumentation (regional anesthesia favoured)
  - short-term prophylaxis with **C1 esterase inhibitor infusions (25 units/kg one time dose), FFP (2-4 units)**
- Treatment of an acute attack
  - Early tracheal intubation, preparation for surgical airway, treatment with C1 esterase inhibitor infusion or FFP

Caesarian Section

1. Potential Emergency - no time for optimization, aspiration risk
2. Pregnancy
   a. potential difficult airway, full stomach
      i. Mallimpatti >1, short neck, receding mandible, prominent incisors (overbite)
   b. physiologic changes including
      i. dec. FRC – rapid desaturation
      ii. anemia
      iii. dec. anesthetic requirements
   c. aortocaval compression
   d. potential massive bleeding
   e. maintenance of fetal oxygenation

3. Complications
   a. Postpartum Hemorrhage - atony, products, accrete, coagulopathy, inversion
   b. Neuraxial - High spinal, Post Dural Puncture Headache (PDPH)
   c. Embolism - PE, VAE, AFE

Anesthetic Goals/Conflicts:

- Determine urgency of situation - Continuous fetal monitoring
- Administer safe, time-sensitive anesthetic with emphasis on mother
- Conflicts
  - Difficult Airway vs. STAT section
  - Hemodynamic instability vs. regional anesthesia

Hx: Urgency of situation; reason for C/S; AMPLE Hx; Ob Hx

PE: airway, cardiopulmonary exam, fluid status and back exam for ease of neuraxial technique

Investigations: CBC, diff, G&S, coags if applicable (PIH or prophylactic anticoagulation)

Optimization: Aspiration prophylaxis; LUD; IV fluids if necessary

Room Setup:

- Standard; emerge drugs and equipment available for GA if neuraxial fails
- Difficult airway cart if difficult airway is anticipated
- Oxytocin, nitro available

Intraoperative Management:

- For neuraxial: frequent BP checks after spinal
- Oxytocin after delivery of neonate
- Good communication with mother and surgeon
- For GA: anticipate potential difficult ventilation/intubation

Post-operative:

- PPH; Aspiration (Extubate awake); pain management

Special:

- Anesthetic complications: Hypotension, high spinal, failed spinal, PDPH, awareness
- Surgical complications: Hemorrhage, atony, difficult extraction

Carcinoid

Carcinoid is the most common GI endocrine tumor (1-2 per 100,000); 2-5% of patients will exhibit carcinoid syndrome: flushing with diarrhea, hemodynamic instability +/- bronchospasm; carcinoid heartdisease is present in 20-40% of patients with carcinoid syndrome

1. Malignancy (mass, medications, metastases, metabolic)
2. Risk of perioperative carcinoid crisis – hypotension & bronchospasm
    - Flushing, diarrhea, hemodynamic instability (serotonin – HTN, histamine -HTN, bronchospasm, hyperglycemia
3. Associated carcinoid heart disease (20-60%)
    - Right-sided valvopathy, 10% L sided valvular disease (MR, AR)
    - constrictive pericarditis, SVT, Intramyocardial metastases
4. Other endocrinopathies
    - Cushing's, acromegaly (bronchial carcinoid)

Anesthetic Goals/Conflicts

- Avoid perioperative carcinoid crisis
    - Avoid triggers: Avoid SNS (hypoxia, hypercarbia, hypovolemia, sympathomimetics), histamine release, pain/anxiety, tumour manipulation
    - Premedicate with octreotide (prevent vasoactive mediator release)
- Treatment of perioperative bronchospasm
    - Avoid B-agonists, epinephrine, theophylline
    - Respond to octreotide, corticosteroids, histamine blockers

Hx: Carcinoid Symptoms (flushing, syncope, headache, hypertension, hypotension, nausea, vomiting, diarrhea, bronchospasm); Mass effect (malnutrition, obstruction – endobronchial, GI); Cardiac dysfunction (palpitations, syncope, edema, HTN); location of tumour; S/S of coshing's, acromegaly; medical therapies

PE: vitals + postural, volume status, Respiratory – Wheeze endobronchial lesion or bronchospasm, CVS - valvularDisease, RVF; Derma: Pellagra (niacin def: dermatitis diarrhea dementia), hyperkeratosis, hyper pigment, venous telangiectasia

Investigations: CBC, coags, lytes, BUN, Cr, Mg, Ca, alb, LFTs, G&S, CXR; ECG +/- ECHO; U/A: 5-HIAA

Optimization: Consult endo/cardio, anxiolysis, pre operative octreotide (50-300 mcg SC 30 minutes pre operative or

C1 Esterase Inhibitor Deficiency (Hereditary Angioedema)

- avoid epinephrine; GA is indicated for symptomatic pts or with tumor manipulation

Room Setup: foley, art line (preinduction), CVP, large bore IV, fluid warmer, Baer hugger. Avoid SNS agents (indirect, beta agonists, reflex activation - epi, norepinephrine, ephedrine, dopamine, isoproterenol); Phenyl, esmolol, phentolamine for HD derangement; octreotide; dilute vasopressin; avoid histamine release

Intraoperative Management: Titrated and deep induction - Goal is stable hemodynamics. Avoid hypotension. Maintain normothermia. Communicate with surgeon and pre-empt hemodynamic shifts following tumour manip with doses of octreotide – 25-50ug bolus (no ceiling – increase. until desired effect); frequent lytes & glucose Bronchospasm is best managed with octreotide (other agents include steroids, antihistamines).

Carcinoid Crisis: stop stimulus, 1.0 FiO_2, fluids, phenylephrine, vasopressin, octreotide 100-200ug boluses titrated to effect; vasopressin, H1 or H2 blockade, serotonin antagonists (ondansetron)

Post-operative: Good multimodal analgesia. Aggressive prophylaxis of N&V. HDU. High risk of delayed awakening secondary to serotonin (decreased MAC …)

Cardiac Assessment for Non-cardiac Surgery

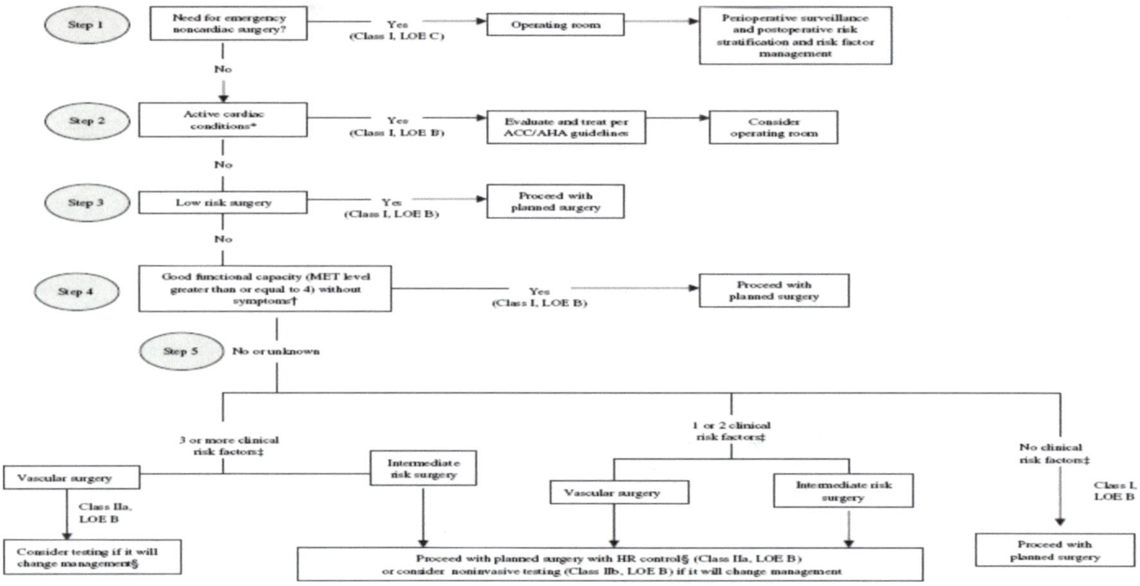

Hx: Stepwise approach

Step 1: Determine urgency of surgery
Step 2: Identify unstable syndromes (5): Recent MI < 30d,Unstable angina, decompensated HF, Severe valvular disease, Severe dysrhythmias
Step 3: If no unstable syndromes and low risk surgery, proceed
Step 4. Assess functional capacity: 1 MET
= ADLS, 4 METs = light housework, i.e., washing dishes, >4 METs = climbing 1 flight of stairs, walking at 4mph or 6.4 km/hr. 1 MET is energy consumed by the body at rest and is equal to 3.5 ml/kg/min.
Step 5: Assess clinical predictors (5): Stroke, stable angina, compensated HF, renal failure, DM.
Step 6: Determine path depending on number of predictors and risk of surgery as per guidelines.

Cardiac Risk: Vascular ~5%, Intermediate 1-4%, Low < 1%
Investigations: Echo Class 1 for CHF, diastolic, continuous, holosystolic, late systolic murmurs, ejection clicks, radiation to neck, or murmurs with infarction, syncope, endocarditis.
MIBI (dobutamine/persantine): More sens/spec than stress test for ischemia
Dobutamine Stress Echo: Best predictor of perioperative cardiac morbidity: cautions with serious arrhythmias, obesity, severe hyper/hypotension.

Optimization: Consult Cardiology, consider angiography, Cancel Surgery, modify surgical procedure (less invasive), consider pre-operative stenting.

For PTCA surgery should be delayed 2 weeks to allow healing, and before 8 weeks (before restenosis) DES may require anti-platelet therapy for 6-12 months, vs BM stents which req 4 weeks.

Cardiac Transplant:

1. **Denervated Physiology**
    - **Pre-load dependent**, **altered response to medications**: direct-acting (+); indirect-acting (-), **pacemaker** in 20%

2. Allograft function
    - **Accelerated CAD**: silent ischemia secondary to denervation, **Rejection**, **Arrhythmogenic**, cardiac transplant vasculopathy

3. **Co-existing end-organ disease**
    - renal dysfunction, HTN (~90%), DM, Malignancy (~30%)

4. **Immunosuppression** therapy
    - steroids (stress dose), cyclosporine, tacrolimus, azathioprine
    - increase. risk of infection; Anemia; Thrombocytopenia; hepato-nephrotoxicity

5. Increased risk of alloimmunization
    - Use irradiated CMV negative blood

Anesthetic Goals / Conflicts

1. Hemodynamic Goals
    - Preload: normal or high preload - transplanted heart increases CO by increasing SV
    - Rhythm: avoid pro-arrhythmic states
    - Afterload: maintain perfusion to potentially ischemic myocardium
2. Use direct-acting sympathomimetics (isoproterenol & dilute epinephrine must be available)
3. Avoid infection — adherence to strict sterile technique

Hx: Heart transplant Hx (indication, surgical & medical compilations, pacemaker)

Functional capacity (rejection, arrythmias, CHF, CAD – dyspnea may be only symptom, no angina) / Medications (immune - Cyclosporine / Tacrolimus: HTN, renal dysfunction, hepatotoxicity, seizure threshold, Azathioprine: bone marrow suppression) / co-existing disease (HTN, DM, renal dysfunction, malignancy) / infections

PE: Vitals / Airway – cushingoid with increase. soft tissue / Respiratory – rule out infection / Cardiac – s/s of CHF (crackles, increase. JVP, hepatomegaly, HJR, edema, S3/S4)

Investigations: Labs - decreased K^+, Mg^{++} (diuretics, dysrhythmias), increased Cr (anti-rejection drugs and renal insufficiency), increase. LFTs (anti-rejection drugs), Pancytopenia (anti-rejection drugs or sepsis), glucose (steroids, DM), coags (dysfunction from drugs) / ECG - RAD, incomplete RBBB, pre- 1994 - two P waves (native P unrelated to QRS), Q waves / CXR – failure / ECHO – LV/RV fxn / Dob stress ECHO for CAD (Exercise Stress Test not useful d/t blunted HR, MIBI not useful d/t diffuseness of disease) / Endomyocardial Bx

Optimization: LV fxn – adequate preload, manage rejection & ischemia / Co-existing dysfunction – HTN, DM CRF / transplant MD to manage transplant medications / Steroids / Abx for prophylaxis if valvopathy

Anesthetic Options: Local / Regional – check coags, maintain preload, direct acting vasopressors / GA – more predictable changes in preload & afterload, caution with renally excreted drugs, assess depthwith BP not HR, avoid hyperventilation (cyclosporine and tacrolimus lower seizure threshold), Azathioprine antagonizes NdMB activity

Room Setup: 5 leads, +- A-line, CVP based on Surgery, TEE based on pre-operative fxn, PNS, crashcart, Drugs - Phenyl, isoproterenol (2-10 mcg/min) and dilute epinephrine (10 mcg/ml)

Intraoperative Management: Aseptic, hemodynamically stable induction, use BP to monitor depth, avoidmyocardial depression with high volatile / Ensure adequate reversal

Post-operative: continue anti-rejection Tx ASAP – consult transplant team Re: levels

Cardiogenic Shock

Cardiogenic Shock: Systolic BP < 90mmHG x 30 mins + Cardiac Index < 2.2L/min/m2 + PCWP >15mmHG

1. Emergency situation with potential for perioperative mortality (>50%)
2. Etiology
   a. Acute MI - maximize myocardial O_2 supply / demand
      i) Medical therapy: ABP, VAD, invasive monitoring
      ii) Complications: CHF/Acute MR/Wall Rupture/Dysrhythmias
      iii) Early revascularization (PCI/CABG)
   b. Systolic and/or diastolic HF, **RVF**, Valvular disease, Arrhythmias
3. Co-morbid illnesses: HTN, DM, hyperlipidemia, Smoking, Advanced age, stroke
4. Risk of bleeding or thrombolytics, GIIb/IIIa inhibitors, LMWH/heparin, clopidogrel
5. revascularization technique given risk of post-operative bleeding

Anesthetic Goals/Conflicts:

1. Resuscitation stabilizing ABC 's, optimizing O2 supply / demand, & maintaining end organ perfusion
   - o Early consideration for Intra-Aortic Balloon bump /Ventricular Assisting Device /Per-Coetaneous Intervention /Coronary Artery Bypass Grafting
   - o Hemodynamic goals: to maintain/augment contractility, avoid tachycardia, reduce afterload, and maintain adequate preload
2. Ventricular interdependence – fluids, inotropes, decrease PVR in RVF
3. Rule out other causes of shock - Hypovolemic, Distributive, Obstructive
4. Diagnose mechanical complications that may necessitate urgent surgical intervention
5. Consult CVT & Cardiology - optimal

Hx: Confirm etiology – cardiogenic vs. others - Focused cardiac history, especially for CHF, dysrhythmias, functional capacity. CRFs: DM/HTN/lipids/smoking, previous therapies/interventions & investigations. Check for contraindications for thrombolytics: previous hemorrhage. Stroke, known CNS neoplasm, active bleeding. Aortic dissection, severe uncontrolled HTN, recent trauma, non-compressiblevascular punctures, recent trauma. Check for contraindications to IAB: Severe vascular dysfunction, AI, aortic aneurysm, irreversible cardiac/brain dmg.

PE: Vitals, U/O, poor pulses and cap refill, cool, cyanotic extremities, increase. JVP, new murmurs S3 +/-S4, pulsus paradoxus from R heart failure; MR – high pitched apical holosystolic murmur; VSD – harsh holosystolic murmur LSB, O2 step-up on PA; Rupture – PEA arrest, tamponade (JVD, muffled HS, pulsusparadoxus)

Investigations: CBC/Lytes/Ca+/Mg+/LFTs (congestion), Troponin, lactate, ABGs, ECG (arrhythmia, ischemia), CXR (effusions edema),

ECHO (valvular, VSD, rupture, effusion, EF), Consider urgent Angiography

Optimization:
Acute MI - Cardiology, MONA), Thrombolysis vs PTCA (90 mins) vs emergent CABG
Shock: Nitrates and BBs contraindicated in shock. Invasive lines, IABP pre-operatively, fluid challenge to PCWP 15-20mmHg for optimal CO, dopamine, dobutamine, Epinephrine, Milrinone. Optimize Hgb. Early intubate to reduce -WOB‖; FFP / octaplex if recently anticoagulated; Aspiration prophylaxis

Room Setup: CAS 5lead + invasive lines (PAC); IABP; crash cart; Inotropes; Perfusion services; blood; TEE

Intraoperative Management: Modified RSI (hemodynamics vs full stomach), ketamine/etomidate/opioid/roc.

Post-operative: ICU, opioid infusions for pain control in ICU vs boluses. Post-operative cardiac monitoring.

Complications: Arrhythmias (A-fib most common >10%), bradycardias, ventricular arrhythmias, V-fib 3- 5% peaks within 4 hours of MI, MR due to pap rupture, Free wall rupture = 2^{Nd} most common cause of death post-MI (15- 30%) pks 1 weak post MI.

Cardiomyopathy

Classification: ***Dilated, Restrictive, Hypertrophic,*** and ***Arrhythmogenic*** *RV cardiomyopathy (fibrofatty replacement of RV myocardium with sparing of LV/septum), risk of sudden death, RHF/unclassified*

1. Risk of peri-operative Systolic/diastolic dysfunction with impaired CO
2. Considerations for underlying etiology
    a. Dilated: Ischemia, HTN, Viral, ETOH, toxins, Idiopathic
    b. Restrictive: Amyloidosis, Sarcoidosis, Hemochromatosis, Idiopathic
    c. peripartum: Autoimmune, Idiopathic
    d. HCM: inherited, idiopathic
3. Risk of perioperative complications:
    a. MI, Ischemia, hypotension, arrhythmia, systemic embolism
4. Risk of dysrhythmias and considerations of pacemaker
5. Risk of systemic embolism, and considerations of anticoagulation

Anesthetic Goals/Conflicts:

- ***Dilated***: Maintain preload / avoid dec. contractility / maintain NSR / dec. afterload
- ***Restrictive:*** Maintain preload / maintain NSR / avoid brady / maintain afterload
- ***Peripartum:*** Maintain preload / avoid decrease in contractility / maintain afterload

Hx: Functional capacity, etiology, type of CM, investigations, signs of CHF, substance abuse (EtOH/ cocaine), medications, pacemakers/AICD settings, history of embolic complications, hx of arrhythmias, conduction defects, valvular dysfunction. Systemic complications related to infiltrative disorders.

PE: Pulse (prominent in HOCM), Displaced apical beat, LV heave (HOCM), S3 for CHF, S4 for infiltrative disorders. Regurgitant murmurs for dilated CM, cresc-decrescendo SEM b/History apex and LSB for HOCM increasing with Valsalva/standing (↓preload). Exam findings of CHF/pHTN. Increased JVP with restrictive and fail 's to fall during inspiration (Kussmaul 's).

Investigations: CBC / Lytes (diuretics) /Cr (hypoperfusion) Coags/CXR (LV/LA enlargement)/ECG – HOCM (LVH, q waves, ST changes, arrhythmias), Dilated LVH/ST changes/BBB 's, PVCs, Restrictive –BBBs, low voltage Echo – HOCM (SAM 25%), Dilated, decreased EF, restrictive, diastolic dysfunction, increased wall thickness, ↓ EF.

Optimization: Cardiology consult, CTU for infiltrative/pacemaker/AICD management/ BB for HOCM

Anesthetic Options: Caution with spinal/epidural with HOCM/consider regional

Room Setup: Crash cart, pacing pads, invasive lines preinduction, 5 Lead ECG, TEE, PAC, inotropic medications

Intraoperative Management: See hemodynamic goals above, consider cardiac induction, avoid SNS with HOCM.

Post-operative: HDU for cardiac monitoring/ischemia/hypotension/arrhythmias. Post-operative pacemaker interrogation.

Peri-partum CM: 4 criteria, develops within 6 months of pregnancy after delivery, no identifiable cause, new diagnosis with no prior heart disease, ECHO shows findings of dilated CM (EF<45%). Unknown etiology, Possible RF – multiple gestation, obesity, advanced maternal age, breat feeding; management similar to any form of HF. 20-80% Mortality.

Carotid End Antrectomy

1. High risk of peri-operative complications:
   a. Ischemic/hyper perfusion neurologic injury
   b. cardiac ischemia
   c. airway obstruction from hematoma / patch disruption
2. Significant peri-operative hemodynamic changes
   a. X-clamp: HTN, tachycardia, increase myocardial O2 demands
   b. Carotid sinus manipulation: bradycardia, hypotension
3. Co-existing medical illness (CAD, DM, HTN, PVD, CKD, smoking, advanced age)
4. Medications (ASA, Plavix, Anti-HTN)

Anesthetic Goals/Conflicts:

- Maintain stable hemodynamics to optimize perioperative cerebral perfusion
- Protect brain and heart from ischemic injury
- Smooth emergence: avoid coughing, bucking, straining on emergence
- Awake patient at end of surgery for neuro assessment

Carotid Stenting

- Remote location, comorbidity, perioperative complications (HD instability, Ischemic injury, MI), monitor for hyper perfusion syndrome postoperatively
- Sedation vs. GA

Hx

- Carotid stenosis: asymptomatic, symptomatic, hx, frequency, manifestations of TIAs/CVAs. Uni vs bilateral
- Comorbidities: CAD – MI is leading cause of peri-op morbidity post CEA, HTN – Increase risk ofneuro deficits after CEA with pre-operative HTN, PVD, DM, COPD, smoking
- Medications for CAD and CVA (anti-platelets, Anti-HTN)

PE: Carotid bruits, pre-existing neuro deficit, baseline BP

Investigations:

- CBC, lytes, BUN, Cr, G&S, EKG, review doppler U/S to assess extent of stenosis

Optimization:

- Beta blockade, continue antiplatelet therapy, consider discontinuing ACEi, ARBs

Anesthetic Options:

- GA, regional, LA + MAC (no diff in postop stroke with RA vs GA)
  Room Setup: CAS (5 lead EKG), A-line, cerebral monitor (EEG, stump, SSEP, transcranial Doppler)

Intraoperative Management:

- Induction / Maintenance: minimize risk of hypoperfusion and cerebral ischemia
- Emergence: minimize coughing (hematoma), IV lido, narcotics, deep extubation. Havenitroglycerin/ nitroprusside infusions, labetalol, hydralazine ready

Post-operative: Complications – thrombosis, intra-operative CNS ischemia, ICH, hyper perfusion syndrome / respiratory depression / airway obstruction – hematoma, RLN injury / hypertension - denervated carotid body / hypotension – baroreceptor hypersensitivity / Peri-operative

Cervical Plexus Block

Indications:

- Neck surgery including carotid endarterectomy

Nerves blocked:

- C2,3,4 nerve roots

Contraindications:

- General: Infection, Coagulopathy, lack of consent, true local anesthetic allergy, lack of resuscitation equipment
- Specific: Contra-lateral recurrent nerve injury (? contralateral phrenic nerve palsy?), severelung disease (FEV1 < 1L)

Equipment:

- Routine monitors and prep supplies
- 1.5-increaseh 25-gauge needle, 1.5 inches 22 gauge needle for insertion

Technique:

- Identify the mastoid process, Chassaignac 's tubercle and the posterior border of the SCM. Draw a line from the mastoid to Chassaignac 's tubercle. The insertion points for C2, C3 and C4 can be estimated as being 2,4 and 6 cm below the mastoid along this line. Then infiltrate the skin under this entire line and then, at each of the three points along the line insert your 22- gauge needle until the transverse process is contacted (perpendicular to skin with a slight caudad angulation). At each level aspirate and then inject 4 cc.

	Onset(min)	Anesthesia(hrs)	Analgesia(hrs)
1.5% Mepivacaine (+HCO3; + epinephrine)	10-15	2-2.5	3-6
2% Lidocaine (+HCO3; + epinephrine)	10-15	2-3	3-6
0.5% Ropivacaine	10-20	3-4	4-10
0.25% Bupivacaine (+ epinephrine)	10-20	3-4	4-10

- Glossopharyngeal branches need to be blocked as well for a CEA. This can be done by having the surgeon infiltrate the carotid (NYSORA).

Complications:

- Direct trauma: pneumo, esophageal perforation, carotid or IJ puncture, hematoma

Local anesthetic effects: inadvertent epidural, brachial plexus, intrathecal, intravenous or vertebral artery injection with associated seizures, phrenic nerve block, bradycardia or RLN dysfunction (60%)

Chronic Obstructive Lung Disease

1. High risk for perioperative respiratory complications including **respiratory failure**
2. Physiologic changes
    a. Chronic hypoxemia / hypercapnia
        i. **Cor pulmonale** and RV failure
    b. Reactive airways disease
    c. Bullous lung disease with the potential need for **lung isolation**
    d. Potential for hyperinflation and pulmonary tamponade
3. Comorbid disease
    a. CAD, DM, HTN, smoking, OSA, Obesity, Cancer, Cystic Fibrosis, Bronchiectasis
4. Increased sensitivity to respiratory depressant effects of anesthetic agents

Anesthetic Goals/Conflicts:

- Ensure optimization of COPD – delay elective cases as required
  - Manage acute infections, steroids, bronchodilators
- Optimize ventilation strategy
  - Prevent dynamic hyperinflation and barotrauma
    - Long I: E, low Pk pressure, low V_T slow rate, permissive hypercapnia
- Minimize peri-operative respiratory complications
  - Avoid use of respiratory depressants
  - Consider neuraxial or regional anesthesia

Hx: Determine disease severity and functional capacity; Dyspnea, wheeze, cough and sputum production; CHF Sx; Fever; Home O2; Meds; Recent exacerbations; ETT; ICU; Steroids; Co-morbidities

PE:

Respiratory: Tachypnea; Barrel chest; Respiratory distress (accessory muscles); A/E bilat; Prolonged Exp; Wheeze; Crackles;

CVS: JVD; HJR; Hepatomegaly; Pedal edema; RV heave; S3 or S4; Loud P2

Investigations: CBC, LYTES, BUN/Cr, CXR, EKG Also consider: ABG, sputum C+S, PFT; ECHO (RV dysfunction)

Optimization: Postpone surgery 4-6 weeks after exacerbation; +/- antibiotics, steroids (stress dose), bronchodilators, d/c smoking in advance (8 week to Decrease the risk), avoid sedatives

Anesthetic Options:

RA preferred but the risk of high neuraxial block will cause Phrenic paralysis → decrease in FEV1 30%;
GA results in decrease FRC, depression of respiratory drive. Consider TIVA

Room Setup: CAS + 5 Leads; Temperature; PNS; Spirometry; A-line (CO_2); TEE, PAC for Cor pulmonale; OLV equipment

Intraoperative Management: Deep GA; Use Ketamine/propofol/Sevoflurane; Lung protective strategies; Bullous disease (SV induction vs standard induction with OLV (unilateral & severe bilat);

Post-operative: Extubate awake; Pain control; PAR; Extubation criteria include: VC > 10 cc/kg, Vt > 6 cc/kg, NIP > - 20 cmH20, pO2/FiO2 > 200, A-a pO2 gradient on 100 % O2 < 350 mmHg

Complications: Auto-PEEP→ D/C from Ventilator; Bronchospasm – volatile, B agonists, Mg^{++}, Ketamine; pneumothorax – chest tube, possible lung isolation; Post-operative respiratory complications

Chronic Renal Failure

1. Increased risk of aspiration
2. Dysregulation of volume status, acid-base, and electrolytes
3. End-organ dysfunction:
    a. Autonomic dysfunction: hemodynamic instability
    b. Cardiac: LV dysfunction, HTN, CAD, CHF, pericarditis
    c. Hematologic: anemia / thrombocytopenia
4. Altered pharmacokinetics
    a. Decreased drug excretion
5. Etiology of renal failure

Anesthetic Goals/Conflicts:

- Optimize electrolytes, volume status, co-morbidities
- Avoid precipitating acute on chronic renal failure (euvolemia, avoid nephrotoxins)
- Coordinate perioperative dialysis if dialysis dependent
- Avoid compromising dialysis access (AV fistulas, indwelling IV lines, PD ports)
- Recognize increased risk of renal failure in certain surgeries (cardiac, aortic, vascular)

Hx: Etiology and co-morbidities: HTN, CAD, DM, severity of CRF, U/O (normal, oliguric, anuric), end-organ dysfunction (exercise tolerance, angina, CHF, palpitations, dialysis (mode, frequency, complications, access, duration, dry weight), GERD, bleeding tendency: GI, epistaxis

PE: Vitals - orthostatic, IV access (avoid subclavian), AV fistulae (avoid IVs and BP cuff), generalized edema, LVH, dysrhythmias, pericardial rubs, volume status, pulmonary edema, tachycardia (autonomicdysfunction)

Investigations: CBC (anemia, dysfunctional platelets), lytes (hyperkalemia, hyperPO4, hypocalcaemia, hypermagnesemia, hyponatremia), serum glucose, serum proteins (hypoalbuminemia), BUN (not a reliable indicator of GFR unless protein catabolism is normal and constant), Cr, ABG (for acidemia)

Imaging: EKG (LVH is common, arrhythmias on the basis of electrolyte abnormalities), +/- ECHO

Optimization: Defer if in ARF, Aspiration prophylaxis, dialysis timing (if chronic, dialyze day before. Ifacute, postop if possible – reduced hemodynamic instability), Empty PD pts, diabetes management, blood conservation strategies (Uremic bleeding: cryoprecipitate, DDAVP (0.3 mcg/kg IV), if borderline function and high-risk surgery for postoperative RF: generous pre-operative hydration, possible use of mannitol intraoperatively

Anesthetic Options: Local, regional, GA OK. Regional may be difficult b/c of AV fistulae, alsodysfunctional platelets. Reflux risk makes sedation or an LMA less attractive

Room Setup: CAS (5 lead EKG), +/- A-line, CVP

Intraoperative Management: Avoid nephrotoxins (aminoglycosides, dye, NSAIDs, ACEi, metformin), careful attention to dose and choice of opioids (avoid Demerol – judicious doses of morphine / hydromorphone – fentanyl OK), Check K+ prior to suxamethonium, NdMB – cis-atracurium, avoid hypervolemia, delayed emergence

Post-operative: postop morbidity (acidosis, hyperkalemia, infections, HTN / HTN, bleeding, dysrhythmias, clotted fistulas). Complications: ARF, volume overload, electrolyte abN, peri-operative CV complications

Cocaine Intoxication / Pregnancy

1. Risk of **Aspiration** – full stomach
2. Multi-system effects
    a. *Airway* – septal necrosis, thermal epiglottis
    b. *CNS* – seizures, hemorrhagic/ischemic stroke, SAH, delirium, paranoia, cerebral edema
    c. *CVS* – HTN, MI, Dysrhythmia, Aortic dissection, cardiomyopathy (chronic use)
    d. *Respiratory* – aspiration, pneumonitis, bronchospasm, pulmonary edema
    e. *Renal* – ARF (infarction, rhabdomyolysis)
    f. *Heme* – thrombocytopenia, DIC

3. **Interaction with Anesthetic** - potential for SNS stimulation (avoid ketamine, atropine), MAC increase. with intoxication, normal with chronic use, variable response to vasopressors (use direct agents, small dose)
4. **Co-intoxicants** - EtOH, MJ, heroin, opioids, amphetamines
5. **Complex pain management**
6. Potential IVDU and blood-bore infections
7. Cocaine effects in pregnancy
    a. Maternal - **placental abruption**, dec. uteroplacental perfusion, spontaneous abortion, premature labor, premature ROM, decreased plasma cholinesterase (decrease cocaine metabolism)
    b. Fetal – increased congenital abnormalities, IUGR, cardiomyopathy, MI, intra-cerebral bleeding, CNS irritability

Anesthetic Goals/Conflicts:

- Supportive and hemodynamic management of acute cocaine intoxication
- Conflicts: Potentially full stomach (RSI) vs hemodynamically stable induction
- Uncooperative patient / Thrombocytopenia with regional techniques

Hx:

Hz/duration of use, co-intoxicants, infectious disease, sequelae of use: stroke, MI, HTN, cardiomyopathy, pulmonary edema, bowel ischemia, renal failure, hepatic failure (hepatitis), bleeding, easy bruising.
+ Obstetric hx: prenatal care, abstinence, spontaneous abortion, abruption, PROM, fetal well-being, anomalies, IUFD, cardiomyopathy. R/o coexisting PIH

PE: Standard PE - vitals, focused on symptoms, FHR

Investigations: CBC, plts, lytes (RF), Coags if suspect liver failure, X-match (risk of abruption), Toxicology, TSH, ECG, CXR (pulmonary edema, dissection), ECHO (cardiomyopathy), fetal U/S, NST, HR

Optimization: - **Delay, if possible, with acute intoxication – duration ~120 min**

HTN: 1st line benzo 's 2Nd line NTG/SNP/alpha blockade (phentolamine 1mg IV q3mins/hydralazine. No BB 's

HD stable VT or SVT: 1st line Benzo's 2Nd line Lido(competes for Na+ channels), $HCO3^-$ 1-2meq/kg shows benefit in animals. CCB is controversial, verapamil 2.5-5mg IV over 2 mins q5-10 max 20 for rate control.

V-fib or unstable VT: Defib/CPR > unknown role for Epi, Vasopressin preferred, Lido + HCO3 as per above, unknown role for amiodarone.

Chest Pain: O_2, monitors, 1st line Benzo 's + NTG 2Nd line phentolamine, ASA. 3rd. considerCCB/ labetalol.

Anesthetic Options: All possible if cooperative, consider thrombocytopenia, hypotension with neuraxial Consider HTN with SNS activation

Room Setup: CAS + 5lead, large bore IV, Arterial line, Temperature (hyperthermia), vasoactive medications, Nitro 0.5-1mcg/kg/min, SNP 0.3-10mcg/kg/min, verapamil 2.5-5mg over 2 mins q5-10mins (max 20).

Intraoperative Management: Increased MAC, deep laryngoscopy, pre-treat HTN, Avoid SNS drugs(ketamine/atropine/potent volatiles), used direct vasoactive meds (smaller dose phenyl)

Post-operative: Ongoing monitoring, risk of arrhythmias, MI, withdrawal, hard to manage pain

CO Poisoning/Smoke Inhalation

1. Potential for evolving respiratory compromise
   - loss of airway from edema/obstruction
   - ALI / ARDS
2. Coexisting injuries - Burns & trauma
3. Complications
   - Sepsis, Rhabdomyolysis, lactic acidosis, Renal failure, Thrombocytopenia, Consumptive coagulopathy, Electrolyte disturbances

Anesthetic Goals/

Conflicts:

1. Rapidly assess need to establish definitive airway - 1 or more are present:
   i) Stridor
   ii) Use of accessory respiratory muscles
   iii) Respiratory distress
   iv) Hypoxia or hypercapnia
   v) Deep burns to the face or neck
   vi) Blistering or edema of the oropharynx
2. Support oxygenation with 100% O2, consider HBO chamber early
3. Volume resuscitation as required

Hx: Events surrounding the inhalation injury, closed-space environment, signs of dyspnea,

PE: Vitals (inaccurate SaO_2 with Carboxyhemoglobin), singed nasal hairs/eyebrows, cutaneous burns on head/ neck/torso. Carbonaceous sputum. Respiratory: edema, wheeze. CVS: dysthymias.

Investigations: CBC, lytes, BUN, Cr, glucose, lactate, ABG: PaO_2, SaO_2, carboxy-Hb level (co-oximetry) CN level. CXR (often initially normal)
FOB (96% PPV of findings if Carboxyhemoglobin >10%, closed-space fire, and carbonaceous sputum. Look for: erythema, edema, ulceration of the airways, and carbonaceous debris.

Optimization: Early intubation, High FiO2, Parkland formula – (4 ml/kg / BSA burned, give ½ in first 8 hrs and the rest over the next 16 hours (underestimates requirements of infants < 10 kg - use 6 ml/kg/% burned per 24 hrs); overly aggressive resuscitation can worsen supraglottic edema, Bronchodilators. Steroids are ineffective and can increase the risk of infection

Anesthetic Options: depends on patient 's condition, often early ETT/↑FiO_2

Room Setup: CAS monitors, uncut ETT, FOB/Difficult Airway cart

Intraoperative Management: ↑FiO_2 for CO treatment
Post-operative: post-operative ventilation until recovery from airway/lung injury and edema

Complex Regional Pain Syndrome

1. Chronic pain with its associated psychological, cognitive, and behavioural effects
2. Requires accurate diagnosis while ruling out other pathology
3. Initial presentation represents a relative medical emergency
   a. Need for early, aggressive, multimodal therapy
4. Medications associated with CRPS
   a. Opiate tolerance

Assessment:

- General Categories: Sensory, Motor, Vasomotor (temperature, colour), and Sudomotor (fluid balance)
- **Hx**: initiating event, severity and duration of symptoms, previous treatments and their impact,rule out other aetiologies (malignancy, infection etc....), functional impact
- **Px**: Vitals, allodynia, hyperalgesia, skin colour and temperature, hyperhidrosis, presence ofskin atrophy, nail and hair changes, edema, joint stiffness, muscle weakness, dystonia.

Etiology: Trauma, neurologic insults, HSV, MI;
Risk Factors: female, trauma, nerve injury, WCB, surgery
Investigations: EMG, sweat tests, 3 phase bone scan, Xray, MRI/CT, diagnostic sympathetic blocks

Treatment:

Early referral to specialist, Multiple modalities with goal of facilitating physio/OT - TCA, gabapentin, opioids, non-opioids (prazosin, clonidine, phentolamine, NMDA antagonists), TENS, IVRA, sympathetic blocks, neuraxial treatment (SCS, intrathecal pumps), surgery (sympathectomy)

Conn's Syndrome (hyperaldosteronism)

1) Hypertension and end-organ dysfunction:
    a. Cardiac dysfunction, stroke
2) Fluid and electrolyte abnormalities
    a. Volume overload
    b. Hypernatremia, Hypokalemia
3) Medications: Spironolactone

Anesthetic Goals/Conflicts:

- Perioperative normalization of fluid and electrolyte status Perioperative control of hypertension

Unstable C-spine

1. Urgent/Emergent airway management with risk of aspiration
2. Difficult airway management: limited cROM, other head and neck trauma
3. Prevention of secondary spinal cord injury
    - Airway management, transfers and positioning
    - Hard collar, manual in-line stabilization, Mayfield pins, full spine precautions
4. Predisposing Comorbidities: Congenital /Acquired / Trauma
5. Acute pinnal cord injury (if appropriate)
    - Neurogenic shock
    - Respiratory insufficiency
    - Succinylcholine contraindicated
    - Loss of thermal regulation

Anesthetic Goals/Conflicts:

1. Adequate pre-operative identification and optimization of unstable cervical spine if elective surgery
2. Safely secure airway with prevention of secondary spinal cord injury through immobilization during airway management, transfers and positioning
3. Potential conflicts: Uncooperative, intoxicated or pediatric patient vs. awake FOI

Hx: Identify etiology and screen for associated comorbidities and aspiration risk
PE: Vitals, airway exam (mouth opening, dentition, TMD, neurological symptoms with neck movement if appropriate), usual cardiovascular and respiratory exams

Investigations: Consider any of lateral neck film (flex/ex if appropriate), 3 views (lateral, AP, open mouth odontoid), CT neck. Ant ADI > 4-5mm abnormal. MRI useful for ligamentous injuries.

Optimization: Aspiration prophylaxis or fasting as appropriate, glycopyrrolate

Anesthetic Options: Spine stabilization during airway management and positioning through manual in-line stabilization (MILS), awake fiberoptic intubation, Mayfield pins (after intubation). FOI with NETT may be technique of choice; DL with MILS also acceptable for emergency cases. DL associated with maximal movement at odontoid-C1/2. Cricoid controversial (risk of aspiration vs. displacement of c-spine).

Room Setup: Difficult airway cart, skilled assistants, consider ENT surgeon present.

Intraoperative Management: Dexamethasone may decrease airway edema

Post-operative: Consider postop ventilation/ICU in head up position or extubation over tube exchanger depending on degree of airway edema, prone positioning and instrumentation

DDx: Congenital (Down's syndrome - 15%, odontoid abn, mucopolysaccharidoses), Acquired (RA-30%, Still's disease, ankylosing spondylitis, psoriatic arthritis, Crohn's/UC, Reiter's Syndrome) and Trauma (odontoid #, other bony #, ligamentous disruption, 5% of TBI have a c-spine injury)
No c-spine imaging acceptable after trauma if: A & O; no head injury; no intoxication; no neck pain; no abn neurology; no distracting injury; neck examination normal

Croup/ Laryngotracheobronchitis

Acute but self-limiting viral infection causing narrowing of subglottic structures and rarely airway compromise requiring intubation

1. Emergency
2. Pediatric patient
3. Complications
   - Association with bacterial tracheitis
   - Airway obstruction

Anesthetic Goals / Conflicts

1. safely secure airway if necessary
2. avoid precipitants of complete airway obstruction
3. r/o other conditions

Hx & Px

6 History /o to 6 History /o; onset 12 hours to 3 days; low grade fever, barking cough; coryza, rhinorrhea

Investigations: AP neck films: -steeplell sign (not specific); CBC, blood cultures

Optimization:

- intubation and Humidified air
- nebulized epi 0.5 ml/kg of 1:1000 max 5 ml (racemic no longer available) q15-20 min
- dex 0.6mg/kg PO
- Can generally be extubated in 4-7 days after confirmation of leak, resolution of other symptoms
- Extubate in OR after visualization

Cushing's Syndrome (hypercortisolism)

- Difficult airway: Obesity / OSA
- Coexisting Disease
  - Cardiac:
    - o HTN / Volume overload (increased renin and glucocorticoid vascular reactivity)
    - o LVH, pHTN/RVF, systolic and diastolic dysfunction
  - CNS: Psychosis
  - Metabolic:
    - o Hypokalemic metabolic alkalosis – mineralocorticoid effects of glucocorticoids
    - o DM – insulin deficiency
    - o Osteoporosis
- Potential difficult IV access
- Perioperative Steroid replacement
- Pharmacologic considerations: Sensitivity to NMB, catecholamines
- Considerations of pituitary tumours (4M 's)

Anesthetic Goals/Conflicts:

Minimize risk of adrenal insufficiency during perioperative stress

Cyanotic Heart Disease

- Right to Left Shunt (Qp: Qs < 1) (Tetralogy Of Fallot's TOF, tricuspid/pulmonary atresia, Transposition od Great Vessels TGV, truncus arteriosus, TAPVR, hypoplastic Lt Heart)

  - Shunt dependent on RVOT obstruction and PVR / SVR
    - o Optimize CO and tissue oxygenation by balancing SVR and PVR
  - **Chronic hypoxemia**
    - o pHTN & cor pulmonale
    - o Polycythemia - risk of thrombosis with HCT > 55, avoid dehydration and Fe deficiency
  - Risk of paradoxical air embolus (prevent air in IV, avoid N_2O)
  - Treatment: Maintain PDA, palliation with BT shunt + Glenn / Fontan vs. primary repair

- Complications
  - General – dec. growth, developmental delay, increased metabolic rate
  - Cardiac - hypertrophy, arrhythmias, RV failure with ischemia, volume overload with CHF
  - Pulmonary
    - o Dec. PBF: TOF, Tricuspid or Pulmonary atresia History /o VSD
    - o Increase. PBF: TGV, hypoplastic L heart, TAPVR, Truncus
  - Heme (polycythemia, hyper viscosity, coagulopathy – dec. Vit K)
  - CNS (brain abscess)

- Assess anatomy/surgical repair/residual shunts and ventricular function
- SBE prophylaxis
- Associated syndromes (Down 's) + defects (craniofacial, skeletal, GI / GU)

ANESTHETIC GOALS:

1. Hemodynamic goals:
   - **o** **TOF**: full preload, high SVR, low PVR, low contractility, low HR, avoid dehydration
   - **o** **BT shunts**: PBF dependent on MAP and PVR – maintain SpO_2 <85% - balance of systemic and pulmonary blood flow – avoid high FiO2 / hyperventilation– pulmonary vasodilation
   - **o** **Fontan**: PBF / CO depends on preload and PVR - **Full preload, low PVR,** normal SVR (prevent R – L shunt), N contractility, and **NSR** (dec. pulmonary venous congestion)

- **Consider factors that increase PVR**: hypercarbia, hypoxia, acidosis, SNS stimulation, lung hyperinflation (PVR is lowest when lung is at FRC → large Vt and low frequency), increased HCT

2. Avoid air bubbles (important for R to L shunts)
3. Avoid hypothermia (left shift of O2Hb curve - less available O2, Platelet's dysfunction, hyperviscosity and metabolic acidosis)

- **Pathophysiology:** Incidence: 8:1000 live births; 25% have other abnormality; 8.5% syndromic(most commonly History / endocardial cushion defect, VSD, TOF)

- **Hx:** Clinical diagnosis, surgical repair, residual lesions; **Functional status**; weight gain if infant; NYHA classification; Prolonged intubation (subglottic stenosis); Strokes (hyper viscosity syndromein cyanotic lesions); Associated syndromes (Down 's, VACTERL, DiGeorge); Medications: inotropes, diuretics, afterload reducers, digoxin (0.8-2 ng/mL therapeutic)

- **Px:** weight, height, VS, SaO_2, cyanosis, clubbing; signs of CHF (elevated JVP, pedal edema, crackles, tachypnea, hepatomegaly in infants), BP discrepancies (coarctation); increase. WOB (nasal flaring, increase RR, chest retractions, accessory muscle use); Shock – cap refill, peripheralperfusion

- **Investigations:** If repaired lesion, doing well, on no medications → only routine investigations dictated by the surgical procedure; If uncorrected lesion:
  CBC Polycythemia in cyanotic lesions (Hb = 200 g/L) - Consider phlebotomy; Thrombocytopenia;
  Coags (coagulopathy 2[Nd] to low levels of vitamin K dependent factors);
  Lytes if on diuretic, digoxin, history of arrhythmia;
  ABG if cyanosis or respiratory failure;
  Imaging: EKG, CXR, ECHO: define anatomy of lesion, exclude other lesions,
  Cath

- **Optimization:** Clear fluids to 2 hrs pre-operatively, optimize preload, SBE prophylaxis, anxiolysis

- **Anesthetic Options:** Local vs. regional vs. general depending on lesion and procedure

- **Anesthetic Setup:** Emergency drugs; CAS monitors; **NIBP and IV on opposite side of shunts;**
- capnography: **dead space will underestimate $PaCO_2$ in R → L shunts;** Consider A-line, CVP

- **Management:**

Regional - Consider the type of cardiac lesion (decreased SVR in TOF undesirable) Improvesperipheral blood flow, decreased DVT, reduced perioperative blood loss; Coagulation status

General anesthesia: Slower inhalation, faster IV induction, potential for overdose in R → L shunts; Ketamine useful: minimal myocardial dysfunction, **maintains SVR, little effect on PVR;** Avoid N2O;Avoid high PAPs and PEEP in patients with decreased pulmonary blood flow; PEEP may be of valuein patients with high pulmonary blood flow (truncus arteriosus, TAPVR); Early extubation may be appropriate in patients with uncomplicated anesthetic and surgical courses

Disposition & Monitoring: Depends on lesion/repair/procedure; Most will require some type of post-operative monitoring

Cyanotic Neonate

1. **O_2 responsive** - Hyaline membrane disease, Meconium aspiration, GBS pneumonia, PTX, Diaphragmatic hernia

2. **Not O_2 responsive** - PPHN, Truncus Arteriosus, TAPVR, TGA, Epstein 's anomaly, Right heart obstruction including TOF (may present late unless severe RVOT obstruction)

3. **PDA dependant lesions**
   - Systemic Flow: Coarctation, interrupted aortic arch, Hypoplastic left heart, Critical aortic stenosis
     a. Shock: Poor distal perfusion with closure of ductus
   - Pulmonary Flow: Tricuspid/Pulmonary atresia, RVOT obstruction (pulmonary stenosis, TOF)
     b. Cyanosis: R to L shunt with ductus closure

4. **Management:** Depends on age of presentation and clinical manifestations
   - R to L shunts - goal is to increase pulmonary blood flow
     a. If duct dependent: start PGE
     b. If not duct dependent; balance between PVR and SVR
   - Shock – goal is to improve systemic cardiac output
     a. If duct dependent: start PGE
   - CHF - Implies L to R shunt with increased pulmonary blood flow and volume overload - need to decrease pulmonary blood flow
   - Supportive – Intubation, Glucose: can become hypoglycemic d/t hepatic congestion, consider bicarbonate to improve metabolic milieu, PGE1

Cystic Fibrosis

1. **Risk of aspiration** – GERD, Mechanical ileus
2. **Risk of perioperative respiratory dysfunction**
   - **Mixed obstructive and RLD with potential for pHTN, RVF, and cor pulmonale**
   - Thick secretions; chronic pneumonia; bronchiectasis; bullous disease
   - Increase. risk of perioperative pulmonary complication: hypoxemia, bronchospasm, PTX, massive hemoptysis, respiratory failure requiring ventilation
3. **Other Co-morbidities**: Malnutrition with anemia or chronic disease
   - Coagulopathy - Vit K deficiency, obstructive hepatobiliary dysfunction
   - Pancreatic insufficiency with DM
   - Meds: O_2, insulin, Bronchodilators, Steroids, mucolytics, Abx
4. Postop: pain management; aggressive respiratory therapy; HDU/ICU

Anesthetic Goals/Conflicts:

- Minimize perioperative pulmonary complications: optimization of pre-operative respiratory function, hydration, and control of secretions; Lung protection ventilation strategies; avoid bronchospasm; pain control
- Minimize lung contamination (hemoptysis or abscess)
- Avoid precipitants of pHTN
- Conflicts: emergency surgery in CF with active infection & regional anesthesia in thesetting of potential coagulopathy

Hx & PE: **severity of Cardiopulmonary disease** – vitals with SaO_2, increase. WOB, dyspnea, cyanosis, Clubbing, orthopnea, adventitia, hyperinflation, infection, pHTN & RV failure (edema, increase. JVP, S3/ S4, P2, heave), functional status; **GI Disease** – cachexia, GERD, hepatic dysfunction (jaundice,

coagulopathy), bowel obstruction; Other Organs – DM
Current Treatment: physio, O_2, bronchodilators, mucolytics, steroids, Abx, insulin/PO hypoglycemics

Investigations: CBC; Lytes; Ur; Cr; Glucose; Coags; LFT; Sputum C/S; ABG; CXR/CT; ECG plus ECHOif evidence of pHTN; PFTs (increase. RV, FRC; dec. FEV_1, PEF, FEV_1/FRC, VC)

Optimization: Consults (respiratory, cardio, endo, peds, ICU); Delay elective surgery if active infection; Pulmonary function – chest physiotherapy and postural drainage, Abx, Bronchodilators, steroids; cardiac medications; correct coagulopathy; aspiration prophylaxis

Anesthetic Options: LA vs RA vs GA or GA/RA

Room Setup: CAS monitors + 5-Lead ECG, PNS, Art line, +/-CVP & TEE if pHTN & RV dysfunction; Meds: vasopressors, pulmonary vasodilators, bronchodilators, large ETT, suction catheter, DLT, FOB, Chest tube Avoid: Anticholinergics; ketamine, nasal intubation

Intraoperative Management: Pre-O_2 with RSI; spontaneous ventilation if bullous disease; use short acting NMB and anesthetics (remi); frequent suctioning; lung protective ventilation strategy (minimize PIP, long E time); Avoid precipitants of pHTN; avoid long-acting respiratory depressants

Emergence: Crisp emergence; completely reversed & suctioned prior extubation; pain control withadjuvants;

Post-operative: HOB 30-40°, resume aggressive Chest physio; Monitor in HDU for perioperativepulmonary complication

Complications: Hemoptysis; PTX; Post induction cardiopulmonary collapse (hypoxemia, PPV, pHTN, RVF); Hypoxemia; High PAP; Failure to wean

Special: 1:30 carrier; 1:3000 births CF: autosomal recessive mutation of CF gene on Ch 7; Abn CFTR(Cl channel→ thick secretion; plugging of Exo glands.

Delayed Emergence

Deferential diagnosis:

- Drugs - absolute or relative overdose
  - Volatile, Hypnotics, Narcotics, Nonaesthetic - Phenothiazines, α_2 agonists, TCA, NdMBs, illicit drugs, ETOH
- Infections
  - Encephalitis, Meningitis, abscess, Sepsis
- Metabolic
  - Hypoxia / hypercarbia, **Hypo/hyperglycemia**, myxedema coma, adrenal insufficiency, Electrolytes (Sodium, Calcium, Magnesium), Toxins (Uremia, hepaticencephalopathy)
  - Hypothermia
- Structural
  - CVA, ICH, Tumor, Cerebral edema, Postictal, hydrocephalus, pneumocephalus, hypoperfusion
- Severe pain

Most frequent causes

- Relative Overdose, Increased sensitivity (extremes of age), Drug interactions, Hepatic/renal disease,
- Consider opioids, MAOi 's, NdMBs, acidosis, Mg, drugs that potentiate NdMBs, recentwithdrawal from EtOH or illicit drugs
- Pediatrics
- Hypoxemia, Ingestion, Meningitis, TBI (abuse)

Management:

- Inform surgeon
- Ensure the patient is hemodynamically stable with adequate oxygenation and ventilation
- Scan monitors for HR, rhythm, $EtCO_2$, SaO_2, cycle BP, Etagent, temperature
- Ensure that all anesthetic agents, volatile and IV are stopped
- Stimulate obtunded patient, restrain combative patient
- Diagnosis and treat metabolic derangement
  - **Blood glucose**, electrolytes, ABG
- Review medications and dosages - Check for syringe or ampule swap
- Consider reversing specific agents
  - Naloxone – 0.04mg IV titrated to effect
  - Flumazenil – 0.2mg q 1 min titrated to effect (max 3mg/hr)
  - Physostigmine – 1mg q 3 min titrated to effect (max 4mg)

- **Hx & Px including neurologic evaluation**
  - collateral history, chart review (drugs, diabetes, lytes, injuries, infection, seizures, endocrinopathy, renal/hepatic impairment); -at risk‖ procedure (bypass, open ventricle, CEA, craniotomy). Anesthetic – duration, drugs, doses
  - Focal neurologic findings - PERL, corneal, gag reflex, Limb reflexes

- **Investigations:** CBC, electrolytes, glucose, BUN, Cr, Mg, Ca, PO4, LFTs, blood/urine culture, tox screen, TSH, fT4, Serum osmolality, lactate, ABGs, ECG, CXR, CT head, consider LP

- **Early consultation with neurology or neurosurgery**

- If no improvement, arrange transport to ICU for continued care

Diabetes Insipidus

1. Etiology and Co-existing Disease
    - Neurogenic - posterior pituitary surgery, tumour, head trauma
    - Nephrogenic - CRF, drug induced (Lithium), fluoride toxicity, hypokalemia, hypercalcemia, sickle cell anemia
    - DDx of hypernatremia- (any cause of excessive water loss, renaldisease, mineralocorticoid excess, hypertonic NG feeds)
2. Hemodynamic instability due to volume depletion
3. Hypernatremia
    - Thirst, altered LOC, lethargy, Seizures, Coma, Hypovolemia, Shock
    - risk of ICH from acute, severe hypernatremia
    - risk of correction (cerebral edema, volume overload, water intoxication)

Anesthetic Goals/Conflicts:

- Pre-operative normalization of serum sodium when possible: correct < 0.5 mEq/hour
    - o IV fluid, DDAVP (neurogenic), Chlorpropamide (nephrogenic)
- Restore intravascular volume
    - o replace ongoing losses with hypotonic IV solution
- Treat underlying etiology

Hx: U/O > 100ml/hr of dilute urine with hypernatremia. Search for etiology: surgical history (esp. pituitary), medications (Lithium, glyburide, ampho B, methoxyflurane), electrolytes (hypokalemia, hypercalcemia, sickle cell anemia), toxicities, renal failure, trauma; symptoms of DI & hypernatremia; previous treatment

PE: Vitals, postural BP, volume status, focused neurological exam for localizing signs, signs of trauma, other pituitary abnormalities

Investigations: Serum and Urine lytes, urine osmolality < 300mOsm/L and serum Na > 150, urine specific gravity < 1.002, Renal function, Calcium (hypercalcemia), Other hormonal deficiencies, CT headfor CNS etiology; Water deficit = TBW x ([Na]/140 – 1)

Optimization: aim for euvolemic but avoid rapid correction (replace water deficit with hypo osmolar fluid (D5W) over 24-48 hrs, not more than 0.5-1 mEq/L/hr), DDAVP for Neurogenic DI (1-3ug IV bid, 5-20ug IN bid), d/c offending drugs. Nephrogenic DI - chlorpropamide 200-500mg/d (potentiates renal effects of vasopressin, A/E hypoglycemia), clofibrate, carbamazepine- enhances vasopressin secretion, HCTZ-potentiates renal effects of ADH

Anesthetic Options: none preferred. Note: higher MAC with hypernatremia

Room Setup: vasopressin (.1-.2U/hr infusion), consider Art line to monitor Na, foley, Consider CVP tomonitor volume status

Intraoperative Management: Fluid management – NS bolus to euvolemia, maintenance plus 2/3 previous hour U/O as D51/2NS, if hourly fluids >400ml, add DDAVP, consider vasopressin infusion

Post-operative: Hemodynamic instability, intracranial hemorrhage, water intoxication from therapy, Cerebral edema

Diabetes Mellitus

1. Potential difficult airway with risk of aspiration
   a. stiff joint, obesity, autonomic neuropathy (gastroparesis)
2. End-organ dysfunction
   a. Macrovascular - CAD, HTN, PVD, CVD
   b. Microvascular - nephropathy, retinopathy
   c. Neuropathy – peripheral, autonomic
3. Increased perioperative risk
   a. Related to end organ dysfunction
   b. Related to DM and its treatment
      i. Hypo/hyperglycemia, DKA, HONK
4. Perioperative management of oral hypoglycemic/insulin

Anesthetic Goals/Conflicts:

- Identify and optimize end-organ dysfunction
- Optimize perioperative glycemic control – 6.5-10 mmol/L
  - hold oral hypoglycemic, ½ NPH dose – 100cc/hr D5W, avoid extremes of hypo-/ hyperglycemia
- Avoid and manage glycemic complications - DKA, hypokalemia, hypoglycemia

OB Considerations: increase. maternal risk (DKA, difficult airway, aspiration, nerve injury, hypoglycemia, PIH, polyhydramnios, preterm, infection c-section, dystocia,); Fetal risk – CVS, CNS, GI

Hx: DM type and duration, meds, insulin, Glycemic control (average BS, HgA1C), Previous episodes ofDKA/ HONK; End-organ disease (CAD, HTN, PVD, CRONIC KIDNEY DISEASE, CVD), **Functional Capacity**, Neuropathy - autonomic (orthostatic HTN, lack of HR variability) and peripheral (burning pain, paresthesia); Retinopathy (have they seen ophthalmology)

PE: VITALS (postural), Airway assessment (Stiff joint syndrome, prayer sign); Focused physical based on history of associated co-morbidities (cardiac / CNS);
Autonomic neuropathy - resting tachycardia, orthostatic hypotension, absent beat-beat variation in HR with breathing, prolonged QT
Inv: CBC, lytes, Ur, Cr (renal insufficiency), fasting glucose, ECG; cardiac work-up as per AHA

Optimization: end-organ dysfunction, Management of meds – stop metformin 48hrs pre-operative, holdhypoglycemic, ½ NPH dose and give D5W pre-operative; glycemic control, 1st case of day, involve endocrine if brittle; consider B-blockers as per AHA

Options: Neuraxial (reduced stress response, but reduced insulin secretion); higher risk of neuropathy with regional (worse with epi); GA

Room Setup: CAS +5 lead; Art line (sampling, neuropathy); Direct acting agents if autonomic neuropathy, glucometer –consider IV insulin infusion to maintain BS 5.0-11 mmol/L; Appropriate airway preparation

Intraoperative Management: Glucose intra-operative monitoring – avoid hypoglycemia; Appropriate padding (prone to neuropathy)

Post-operative: dependant on case and comorbidity

Complications: Perioperative MI, ARF, hypoglycemia, DKA, HONK, autonomic instability, infection, sepsis

Diabetic Keto Acidosis & HONK

DKA in type I DM, NKH in type II DM - Both due to precipitating event: hypovolemia, trauma, infection, MI, CVA, pancreatitis, drugs (diuretics). HONK - no ketones due to residual basal insulin secretion which impairs lipolysis.

1. Emergency situation
    a. aspiration risk, limited time for optimization
2. Metabolic derangement
    a. Hyperglycemia with dehydration, hyperosmolarity and coma
    b. Metabolic acidosis
    c. Electrolyte disturbances – hypokalemia, hyponatremia
3. Considerations of DM (neuropathy, nephropathy, airway, CAD)
4. Risk of cerebral edema with rapid reduction in serum osmolality

Anesthetic Goals/Conflicts:

- Volume replacement with NS until end-organ perfusion restored
    - 1-2 L in DKA; 3-8L in HONK
- Humulin R 0.1U/kg bolus then Humulin R 0.1U/kg/hr infusion
- Continue insulin until anion gap resolved – switch to D51/2NS when BS 15 mmol/L
    - Monitor Na & replace total water deficit over 24-48 hr – urine output as a guide
- Start KCl infusion (40mEq/L) when U/O > 0.5ml/kg/hr, and K < 4.5
- Monitor glucose q30-60min; lytes, AG and Phosphate q 60 min – phosphate will need repletion
- Identify etiology (sepsis, MI, poor compliance, new diagnosis)

Hx: Standard DM history when applicable; usually precipitated by poor patient compliance with insulin; hxof any precipitating factors; symptoms – polyuria, polydipsia, weight loss, lethargy, visual changes, stupor, coma, Sz, N/V, abdominal pain, fruity odor on breath

PE: Vitals (postural BP - osmotic diuresis and vomiting); Kussmaul's respirations (severe acidosis);Decreased LOC, coma

Investigations: CBC (polycythemia), lytes (Hyperglycemia (HONK > DKA), metabolic acidosis withanion gap (pH< 7.3, HCO3 < 15) hyponatremia with hyperosmolarity, hyperkalemia initially → hypokalemia with treatment, hypophosphatemia), Cr (ARF), osmolarity, urine ketones,

Optimization: treat the DKA before O.R. unless an emergency

Intraoperative Management: continue to manage the DKA

Post-operative: HDU for intensive monitoring of electrolytes

Complications: Hypokalemia, Hypophosphatemia, Cerebral edema

Disseminated Intravascular Coagulation

Widespread systemic activation of coagulation intravascular thrombosis & consumptive coagulopathy

1. Emergency situation with high mortality requiring urgent evaluation and management
2. Multisystem complications
   a. Bleeding (ICH, tamponade, hemothorax, hematuria, surgical wounds etc.)
   b. Thromboembolism (CNS ischemia, ARF, ARDS, PE, liver failure)
3. Considerations for underlying etiology

Anesthetic Goals/Conflicts:

- Diagnose and treat underlying cause
- Replace consumed coagulation factors/platelets and lost RBCs as required
- Support multi-organ system failure

Hx: AMPLE, details of critical illness

PE: Vitals, GCS, Airway, Cardio-Respiratory exam, look for bleeding, end-organ failure – decreased level of consciousness, shock, ARDS, Acute renal failure, liver dysfunction

Investigations: CBC, coags, fibrinogen, FDPs, D-dimer, ABGs, ECG, CXR; DIC is suggested by aclinical condition consistent with DIC, thrombocytopenia (< 100 x 109/L), prolonged PT and a-PTT, presence of FDP/D-dimer

Optimization: Correct underlying etiology and physiologic derangement, Platelets >50, FFP to keepINR<1.5-2, Cry to keep fibrinogen>1.5, PRBC to maintain perfusion

Room Setup: Standard CAS, large bore IV, fluid warmer, +/- Artline & CVP

Intraoperative Management: GA, Neuraxial contraindicated. Potential conflict of need for RSI with possible hemodynamic collapse on induction. Need for continued supportive management, keep up with consumptive coagulopathy, keep warm, repeated intra-operative bloodwork. Replacement of factors/bloodwhen needed.

Post-operative: Ongoing coagulopathy, likely need SPAR/ICU setting

Special: Complications include massive hemorrhage, ongoing bleeding, and multi-organ failure

Difficult Airway

Expected difficult intubation 2° to history and/or physical

- Previous anesthetics, Hx of OSA, radiation to head and neck, tumours of head and neck, previous long- term intubation (stenosis); short -bullll neck, prominent incisors, limited ROM of neck or TMJ, pregnancy, congenital syndromes, airway infections, trauma, anaphylaxis, morbid obesity, obvious anatomical abnormalities, stridor, subcutaneous emphysema, blood in oro/nasopharynx

- Assess for difficult airway (obesity, tumor, burns, dec. neck mobility)

- Consider alternatives to GA
  - Airway management will still be a problem if complications arise

- Prepare basic airway equipment plus contingency plan
  - Multiple blades and ETT sizes, stylet, bougie, light wand, glide-scope, LMA +/- Fastrack,
  - Equipment for transtracheal jet ventilation
    - Readily available and connected to O_2 source
  - FOB; Cricothyrotomy set and skilled clinician; Consider CPB standby

- Perform awake intubation
    - Judicious IV sedation
        - Conflict between cooperative patient and awake patient
    - Topicalize airway
        - 0.2 mg glycopyrrolate5cc 4% cocaine with 15cc 4% lidocaine in atomizer
            - Base of tongue, tonsillar pillars, posterior pharyngeal wall, hypopharynx
        - Lidocaine to vocal cords
    - Awake direct laryngoscopy - If adequate view, induction, paralytics, intubate
    - Fiberoptic laryngoscopy - Induction once ETT confirmed in position
    - Light wand - Upright patient

Failed intubation – two failed attempts by experienced clinician

- Emergency situation
- Call for help and difficult intubation cart
    - Multiple blades and ETT sizes, stylet, bougie, light wand, glideslope, LMA +/- Fastrack,
    - Equipment for transtracheal jet ventilation
        - Readily available and connected to O2 source
    - Fiberoptic
    - Cricothyrotomy set and skilled clinician
- Attempt to mask ventilate with 100 % O_2
    - Adequate
        - wake patient and either cancel or proceed as with expected difficult intubation
        - if NdMR given optimize position, equipment, and clinician
- Inadequate mask ventilation (oral airway, two person)
    - LMA placement → adequate?
    - If inadequate move to emergency cricothyrotomy, or tracheostomy

Complications: damage to airway, bleeding, airway obstruction, hypoxemia, esophageal intubation, gastric distention and regurgitation/aspiration, C-spine injury

Down's Syndrome

Incidence: 1 in 800 livebirths.

1. Airway abnormalities
   a. Difficult BMV — macroglossia, Choanal atresia / narrow nasopharynx, prominent tonsils & adenoids (population risk of difficult intubation – 0.5%)
   b. Subglottic stenosis — require a half-size smaller ETT than predicted by age
   c. Possible unstable C-spine — 31% A-A (20% asymptomatic) and Atlantoaxial instability
2. Congenital Heart Disease (40%)
   a. AV canal defects (50%), VSD (~25%), secundum ASD, PDA, Tetralogy of Fallot (4%)
   b. Accelerated CAD, adult-onset valvular disease, SBE prophylaxis, Bubble-free IVs
3. OSA — sensitive to respiratory depressants; risk of pHTN and RV failure
4. Uncooperative patient — Developmental Delay, Early onset Dementia
5. Associated conditions: DM, Hypothyroid, Obesity, Cataract 's, Recurrent Otitis Media, Immune Deficiency, Duodenal atresia, difficult IV access

Anesthetic Goals/Conflicts:

- Identify presence of A-A instability and manage the safely
- Identify and manage comorbidity that increase. perioperative risk
  - OSA, post-operative stridor – minimize respiratory depressants, post-operative monitoring
  - CHD, pHTN, DM

Hx: History of OSA, C-spine instability (neck pain, altered fine motor, gait, B&B, vertigo, syncope).

Cardiac evaluation, functional capacity, mental capacity, previous surgeries. Co-existing disease: Cataracts, recurrent OM, hypothyroid, DM, Duodenal Atresia, TEF, Hirschsprung 'sdisease, leukemia, GERD/aspiration

PE: examination, AAI > neurologic symptoms (spasticity, gait, neck tenderness), cardiac exam: heartfailure, **pHTN** (Loud P2, RV Heave, JVP), **PDA** – Harsh Holosystolic murmur LSB (VSD) vs continuous at LSB. **TOF** – Cyanosis, clubbing, palpable LSB heave (RVH), systolic ejection murmur (LUSB), loud A2, IV Access

Investigations: BW & TSH as dictated by Sx, Flex/ex c-spine (no screening, new symptoms, ENTprocedure), ECG, ECHO

Optimization: Cardiac Consultation, Respiratory consult for sleep study/overnight oximetry. Neck Xraypre-perioperatively; if neuro symptoms – delay and refer for consultation.
Midazolam (0.5mg/kg max 20mg) may have unpredictable response – monitor for obstruction, IM Ketamine for uncooperative patient, anti-sialagogue (glycopyrrolate 0.01mg/kg), EMLA creamfor IV placement, SBE Prophylaxis.

Room Setup: Based on medical condition, airway adjuncts (Macintosh maybe better than miller for tongue management) smaller ETT tubes for subglottic stenosis. Invasive monitoring for CHD

Intraoperative Management: Regional probably not feasible with uncooperative patient, IH vs IV, c-spine precautions – manual inline stabilization, Bubble-free IV 's, Prone to Bradycardia – Atropine 20ug/kg, MAC unchanged in Down 's Syndrome. Careful head / body positioning (lax joints) Avoid long-acting opioids, use multimodal analgesics, full reversal.

Post-operative complications: high incidence of agitation – family presence, Monitoring forOSA, airway obstruction, stridor, bronchospasm, Severe bradycardia

Drowning

1. Trauma
   - C-spine injury & aspiration, occult life-threatening injuries, hypovolemia, hypothermia, Intoxication
2. Hypothermia: Rewarming, Arrythmias, Hypovolemia, Coagulopathy
3. Multi system organ dysfunction
   - Acute Lung Injury /ARDS
   - Hypoxic brain injury
   - Hypoxic cardiomyopathy, shock, arrhythmias
   - Acute renal failure (ATN)
   - Electrolyte abnormalities (hypo/hyperkalemia)
4. Mechanism of drowning: Trauma / Intoxication
   - Children: Lack of supervision, Abuse,
   - Adults: MI, arrhythmia, hypoglycemia, CVA, Seizure, intoxication

Anesthetic Goals/Conflicts:

1. Primary Resuscitation to ensure adequate oxygen exchange and perfusion pressure
2. Prevent secondary injury: C-spine precautions
3. Correct hypothermia

Hx: mechanism of drowning (trauma, stroke, MI, intoxicants etc.), location and duration of drowning (water temperature), arrest time and resuscitation measures to date

PE: Vitals including temperature, airway, Respiratory (aspiration, contusion, ARDS), Cardiac (arrhythmias), neurological (hypoxic brain injury, intoxication)

Investigations: CBC, electrolytes (hypokalemia d/t shift), Ca/Mg (hyper in salt water near drowning), CK (Rhabdo), coagulation profile, Toxin's screen, ABGs, ECG, CXR

Optimization: Resuscitation –ventilation, correct acidosis and electrolytes , re-warming

Room Set-up: CAS monitors + 5L ECG + arterial line + CVL (for vasopressors/inotropes), large bore IV access (coagulopathy, bleeding), core temperature monitoring, warming devices (see below)

Intraoperative Management: Consider RSI for aspiration risk but watch for increased ICP, continue rewarming, lung protective ventilation

Post-operative: HDU, likely post-operative ventilation

Extra Corporeal Membrane Oxygenation (ECMO)

1. Critically ill patient with multi-organ system failure, at high perioperative risk
   - hypoxia and hemodynamic instability prior to bypass
2. Indications and underlying pathologicprocess
   - Etiology of respiratory or cardiac failure
3. Anatomy of ECMO circuit (VA / VV)
   - Contraindications to ECMO
4. Complications related toECMO
   - Embolism: air, MI, CVA
   - Tamponade
   - Atelectasis, pneumothorax
   - Acute Renal Failure
   - Sepsis
   - Hemorrhage, consumptive coagulopathy
5. Intensive monitoring for complications, adequacy, and weaning from ECMO

Anesthetic Goals/Conflicts:

1. Avoidance of complications; specifically bleeding
   - Minimize procedures, avoid removing lines
2. Close monitoring of all body systems and avoidance of secondary injury
3. Others as determined by underlying pathologic process

Hx: Identify indications for ECMO (acute, reversible, severe hypoxemia with failure of conventical therapy, failure to wean from CPB, neonatal PPH/RDS/CDH/meconium asp, post-traumatic respiratory failure, post lung transplant), identify multi-organ dysfunction, Identify contraindications to ECMO (mech. Ventilation > 7d, irreversible underlying disease or cardiac fxn, severe pulmonary HTN, cardiac arrest, age >60 or <34 weeks or <2kg, immunosuppression, contraindication to anticoagulation)

Contraindications: Gestational age <35 weeks, Weight <2000 g, Pre-existing intracranial hemorrhage, Congenital or neurologic abnormalities incompatible with good outcome, >1 week of aggressive respiratory therapy, congenital heart disease

PE: Vitals, ECMO settings, Ventilator settings (when applicable), neurological, CVS, RESPIRATORY

Investigations: Full labs, coags, recent ABG, CXR, echocardiogram

Anesthetic Options: May be cannulated in OR (post-CPB), under local or sedation in ICU

Room Setup: ICU setting with full invasive monitoring.

Anticoagulation: Heparin 100-150 U/kg, target ACT of 200, keep platelets >100.

Complications: Hemorrhage, ICH, seizures, coagulopathy, multiorgan dysfunction, PTX, tamponade, sepsis.

Special: V-V ECMO has better outcomes in adults than V-A ECMO and is preferable whenever the patient does not require CVS support. Neonatal ECMO is most often VA.

1. Reversal of chronic L-R shunt caused by increased PVR to a level that equals or exceeds SVR
    a. Occurs in approximately 50% of pts with untreated VSD, 10% of pts with untreated ASD
    b. High risk of morbidity and mortality
2. Pathophysiology
    a. Risk of hemodynamic collapse with profound hypoxemia on induction / PPV
        i. Increase. PVR, increase. R to L shunt, RV dilation, LV impairment, hypoxemia
    b. Polycythemia – with thrombosis
    c. Arrythmias – A-fib / flutter
    d. Sudden Death
3. Risk of paradoxical emboli
4. Medications
    a. pHTN medications
    b. anticoagulation
5. SBE prophylaxis

Anesthetic Goals / Conflicts

- Hemodynamic Goals
    a. **Maintain SVR**, Avoid Increase. in PVR (limit PAWP, avoid PEEP, early extubation, avoid hypoxia/hypercarbia/acidosis), Full preload, Maintain NST(reduce pulmonary venous congestion)
- Meticulous de-airing of IV tubing

Hx: Establish severity and etiology of disease - functional capacity; syncope, current treatments; hemoptysis;

Px: RA SaO_2; Respiratory - increase. WOB, cyanosis, clubbing, Cardiac – pHTN (P2, RV Heave) RVF (peripheral edema, hepatic congestion); ASD/VSD murmur disappears when Eisenmenger 's develops

Investigations: CBC (polycythemia) lytes, Ur, Cr, Coags (anticoagulation), CXR, ECG (signs of RVH, pHTN), ECHO

Optimization: Consult respirology and cardiology; high risk of mortality with anesthesia – defer surgical treatment if at all possible; may benefit from normovolumic hemodilution with phlebotomy pre-operatively for polycythemia; treat pHTN

Warming ATLS recommendations:

Limit to 1 shock for pulseless VF/VT if temperature < 30˚C, give meds with longer intervals 34-36˚C: passive rewarming, active external rewarming

30-34˚C: passive rewarming, active rewarming of truncal areas only –electric warming devices, hot water bottles, heating pads, radiant heat sources, warming beds/blankets)

<30˚C: Active internal rewarming > Warm IV fluids, humid oxygen, peritoneal lavage (KCL-free fluid), Extracorporeal rewarming, esophageal warming tubes>> discontinue when core temperature > 35˚C

Options: Dependant on surgical procedure; Irreversible increased PVR contraindicates surgical correction of original defect; minimally invasive with LA preferred, Regional with titrated epidural – no epinephrine to avoid dec. SVR (avoid sedation); GA as required (high risk); Laparoscopic procedures are contraindicated

Monitors: CAS, 5 lead, preinduction Artline and CVP, available TEE

Anesthetic Management: Absolute maintenance of SVR to prevent increase/ R to L shunting with hypoxemia; Early tracheal extubation is preferable

Pregnancy: vaginal birth is the goal; labor analgesia with a slowly titrated epidural (avoid epi), maintain SVR. C/Scan be accomplished with GA or epidural. IV drugs have rapid onset while IH is slow down the R to L shunt

Eisenmenger's Syndrome

1. Physiological changes from ECT
   a. HD instability, risk of arrhythmia, increase ICP, IOP, intragastric pressure
2. Potentially uncooperative psychiatric patient
   a. psychotropic meds: management & altered response to sympathomimetics
3. Contraindications
   a. Pheochromocytoma (absolute), increase. ICP, intracranial tumor, recent CVA, cardiovascularconduction defects, high-risk pregnancy, and aortic and cerebral aneurysms
4. Out-of-OR location
5. Complications
   a. headaches, myalgias, confusion, memory loss, CVA, malignant arrhythmias, myocardial infarctions (67% of ECT mortalities), pulmonary edema, emboli, obstructions, aspiration

Anesthetic Goals

- Attenuate hemodynamic and autonomic response
- Prevent awareness & injury
- Optimize seizure
- Rapid emergence

Hx: Standard anesthetic history (may be difficult to obtain), Indication, Old anesthetic records & previous ECT treatments & doses required, Assessment of cardiopulmonary and neurologic status, **Review medications**: TCAs – block reuptake of Catecholamines → deplete central adrenergic stores → unpredictable response to indirect agents, direct-acting may cause exaggerated response; anticholinergiceffects, MAOIs – irreversible complex with MAO → prevents breakdown of norepinephrine, 5-HT, dopamine → indirect agents can cause HTN crisis, direct acting may cause exaggerated response, Lithium – prolongs effects of depolarizing MR, certain NdMR, and sedatives (barbiturates); **R/O contraindication to ECT** - CAD, pacemakers/ICDs, a-fib

Px: vitals including postural BP. ease of intubation & BMV, increase. ICP, CHF

Inv: labs as directed by comorbidity, ECG (previous MI, arrhythmia), CT if query increase. ICP

Optimization: Aspiration prophylaxis, disable ICD (clinic, magnet), asynchronized pacemaker

Equipment: CAS, PNS, equipment, Emergency drugs (atropine, vasopressors, vasodilators)

Induction: Preoxygenation, Mild hyperventilation (hypoxia, hypercarbia reduce seizure), Bite block, consider management of Hemodynamic instability (atropine, esmolol), **Thiopental** 2mg/kg (↑ seizure threshold, delayed awakening), **Propofol** 2-3 mg/kg (↓ seizure duration, rapid awakening but no difference in outcome, pain on injection), Etomidate may prolong seizure duration **Ketamine** prolongs seizure duration but exacerbates sympathetic response, avoid benzodiazepines, **Suxamethonium** (0.5mg/kg), **NdMR** if Suxamethonium contraindicated (intubate and ventilate)

Post-operative: monitor in PACU, Supplemental O_2, acetaminophen, NSAIDs may alleviate ECT-induced myalgia

Complications: Confusion, agitation, amnesia, headache, Rare - Aspiration, myocardial ischemia, neurological vascular events, fracture/dislocation, status epilepticus, death (Current mortality rate is 1 in 10,000-30,000 treatments.

Epiglottitis

1. Emergency with potential for complete airway obstruction
    a. ENT, difficult Airway cart, urgent transport to OR, avoid agitating patient
    b. Risk of aspiration
2. Potential sepsis with need for fluid resuscitation
3. pediatric patient
4. Postoperative management
    a. disposition, treatment of infection, need for specialized pediatric care

Anesthetic Goals/Conflicts:

- Rapid assessment and diagnosis transport to OR
- Safe and timely airway management, **avoiding precipitants of airway obstruction**:
    - position changes, crying, airway exam
    - KEEP CHILD CALM
- Early antibiotics once IV access secured (this may have to wait until airway secured)

Conflicts:

- Need for fluid resuscitation vs need to avoid agitating child
- Risk of aspiration vs need

Differential diagnosis: croup, foreign body, abscess, caustic aspiration, anaphylaxis

Assessment: Classic presentation of "Toxic, drooling child", often maintaining upright sniffing position (tripod); Generally, age 2 – 7; Acute, rapidly progressive onset: 2-4 hrs; Fever, sore throat may be initial symptoms; If high suspicion - immediate transport to the OR

Px: signs of fatigue, impending failure which would precipitate urgent transfer to OR. Assessment of volume status

Investigations: Diagnosis is clinical. If any concern goes to OR; if stable and no signs of impending airway obstruction – CBC, blood cultures, lateral neck Xray

Optimization

Oxygen, Fluid resuscitation; Antibiotics to cover HiB and beta-hemolytic strep; Steroids; ENT; PICU

EARLY TRANSFER TO OR, ENT, DIFFICULT AIRWAY CART, TRACH/CRIC KIT AVAILABLE

Management:
Moribund: awake DL;
Stable child: SV GA, IH – 4% ET Sevoflurane, TIVA – Propofol infusion at 200 u/k/m, Remifentanil 0.1-1.2 u/k/m; DL when unresponsive (may take ~10min); ETT placed (use 0.5-1.0 size smaller); Topicalize airway prior to rigid bronchoscopy (lido 3mg/kg)

Disposition: Keep intubated for 2 days or until response to medical Rx observed and cuff leak/ETT leak occurs. Extubate in OR using same spontaneously ventilating technique and direct observation of larynx

- to maintain spontaneous ventilation

INCREASED $EtCO_2$

DDx

- Decreased Elimination
  - Rebreathing
    - Rebreathing Increased Dead-space
    - Inspiratory valve failure (if PPV, if SV, could be either IV or EV)
    - CO2 absorber exhaustion
  - Alveolar hypoventilation

- Increase. Production
  - Sepsis
  - MH / NMS / Serotonin Syndrome
  - Thyrotoxicosis
  - Cocaine
  - Pheochromocytoma
  - Transfusion reaction
  - Hyperthermia
  - Reperfusion

- Exogenous (e.g., laparoscopy)

Anesthetic Management:

- Emergency situation - simultaneous diagnosis and treatment
- Inform the surgeon and call for help
- Scan my monitors: rate, rhythm, BP, $EtCO_2$, SaO_2, temperature
  - CO_2 waveform
  - eliminate rebreathing as etiology
    - high fresh gas flow
    - hand ventilates
- Ensure adequate minute ventilation - decompress belly if required
- Rule out another etiologist

Femoral Nerve Block (L2,3,4)

Indications: Analgesia for hip or knee surgery. Combined with Sciatic for entire lower extremity.

Contraindications: Usual + possible compartment syndrome

Anatomy: Lateral to femoral artery, beneath Fascia Lata and Iliaca, anterior to iliopsoas. Ant branch gives of sensory to anterior, anteromedial and medial aspects of thigh. Posterior branch gives motor to quads and sensation to knee, and medial leg (saphenous).

Complications: Vessel puncture, nerve injury, infection, LA toxicity

Technique: Standard CAS Monitors, Supine, along femoral crease, lateral to femoral artery, 5cm needle, perpendicular to skin, goal is patellar twitch, inject 20 ml LA. If Sartorius twitch, go slightly lateral and deeper. 3 in 1 block is the same approach, but needle insertion slightly cephalad, 40 ml LA History / distal pressure.
Unreliable in blocking LFCN 62% and obturator 52%. Fascia Iliaca block: Trisect inguinal ligament, insertion site is 1cm caudal to the point bw lateral and middle third, 5cm blunt needle, feel for 2 pops.,inject 30ml. LFCN History / FI block ~90%, Obturator 38%.

LFCN block: Supine, 2.5cm inferior and medial to ASIS, 4 cm needle inserted perpendicular to skin, 1 pop through fascia lata, 10 ml injected above and below Fascia Lata in a fan wise approach.
For sensory block of anterolateral thigh to knee.

Obturator Nerve: Pt is supine, leg slightly abducted. Landmarks 1.5 cm inferior and lateral to pubic tubercle. 10 cm needle, perpendicular to skin, contact bone (inferior ramus of pubis), withdraw, redirect slightly laterally and caudad to enter obturator foreman, advance 2-3 cm, look for adductor twitch.

Lumbar Plexus Block (Psoas Compartment Block): *Analgesia for hip and knee surgery*
Contraindications: Usual
Technique: Pt is lateral, knees flexed. Landmarks are 1. Midline 2. Parallel line along PSIS 3. Line between iliac crests. Insertion site 2/3 from midline to PSIS along iliac crest line. Nerve roots lie at a depth of 7-10cm almost always 2 cm past transverse process. Fascial click into perineural sheath. Patellar twitch at 0.5-1 mA. Inject 40 ml.

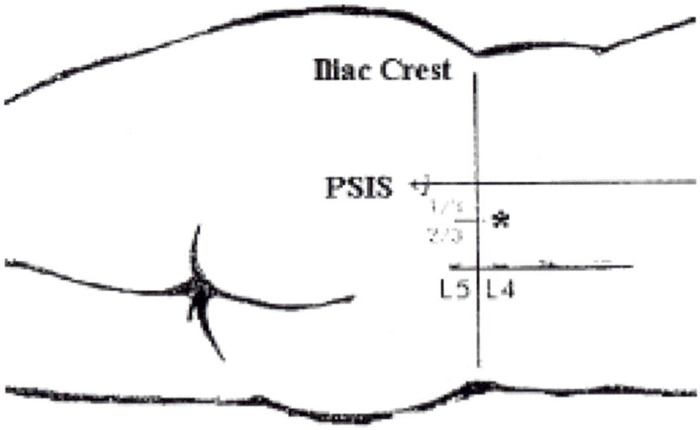

Trouble Shooting: If hit TP, redirect cephalad and go 2 cm deeper. If no twitch fan in cephalad-caudad plane. If paravertebral muscle twitch, go deeper, if psoas stims, pull back. If hamstrings, too caudad.

Complications: Nerve injury, retroperitoneal hematoma, injury to structures deep to LP (kidney, majorvessels, GI). IV, Subarachnoid, epidural, LA toxicity.

Fetal Distress

1. Emergency situation requiring immediate maternal and IU fetal resuscitation
2. Etiology of the fetal compromise:
    a. Aortocaval compression
    b. Maternal morbidity (Abruption of the placenta, Uterine rupture, Pregnancy Induced Hypertension , Shock, Sepsis)
    c. Fetal morbidity (Cord prolapsed/Ut hypertonus/IUGR)
3. Anesthetic plan for C/S — based on degree fetal compromise and maternal condition
4. Preparation for neonatal resuscitation — Pediatrician present

Anesthetic Goals/Conflicts:

1. Resuscitation of mother to optimize UPP (O_2, iv fluid, LUD, stop oxytocin, tocolytics)
2. Clear communication between services (anesthesia, OB, pediatrics)
    - Rapid assessment & initiation of delivery plan
    - Facilitate prompt delivery without compromising maternal safety
3. Be prepared for neonatal resuscitation (pediatrician, etc.)
    - Hypotension with RSI (hypovolemic) vs. Aspiration with titrated induction
    - Difficult Airway vs. STAT C/S

Immediate Resuscitation: O_2, LUD, Fluid Bolus, vasopressors, Stop uterine contractions (oxytocin, NTG 50- 100 ug bolus)

Hx: Etiology of distress – Maternal, fetal (Cord prolapsed, footling breech, massive abruption, Uterine rupture, Increased uterine tone, PIH, Hypotension/ shock/ sepsis); AMPLE Hx; obstetric hx

PE: maternal VS, FHR (baseline, variability, and decelerations), maternal airway, uterine tone

Investigations: don 't wait if severe distress – CBC, x-match, coags and fibrinogen for DIC

Optimization: Continued maternal resuscitation as directed by etiology; Asp. Prophylaxis, topicalize airway as indicated, continuous fetal heart rate monitoring

Anesthetic Options: GA vs SAB vs insitu Epidural; Normal airway - RSI GA; Diff. airway - AFOI

Room Setup: NTG for uterine relaxation, pressors, oxytocin, hemabate; Difficult airway cart, large bore IV, continuous FHR, OB/paediatrician in room

Induction: Position Pt to optimize airway management; De-nitrogenate with 100% FiO_2; prepped and draped, surgeon scrubbed, Cricoid, Thiopental 3-5 mg/kg (Ketamine 1-1.5 mg/kg), Suxamethonium \ 1.5mg/kg

Intraoperative Management: consider TIVA/NO_2 after the baby is out (decrease volatile after delivery); orogastric tube prior to emergence

Post-operative: Extubate when awake; HDU/ICU/NICU; Postop pain – NSAIDS, PCA

Complications: Aspiration; Failure Intubation (BMV +- LMA, optimize and re-attempt, wake patient vs. continue with LMA); HD compromise; Neonatal resuscitation Pregnant Patient considerations

Fontan's Circulation

1. Univentricular physiology – completed repair around 3 years of age
    a. Passive pulmonary flow (dependent on venous pressure - PVR)
2. Cardia Dysfunction
    a. arrhythmias: **SVTs**, VTs - defib pads pre-operatively
    b. Ventricular dysfunction - 70% by 10yrs (pericardial and pleural effusions)
    c. Late forming pHTN – d/t elevated pulmonary perfusion pressures
3. Risk of hypoxia with fenestrated Fontan – R to L shunt
    a. Paradoxical emboli - airless IV 's
4. Co-morbid illness: Protein losing enteropathy, Thromboembolism (30% at 10yr - anticoagulation)
5. Consideration of SBE prophylaxis

Anesthetic Goals/Conflicts:

- Maintain full venous return, avoid pHTN triggers, avoid dehydration
- Hemodynamic goals:
    - **Full preload**
    - normal SVR – prevent R – L shunt
    - low PVR – avoid hypercarbia, excessive PPV
    - normal contractility, and **sinus rhythm** (dec. pulmonary venous congestion)
- Treat hypotension with phenylephrine (increase SVR > PVR)

Foreign Body

1. Potentially life-threatening emergency
    - Potential perioperative airway obstruction
    - Barotrauma (ball-valve phenomena)
    - Bronchospasm
2. Co-morbid disease
    - Neurologic disease (aspiration risk)
    - Intoxication
    - Post-obstructive pneumonia (if delayed)
3. Rigid bronchoscopy
    - Shared airway
    - Maintenance of anesthesia
    - Ventilation and oxygenation during bronchoscopy
4. Pediatric patient

Anesthetic Goals/Conflicts:

1. Minimize risk of aspiration (prophylaxis, fasting)
2. Minimize risk of airway obstruction
    - Minimize distal displacement of FB through avoidance of PPV
    - Minimize ball-valve obstruction
3. Facilitate retrieval of FB (Immobile patient with minimal coughing)
4. Effective communication with Surgeon

Hx: Aspirated object/substance (if known; sharp vs. organic/inflammatory), time of aspiration, symptoms of airway obstruction or compromise (stridor, drooling, tachypnea), signs of infection (fever, productive cough, hypoxemia); risk for aspiration, last meal

PE: Vitals – including RR/O_2 sat (respiratory distress) + temperature (infection) + weight, airway exam, respiratory exam for distress (retractions, tracheal tug, stridor, wheezing, crackles) and CVS exam.

Investigations: minimal if obstructing. Consider CXR (90% of objects are radiolucent, so not sensitive), CBC (infection), ABG (unwell, pneumonia)

Optimization: O_2, ENT immediately available; Aspiration prophylaxis if urgent – delay for fasting guidelines if not acutely obstructed; Heliox, bronchodilators, racemic epi to temporize; Anti-sialagogue for pediatric; IV antibiotics if infection; Position: Upper airway - position of comfort/sitting upright/leaning forward; Distal airway: affected lung down, to protect normal lung

Anesthetic Options: May do adults under sedation local if flexible FOB. Peds and rigid bronchoscopy must be done under GA. With adults, obesity or other conditions which make SV difficult/impossible under GA, consider intubation History / PPV, may have to leave bougie, extubate during brief periods for rigid bronchoscopy

Room Setup: Difficult airway cart, FOB, jet ventilator and help available. Warming if peds. Resuscitation drugs.

Intraoperative Management: ENT in room; IV vs. IH induction with SV; PPV may be necessary. TIVA does not depend on surgical technique. Consider intubating after retrieval of FB prior to emergence (minimize risk of aspiration).

Post-operative: risk of laryngeal edema x 24hrs – O_2, racemic epinephrine, steroids, chest physiotherapy, possible postoperative ventilation

Complications: Bronchospasm (Ventolin, deepen anesthetic); inadequate ventilation , airway obstruction (push FB distal, thoracotomy); PTX; tracheobronchial trauma with hemorrhage; pneumonia.

Foreign Environment

1. Three step approach
    a. Patient – ASA, comorbidity, airway, monitoring requirements
    b. Procedure – Duration, invasiveness (pain), special requirements (monitoring, paralysis), complications
    c. Environment – equipment, patient access, personnel, hazards (radiation, magnet), temperature, interference

Anesthetic Goals

- Provide same standard of care of patient in the OR
    - anesthesia equipment, monitors and procedures
- Identify and mitigate all environmental hazards
    - Ionizing radiation, ferromagnetic radiation, contrast media
- Identify reasons why the patient requires GA or anesthesia-administered sedation
- Familiarize yourself with the remote environment, staff and location of all necessary emergency equipment and drugs

Preparation: ensure the presence and proper function of all necessary equipment – central O_2, cylinder, suction, lighting, gas scavenging, electrical outlets, resuscitative equipment; Identify bulky and immobile equipment, assess need to monitor the patient remotely

Hx & Px: Assess patient for comorbidities, potential complications and conflicts with procedure (Sedation vs. GA, paralysis, limited access to patient, remote monitoring)

Monitors: CAS monitors + those dictated by the procedure and the patient

Specific Procedures:

Angiography/intervention – minimal sedation vs. GA, contrast agents (nephropathy, allergic rhinitis – fish allergy), ensure lines / tubes free to allow the table to move

CT – trauma, acute situations, resuscitate prior to scan, oral contrast

Radiofrequency Ablation – Rx for tumors (liver, lung, adrenal etc..) likely end-stage disease (4Ms), beware of complications (PTX, BPF, Hemorrhage), pacemaker contraindicated (heat / burns)

MRI – Peds, limited access, remote monitoring, need to exclude ferromagnetic components, interferences with monitors (ECG artifact – place electrodes close together), pacemakers contraindicated, burns possible from various monitors – run cables in straight lines (no coils), if emergency – stop sequence, rapidly remove patient from MRI/scanner room (need for resuscitative equipment that is not magnet safe)

G6PD deficiency is an enzymopathy that can result in hemolysis secondary to oxidative damage to susceptible red blood cells; X-linked; common in African Americans, Africans, Asians, and Mediterraneanpopulations

1. Chronic hemolytic anemia
2. Need to **avoid precipitants of hemolysis**
    a. Oxidative drugs
    b. Infection
    c. Metabolic abnormalities (e.g., DKA)

Avoid precipitants of hemolysis:

- Acetaminophen – safe in therapeutic doses
- Salicylates – safe in therapeutic doses
- Antibiotics: Nitrofurans; Penicillin; Streptomycin; Chloramphenicol; Isoniazid
- Sulfonamides
- Antimalarial Drugs
- Miscellaneous: **Probenecid; Quinidine; Vit K analogues; Methylene Blue; Nitroprusside**

Hx: episodes of acute hemolytic anemia (usually asymptomatic in steady state; triggers can ppt hemolysis); History of neonatal hyperbilirubinemia, Favism (d/t ingestion of fresh fava beans)

PE: Pallor; Jaundice; hepatomegaly

Investigations: CBC, Diff; Blood film (Heinz bodies-clumps of patient; With hemolysis: microsporocytes; eccentricates –bite cells; reticulocytotic)

Optimization: Hematology consultation

Anesthetic Options: No limitations

Room Setup: CAS monitors

Intraoperative Management: avoid oxidant drugs; Anesthetic agents are not known to ppt hemolysis

Post-operative: standard

Complications: Acute hemolysis: early post-operative (2-5 days) evidence of hemolysis may indicate G6PD; self-limited as only older RBCs are affected

Special: Avoid drugs that can result in methemoglobinemia (prilocaine, Lidocaine, benzocaine) because treatment with methylene blue is contraindicated

G6PD deficiency

Guillain Barre Syndrome

Acute idiopathic inflammatory demyelinating polyneuropathy characterized by ascending progressive muscle weakness and areflexia, usually associated with spontaneous remission.

1. Risk of **aspiration** – weakness of pharyngeal muscles
2. **Respiratory failure** – intercostal muscle weakness/post-operative ventilation
3. **Autonomic instability** – compensatory CV responses may be absent, exaggerated response to stimuli or hypovolemia, tachycardia, hypo/hypertension, arrythmias
4. **Altered response to NMB** - Hyperkalemic response to succinylcholine - NdMB sensitivity
5. Increased risk of venous **thromboembolism**, raised ICP (rare)
6. **Acute Medical therapy**: IVIG / Plasmapheresis (Steroids not helpful!)

Anesthetic Goals/Conflicts:

- Minimize aspiration risk
- Maximize respiratory muscle strength (minimize / avoid NdMB)
- Maintain hemodynamic stability
- Conflicts: RSI without Suxamethonium /decreased NdMB vs hemodynamically stable induction

Hx & PE: Onset of symptoms, respiratory compromise, cough, bulbar symptoms, cardiovascular instability, a`rrhythmias. Treatment. Functional capacity. AMPLE Hx, Focused cardiorespiratory exam, neurologic exam.

Investigations: Usual investigations, PFTs / VC, ECG, CXR

Optimization: Delay elective surgery, Neurology consult, aspiration prophylaxis, DVT prophylaxis.

Anesthetic Options: GA, and Neuraxial are plausible.

Room Setup: CAS / PNS / consider invasive monitors, vasopressors for hypotension, assistance for cricoid.

Intraoperative Management: Consider RSI, avoid suxamethonium, judicious NDMRs, ensure reversal direct acting agents for hypotension, avoid stimulants on induction.

Post-operative: Arrythmias / DVT / PE / Respiratory embarrassment.

Special: M > F, bimodal distribution in young adults and elderly, 1:33,000, starts in legs, ascending flaccid paralysis, 5% mortality, children less severely affected. Rx: IVIG 0.4mg/kg x 5days, plasmapheresis, steroids not useful.

Hypertrophied Cardiomyopathy

Myocardial hypertrophy resulting in a small and hyperdynamic left ventricle - risk of ischemia, sudden cardiac death and fixed or dynamic LVOT obstruction

1. Potential for dynamic outflow obstruction in 25%
    a. Precipitated by increase. contractility, decreased preload, and/or decreased afterload
2. Complications
    a. Tachyarrhythmias
    b. Hypertrophy, diastolic disfunction and increase. MVO_2 – myocardial ischemia
    c. Mitral regurgitation
3. Associated medications – BBs, antiarrhythmics, anticoagulants, diuretics
4. Pacemaker or AICD

Anesthetic Goals/Conflicts:

1. Avoid acute LV outflow tract obstruction
    a. Maintain **full preload** and adequate afterload to stent LVOT open while **avoiding any increase. in myocardial contractility**
2. **Avoid tachycardia** while maintaining **strict NSR** (diastolic dysfunction)
3. Be prepared to treat lethal arrhythmias and avoid precipitating arrhythmias
4. Maintain myocardial oxygenation and **monitor for ischemia**
    a. Optimize oxygen delivery
    b. Maintain **adequate afterload**
    c. Consider invasive monitoring

Hx: Many patients are asymptomatic - Hx of SOB on exertion (90%), angina (~30%) presyncope, syncope. A-fib /flutter/SVT (25%), PVCs/VT/brady (20%), MR, Hx of CHF. Prior cardiac arrest, pacemaker settings. Assess for risk of SCD and need for AICD (pts with prior cardiac arrest, sustained VT or 2 or more risk factors:
family hx of SCD, <45 years, Flat (failure to increase SBP by 25mmHG) or hypotensive (decrease SBP > 15mmHg) response to exercise in patients, <40years, non-sustained VT during 48hr Holter monitoring, LV wall thickness >30, resting peak instantaneous gradient >30mmHg.

PE: Displaced apical beat, S4, Harsh SEM bw apex/LSB (worse with Valsalva and standing) radiates to axillae. CHF, ↑JVP, R sided S4 with R heart involvement. Murmur of MR.

Investigations: CBC/Lytes, ECG – arrhythmias, BBB, LVH (Deepest S in lead V1 or V2 + tallest R in V5 or V6 > 35 and or a R wave in lead AVL >12), LAD, q waves, -Giant t-wave syndromeǁ = sharply negative T- waves in V3-5 are typical of apical HCM. CXR may demonstrate LV/LA/RAenlargement. ECHO: asymmetric hypertrophy, SAM, gradient, systolic & diastolic dysfunction, MR, LA size, check for provocable LVOT obstruction, MIBI, angiography.

Optimization: Ensure adequate volume status. Cardiology consult, consider AICD/Pacemaker placement, consider septal alcohol ablation prior to elective procedure. If systolic dysfunction, evaluate for transplantation. BB / CCB (verapamil 75mcq/kg, may repeat 150mcq/kg in 15-30mins, max dose 20mg) for LVOT obs, consider anxiolytic for tachycardia. Diuretics for CHF, antiarrhythmic therapy to restore NSR or cardioversion.

Anesthetic Options: GA generally well tolerated. Neuraxial techniques are acceptable and welltolerated if HD goals met - OB: GA, epidural, CSE with intrathecal opioid (spinal contraindicated), avoid oxytocin bolus

Room Setup: Invasive lines, alpha agonists, BBs/CCBs, antiarrhythmics, pacer, TEE/PAC in high-risk patients.

Intraoperative Management: See hemodynamic goals above. Deep plane of anesthesia prior to airway manipulation, consider phenylephrine infusion and volume preload. Avoid ketamine. Consider arrhythmias with CVP/PAC placement

Post-operative: Avoid tachy/pain on emergence, observe in HDU, maintain hemodynamic goals.

Complications: Hypotension, acute LVOT obstruction, arrythmias

Hemophilia A (F VIII), B (IX), & Von Willebrand disease

1. High risk of perioperative bleeding associated with specific factor deficiency
   a. F VIII – Hemophilia A (Classic) – sex linked recessive
   b. F IX – Hemophilia B (Christmas Disease) – sex linked recessive
   c. von Willebrand Disease
2. Sequelae of bleeding in enclosed spaces: Joints, Intracranial, Pericardium, Thorax
3. Potential contraindication to neuraxial anesthesia and analgesia
   a. Labour Epidural in parturient ok if FVIII & vWF >50%
4. Consultation with hematology for factor optimization, identification of inhibitors, difficult cross match
5. Coexisting viral infections: HIV, HBV (less now with recombinant products)

Anesthetic Goals/Conflicts:

1. Optimize factor activity and coagulation profile in perioperative period
   - DDAVP / Humate P / cryoprecipitate
2. Techniques for minimizing perioperative blood/Factor loss.
3. Manage bleeding episode with appropriate Factor replacement.

Hx: Bleeding Hx – easy bruising, petechiae, mucosal bleeding, epistaxis, menorrhagia, family bleeding Hx, hx of cancer or collagen vascular disease. History of prolonged bleeding after Sx (dental work, tonsillectomy)

PE: Bruises, petechiae, oral mucosa, lymph nodes, hepatosplenomegaly. Airway – hematoma MSK – Joint deformity

Investigations: CBC, INR, PTT, cross match. Assay for activity level of factor, factor antibodies (anti- FVIII). Most sensitive test for vWD is rustication cofactor activity. Other Inv. as dictated by procedure and patient co-morbidity

Optimization: Consult hematology. Plan OR early in the week/day. Consider antifibrinolytics perioperative

Hemophilia: Assay factor levels **48h** prior to OR and restore levels to >50% for major surgery (maintain 5-10 d), dental extraction (maintain >12hrs), delivery/puparium (maintain 3-4 d). > 30% for minor surgery (maintain 2-4 d).

Rpt factor assay after administration and within 2h of OR to confirm factor activity. Monitor levelintra-operative as dictated by clinical situation. No anti-platelet meds.

Hemophilia A: Severe <2%, Mod 2-10%, mild >10%. ↑PTT, Normal INR. DDAVP (may ↑FVIII), Recombinant F VIII (1U/kg ↑FVIII 2%), Recombinant F VIIa for inhibitors, Cryo if nothing else available (the only fractionated blood product containing meaningful amounts of F VIII and vWF, FFP has ~.7-.9u/ml FVIII). VIII T½ = ~12hrs in adults, ~6hrs in Peds

Hemophilia B: ↑PTT. rFIX (1U/kg ↑FIX 1%, half is absorbed by collagen in the vasculature), rFVIIa (for inhibitors), FFP if nothing else available (cryo does not contain FIX). FIX T½ = 8-24 hours.

Pregnancy: Consider fetus affected in carriers and minimize trauma to fetus especially if male

vWD Subtype 1 (70-80%), Nstructure, dec. quantity; Responds to DDAVP (3-5-fold increase. in vWF; dose = 0.3 mcg/kg (max 20 mcg/dose and rpt 24h). Subtype 2a (20-30%) Abnormal structure, normal or dec. quantity; Requires F VIII- vWF concentrates (Humate P) in addition toDDAVP.

DDAVP contraindicated in subtype 2b, as this promotes thrombocytopenia. Subtype 3 (rare) Little orno vWF. Bleeding pattern same as Hemophilia A. Require treatment with F VIII-vWF concentrates, platelets if thrombocytopenic. DDAVP no benefit. Emergency: 1st humate P (50iu/kg →consult hematology), cryo, Platelets concentrates.

Pregnancy: Factor VIII, vWF, ristocetin cofactor early in pregnancy and at 34 weeks. During pregnancy, prophylactic Tx if FVIII level <25%. During labour, maintain levels 50% of normal, if c- sec 80% normal. Post-partum, follow levels and Tx if <25% or significant hemorrhage. **vWF:** Type I or IIA, DDAVP 0.3ug/kg with labor q12h. Non responders, Tx with humate P (40iu/kg). Regional: LEA OK if FVIII and vWF > 50%.

Anesthetic Options: surgery done in ctr capable of rapid Factor assays. Neuraxial – requires 70-100%of Factor activity, reasonable platelets: vWD: >50 % activity of F VIII/vWF

Room Setup: CAS, Large bore IV, Temperature probe, blood warmer, rapid infuser, cell salvage, Arterialline for sampling, Factor (recombinant, human derived) available, X-match prior to OR – may be delays for antibody investigation

Intraoperative Management: Careful positioning/laryngoscopy.

Post-operative: Mild Hemorrhage (early joint/muscle, epistaxis, hematuria, dental bleed) target 20-30% activity. Major Hemorrhage (advanced joint/muscle, hematoma neck/tongue, prophylaxis after severe trauma) target 40-50%. Life- threatening Hemorrhage (intracranial, surgical, GI bleed, major trauma bleed)target 50-100%.

HIV

1. **Multisystem disease:**
   - CNS: Dementia, peripheral neuropathies, myopathies, visual loss, mass lesions with increase. ICP
   - Airway: upper airway obstruction with Candida, possible difficult intubation
   - Respiratory: Pneumonia, Lymphoma, Primary pHTN, pleural effusions
   - CVS: Autonomic neuropathy, pancarditis (IE in IVDU), accelerated CAD
   - Renal: End stage nephropathy
   - Heme – Anemia, coagulopathy (ITP), lymphopenia

2. **Immunocompromised:**
   - Opportunistic infections - Meningitis, encephalitis, pneumonia/TB, esophagitis, enteritis
   - Malignancy – Lymphoma, Kaposi Sarcoma

3. **Medications:** Bone marrow suppression, renal failure, peripheral neuropathy, p450 activation
4. **Chronic pain / Substance Abuse**

5. **OB and HIV:** dec perinatal transmission with AZT (25% - 8%), elective C/S, Regional OK (document peripheral neuropathy, coagulation, strict sterile technique, blood patch OK – airway patent)

Hx & Px: duration Drug Hx, Current treatment (prophylaxis), Screen for comorbid disease: opportunistic infections (CNS – Dementia Respiratory – CD4 < 200 PCP, Cryptococcus, CMV), Vital increased temperature, focused respiratory (SpO_2, cough, crackles), CVS (chest pain, rub, decreased exercise tolerance), peripheral neuropathy, GI disturbance (dysphagia, diarrhea)

Inv: CBC, E7, CD4, ECG, CXR, Consider PFTs, ABG, ECHO, MRI/CT Head

Optimization: Adequate prophylaxis, treat infections

Options: GA or regional OK

Anesthetic Setup: CAS monitors, strict asepsis, otherwise as required by comorbidities and procedure

Complications: As described by comorbidities

Hyperkalemia

1. Underlying etiology
   - Shift - acidosis, meds
   - Impaired excretion - renal failure, ureteric obstruction, Addison 's, lupus
   - Excess intake or release - rhabdo, hemolysis, transfusions, burns, tumour lysis
2. Physiologic sequelae of hyperkalemia: weakness, arrhythmias which may progress tomalignantarrhythmias
3. Need for continuous monitoring

Anesthetic Goals/Conflicts:

- Prevent/treat arrhythmias
- Reduce serum potassium levels
- Reduce total body potassium if elevated

Hx: Meds, Past Med Hx, allergies, fatigue, weakness, paresthesia, palpitations, pain or history of trauma (rhabdomyolysis), recent transfusions.

PE: Vitals, cardiorespiratory exam, neuro (decreased DTRs, weakness), evidence of renal failure(bruising, petechiae, edema, presence of fistulae), palpate compartments.

Investigations: 12 lead EKG, Lytes, BUN, Cr, Mg, Ca, Dig level (if on dig), ABG, urine myoglobin, urine R&M
Peaked Ts, QT shortening, ST depression
Increased PR, BBB, decreased P wave
Widening of QRS eventually to sine wave then V-Fib, Asystole

Treatment: Calcium chloride 5-10cc (stabilize myocardium), glucose/insulin 25-50g and 10 units (shifts intracellular), Lasix 1 mg/kg (increase K^+ excretion), B agonism – Ventolin 5-20 mg (shifts K intracellular), alkalinize – bicarb 1 amp or 3 amps in 1 L D5 (shifts K intracellular), kayexalate 15-30 g po or 30-60 g pr or calcium Risonium (exchange resin to remove potassium from body – note kayexalate results in increased sodium which may not be desirable if CHF, renal failure or hypernatremia are part of clinical picture). Failure to respond to above medical therapy or severe hyperkalemia (> 7 or >6 with physiologic derangement) should prompt consideration of urgent dialysis.
Meds which can cause hyperkalemia include: Amiloride, Angiotensin II inhibitors, ACE Inhibitors, Pentamidine, Spironolactone, Succinylcholine, Triamterene, Trimethoprim, NSAIDs, Heparin

Hyperparathyroidism

1. Underlying etiology (parathyroid tumour, PTH producing tumour, chronic hypocalcaemia & hyperphosphatemia - CRF, acute pancreatitis)
2. Potential difficult and dangerous airway secondary to mass effect and osteopenia bone
    a. pathologic fractures mandible and vertebral bodies, increase. aspiration risk
3. Physiologic changes of Hypercalcemia
    a. CNS: ↓LOC, hallucinations, psychosis
    b. CVS: HTN, hypovolemia, conduction blockade, long PR, Short QT
    c. Respiratory: potential respiratory muscle weakness with RLD, poor clearance of secretions
    d. Other: Renal failure - nephrolithiasis (70%); N/V, abdominal pain, pancreatitis; weakness (titrate NdMB to effect); anemia
4. Considerations of cancer and associated syndromes
    a. MEN 1: hyper parathyroid, pancreatic islet cell tumors, pituitary hyperplasia or tumor
    b. MEN 2A: hyper parathyroid, medullary thyroid CA, pheochromocytoma
5. Prevention of pathologic fractures during positioning
6. Post-operative airway obstruction after parathyroidectomy
    a. hematoma, laryngospasm, hypocalcaemia, RLN injury, tracheomalacia

Anesthetic Goals

- Management of hypercalcemia
- Monitor ECG and Ca concentrations perioperatively
- Prevent pathological fractures
- Airway vigilance

Hx: Underlying etiology, symptoms of hypercalcemia; symptoms of neck mass (positional dyspnea, stridor)

Px: Vitals; volume status, airway (mass effect), muscular atrophy; fractures/deformities

Investigations: Ca, Lytes, Cr, PO4, Mg, albumin, PTH, ECG (long PR, QRS, short QT, arrhythmias), +/- CT neck

Optimization: Endocrine consult; Management of hypercalcemia - IV rehydration (2-6L) followed byLasix (40- 80mg) after euvolemia - goal of 3-5 L urine/day; If severe add - Bisphosphonate (etidronate7.5mg/kg IV OD or 20mg/kg PO OD); Calcitonin 200 IU nasal spray/day; IV steroid (inhibit GI Ca absorption); Phosphate repletion; Mithramycin to antagonize PTH (prompt dec. in Ca) – results in thrombocytopenia, hepatotoxicity, nephrotoxicity; Hemodialysis if CRI/RF

Options: No particular anesthetic technique is indicated

Management: AFOI if difficult airway or significant osteopenia; watch for hypotension with induction; MAC may reduce with CNS symptoms; careful positioning; unpredictable response to NdMB – use a nerve stimulator; maintain normocarbia (acidosis results in increase. ionized Ca, alkalosis results in dec. ionized Ca & hypokalemia – unopposed Ca)

Complications: Cardiac arrhythmias 2'to hypercalcemia – serial monitor Ca, Mg, PO4; airway obstruction – B/L RLN injury, tracheomalacia, hematoma; Hypocalcaemia - laryngospasm, arrhythmia, Sz; Hypomagnesemia, pneumothorax

Hypoparathyroidism

1. Etiology (thyroidectomy, parathyroidectomy, DiGeorge, hypomagnesemia, excess phosphate)
2. Physiologic changes of hypocalcaemia
    - CNS: decreased LOC, **seizures**
    - Respiratory: **laryngospasm**, **bronchospasm**
    - CVS: **decreased contractility**, **dysrhythmias**, hypotension
    - MSK: **muscle spasms**, altered response to NdMB (use PNS)
3. Hyperventilation induced alkalosis causes ↓ serum Ca (↑ Ca protein binding)

Hx: identify cause and look for symptoms of hypocalcaemia (decreased LOC, confusion, delirium, seizures, perioral paresthesia, laryngospasm, bronchospasm, hypotension, syncope/presyncope, palpitations. Cramps, spasms, heterotopic ossification

Px: Vitals (orthostatic), Respiratory – bronchospasm; CVS – CHF, hypotension, Muscle spasm - Chvostek 's (masseter twitch with facial tap), Trousseau 's (muscular contraction of the hand with BP cuff inflation)

Investigations: CBC, Lytes, Ca, Mg, PO4; ECG – prolonged QT

Optimization: Consult endocrine; replete serum Ca & Mg; dec. dietary PO4, PO4 binders early

Intraoperative management: No particular anesthetic technique is indicated.Unexplained intraoperative hypotension should either prompt laboratory testing or empirictreatment for hypocalcaemia in addition to your normal approach to hypotension

Most common perioperative comorbidity in surgical pts (~20-25%), and causes accel end-organ dysfunction (CAD/PVD/CVD/CRONIC KIDNEY DISEASE) and increased peri-operative morbidity

1. Increased perioperative morbidity
2. Potential for end-organ dysfunction
   - CAD +/-LV dysfunction
   - CRF
   - PVD
   - CVD
3. Labile perioperative hemodynamics
   - Exaggerated response to endogenous and exogenous catecholamines
   - Relative intravascular volume depletion-hypotension on induction
4. Perioperative medication management
5. Potential secondary causes of hypertension
   - Renal (CKD, renal artery stenosis), OSA (30%), Endocrine (pheochromocytoma, Cushing 's, hyperaldosteronism, hyper/ hypothyroid, hyper parathyroid)

<u>*Anesthetic Goals/Conflicts:*</u>

- Maintain perioperative BP within 20% normal
- If SBP > 180, DBP > 110 – try and delay for History /o of secondary causes / optimization

Hx: Document baseline, severity, duration, lability and control of HTN. Determine end-organ complications of severe HTN (CAD/CRONIC KIDNEY DISEASE /CVD/CHF). Inquire about secondary causse (**Pheo**/Thyroid, Hyperaldosteronism, Cushing's). Medical Rx and compliance. Co-morbid illnesses (DM/Smoking/OSA).

PE: Vitals, BP both arms, postural. Carotids for bruits. LVH >> displaced apex, loud S2. CHF >> audible S4, basilar crackles, raised JVP. Renovascular bruits.

Investigations: Lytes if on diuretics or co-morbid CKD, Hypokalemia? hyperaldosteronism. 12-lead ECG (associated LVH / ST changes, q waves).

Optimization: Endocrinology/Cardiology consult if concerned about secondary causes of HTN. Consider cancelling elective surgery if evidence of end-organ dysfunction or SBP > 180/110. If untreated HTN consider IV/PO medications perioperatively (note POISE study results). Hold ACEi ~ 48hrs for cases with anticipated major hemodynamic shifts/CPB. Consider holding diuretics for procedures associated with bowel prep/major fluid shifts. Continue all other antihypertensives and resume post-operative.

Anesthetic Options: Any

Room Setup: 5 leads, consider invasive monitors, antihypertensives: BBs/NTG etc. Usual vasopressors Vasopressin for refractory hypotension with patients on ACEi.

Intraoperative Management: Any, observe intravascular depletion and sens to exo/endogenous catecholamines
Minimize intubation time < 15s, generous opioids, anticipate lability, avoid ketamine.
Maintain BP ~20% of baseline.

Post-operative: Monitor for ischemia, adequate analgesia, r/o bladder distention, continue antihypertensive ASAP

Hypertension

- Inform the surgeon and ensure no surgical factors
- My initial differential diagnosis includes:
    - Hypoxemia / hypercapnia
    - Drugs: administered, illicit, errors and withdrawal
    - Pain / light anesthesia
    - Patient factors including endocrine
- I would scan my monitors for HR, ECG, rhythm, CO_2 tracing and **temperature**
- I would deepen the anesthetic and do a target physical examination:
    - Pupils (increase. ICP)
    - Diaphoresis and flushing (carcinoid, pheochromocytoma, thyroid)
    - Rigidity (MH, serotonin syndrome)
    - Peripheral perfusion
    - Bladder distention (autonomic dysreflexia)
    - Hyperthermia (thyroid storm, MH, serotonin syndrome)
- Scan machine, infusions and recent meds administered
    - Drug error (bolus or infusions)
    - Awareness – TIVA disconnect, circuit disconnect
    - tourniquet

Hyperthyroidism

1. Goiter - Difficult airway
2. End-organ dysfunction of Hypermetabolic state
   - CVS: tachycardia, high output CHF, atrial fibrillation
   - Respiratory: respiratory muscle weakness
   - CNS: anxiety, hyperactivity
   - MSK: skeletal muscle weakness, fatigue, tremor
   - Other: exophthalmos (graves); Electrolyte disturbances; Altered pharmacokinetics
3. Thyroidectomy - Postoperative complications:
   - Tracheomalacia, Hematoma, RLN palsy, pneumothorax, Hypocalcaemia from hypoparathyroidism (tetany, laryngospasm)
   - Risk of AMM with retrosternal goiter – positional dyspnea
4. Antithyroid drugs and their adverse effects
   - Agranulocytosis, thrombocytopenia, aplastic anemia, Lupus-like syndrome, hepatitis, cholestatic jaundice, hypoglycemia
5. Risk of thyroid storm (see below)

Anesthetic Goals/Conflicts:

- Render patient euthyroid before elective surgery – resting HR should be < 85
- Avoid SNS stimulation

1. Medications - pancronium, ephedrine, atropine, epinephrine, ketamine

- Monitor for signs of thyroid storm (temperature, hemodynamics)
- Diagnosis and management of thyroid storm

Hx: Etiology - Graves 'disease (thyroid stimulating autoantibodies), excess TH replacement, toxic nodular goiter, thyroiditis, TSH-secreting tumors (rare); Symptoms of hyperthyroidism - anxiety, emotional lability, weakness, tremor, palpitations, heat intolerance, increased perspiration, and weight loss despite a normal or increased appetite

Px: Vital+ temperature & postural (HTN, tachy, hyperthermia); airway for BMV, intubation, surgical (masses); CNS - hyperactivity, agitation, confusion, lid lag; CVS – arrhythmia, CHF (high output), volume status, shock; MSK – proximal muscle weakness, tremor

Inv: CBC, lytes, Cr, Calcium, TSH, free T4 & T3, ECG (sinus tachy, A-fib, prolonged QTc), CXR +/- CT chest (neck mass); ECHO

Optimization: euthyroid prior to elective surgery; if emergent – esmolol infusion (100-300ug/kg/min),propranolol, PTU, steroids, sodium iodide; Endocrine consult; continue antithyroid meds; benzodiazepines for anxiety

Options: local, regional, GA

Room Setup: CAS +5 lead, temperature, Art line, foley +/-CVC (volume status); TEE for LV dysfunction;protect protuberant eyes

Anesthetic Management: avoid SNS - Deep anesthesia prior to stimulus, avoid ketamine, pancuronium,ephedrine, hypercarbia; AFOI if neck mass (consider armoured ETT); judicious NdMB (weakness); monitor for thyroid storm; treat hypotension with direct acting agents (phenylephrine); ensure reversal prior to emergence

Disposition: HDU/ICU if high risk for thyroid storm

Complications: Thyroid Storm – usually presents 6 to 18hrs post-operative – 72 hr duration; Arrhythmia: beta blockers, lidocaine, digoxin; CHF – digoxin; Airway obstruction (thyroidectomy): hematoma, tracheomalacia, RLN; Hypoparathyroidism – Hypocalcaemia (stridor, neuromuscular excitement)

Thyroid Storm

1. Emergency situation with a high mortality
   - Supportive measures: fluid resuscitation, Cooling
   - Esmolol 0.1-0.3 mg/kg/min, Propranolol 10-40mg ng, 1 mg/min IV
   - Propylthiouracil 100 – 400 mg po/ng/pr q6h
   - Potassium iodide 5 gtts po/ng q6h or Sodium iodide 0.25g IV q6h
   - Hydrocortisone 100-200 mg IV q8h

2. End-organ dysfunction
   - CNS: decreased LOC (may require airway management), CVA
   - CVS: high output CHF, A. fib, MI
   - Respiratory: muscle weakness and hypercarbia
   - Metabolic: hypermetabolic state and electrolyte abnormalities

3. Differential diagnosis
   - pheochromocytoma, MH, NMS / serotonin syndrome, sepsis, light anesthesia, cocaine toxicity
   - rhabdo distinguishes MH from thyroid storm

Anesthetic Goals/Conflicts:

- Restore intravascular volume, cool, invasive monitoring
- Excess Sympathetic – Esmolol, Propranolol
- Reduce peripheral conversion – PTU, Steroids
- Reduce release of thyroid hormone – Steroids, iodide Sodium iodide: 0.25mg IV/PO/NG q6h
- Reduce synthesis of thyroid hormone (PTU, methimazole, steroids)

Hx: Precipitants of thyroid storm - surgery, sepsis, anesthesia, labour, I-131 therapy, DKA, withdrawal of anti- thyroid meds, trauma, PIH; DDx: MH (rhabdo - CK, plasma and urine myoglobin, elevated K), Sepsis (Blood C+S)

PE: hyperthermia, tachycardia, hypercarbia, CHF, dehydration, hyperglycemia, changes in LOC, shock and death

Inv: CBC, lytes, Creatinine, TSH, fT4, T3, TSH, ECG, CXR, +/- echo

Management: Rapid diagnosis; Increase. Monitoring; Supportive management – active cooling (Demerol for shivering, IV fluid replacement (art line, CVC), glucose and electrolyte replacement, oxygen, Steroids – hydrocortisone 100mg IV q8h; PTU – 200-400mg PO/PR q6h; methimazole 20-25mg PO (60-100mg PR) q6h; Iodine one hour after PTU - Na Iodide 1gm IV, lugol 's solution 4-8 gtts PO, PR q6h; B-blockers for SNS – Esmolol 100-300ug/kg/min, propranolol 10-40mg ng (1mg/min IV); plasmapheresis; Digoxin IV for CHF – amiodarone may make crisis worse (especially if given prior to PTU)

Post-operative: ICU setting, most likely to occur 6-18 hr post-operative

Hypotension

Main DDx of Intra-operative hypotension:

- Hypoxemia
- Hypovolemia (Preload) – Hemorrhage, surgical obstruction to venous return, ischemic reperfusion
- Cardiogenic – rate (vagal), rhythm, contractility, ischemia, valves
- Obstructive - PE, AFE, VAE, pHTN, PTX, tamponade
- Distributive - anaphylaxis, SIRS, neuraxial, neurogenic
- Drugs - relative anesthetic overdose
- Less common etiologist:
    - Endocrine (Addison's, Myxedema, Carcinoid), Metabolic (hypo CA, hypoglycemia)

Anesthetic Management

- Emergency - simultaneous diagnosis and management - Inform the surgeon and call for help
- Decrease anesthetic, hand ventilate with 100% O_2 and temporize with vasopressors +/-fluid, inotrope
- Cycle BP and scan the monitors for HR, rhythm, ST segment, SaO_2, $EtCO_2$, PAP
- **Check pulse:** if no pulse → ACLS protocol. If pulse present → targeted physical exam
- Reassess DDx based on findings

Targeted PE: Urticaria, flushing, angioedema, tracheal deviation, s/c emphysema, air entry, JVP, CVP, PCWP, peripheral perfusion, check surgical field for blood loss, IVC compression etc.

DDx

Post-induction hypotension:

Anesthetic: relative overdose, relative hypovolemia, anaphylaxis, arrhythmia **Patient**: cardiac compression due to mediastinal mass, PTX, tamponade

Obstetrical Hypotension: hemorrhage, High/total spinal, AFE, PE, aortocaval compression, Cardiomyopathy

Medications (oxytocin)

Neurosurgery Hypotension: Arrhythmia (posterior fossa or brainstem surgery), Hypovolemia(mannitol, Lasix), Hemorrhage, VAE, Neurogenic (if SCI);
Management: lower HOB, flood field, Bone wax

Trauma Hypotension: Hemorrhage (Occult), Tension PTX, Tamponade, Fat embolus, Cardiac contusion, Pulmonary contusion, Neurogenic shock, Drug intoxication (cocaine), Rare: Anaphylaxis,arrhythmia, sepsis

Post-pneumonectomy Hypotension: Surgical – Hemorrhage, Cardiac herniation, Tension PTX (stump disruption, BPF); Anesthetic - High TEA, Sedation; Patient -Arrhythmia (A-fib), MI, pHTN/RVF; **Management:** Operative side UP, physical exam: airway, PTX, CVP, check chest tube for blockage, turn of TEA, sedation, CXR, ECG, CBC, ABG. Cardiac herniation: to OR, d/c PEEP, minimize Paw, turnoff suction to CT, 1-2L of air into thorax, inotropes prn

Laparoscopic Hypotension: Vagal response to peritoneal distension, Compression of IVC, Hemorrhage, VAE, Tension PTX, Hypercarbia-induced arrhythmia

Refractory Shock: Ingestion/toxidrome, Adrenal insufficiency, Hypocalcaemia, Hypovolemia (severe)

Hypothyroidism

1. Etiology of hypothyroidism and adequacy of treatment
    a. associated AI disease, previous radiation, surgery, hypothalamic / pituitary dysfunction
2. Potential difficult airway - Enlarged tongue +/- goiter from chronic thyroiditis (Hashimoto 's)
    a. Decreased gastric motility with risk of aspiration
3. Multisystem effects
    a. **CNS**: exaggerated effects of sedatives & NdMB
    b. **CVS**: hypodynamic circulation, ↓CO, CHF (diastolic and systolic), pericardial effusion, increase. QT
    c. **Respiratory**: Potential for mass lesion, pleural effusions, impaired ventilatory response to hypoxemia & hypercarbia, exaggerated ventilatory-depressant response to drugs
    d. **Metabolic**: hypothermia, hyponatremia (SIADH), hypoglycemia
    e. **Endocrine**: adrenal suppression (cortical atrophy)
4. Potential for myxedema coma → may develop in previously asymptomatic patients
    a. mortality >50%, precipitated by stress (surgery, infection, trauma, MI, CVA)
    b. Exaggerated features of hypothyroidism
        - Dec. LOC, increase. sensitivity to NdMB & sedatives, myocardial & respiratory depression
        - High risk for delayed emergence and need for post-operative ventilation
    c. Treatment of myxedema coma
        - IV T3 0.2mcg/kg q6h (onset 6-24 hrs) or T4 300-500 mcg IV load then 100mcg IV q24
        - Hydrocortisone 100mg IV then 25mg q6h (common association with adrenal suppression)
        - Risk of myocardial ischemia with IV T3/T4 supplementation in those with CAD

Hx: Inquire about etiology - autoimmune diseases, RAI, radiation, thyroidectomy; Determine cause. Look for symptoms of over or undertreatment (hyperthyroid = palps, anxiety, weight loss, heat intolerance, diarrhea; hypo = dry skin, brittle nails, brittle hair, cold intolerance, constipation, fatigue, depression, weight gain, edema). Evaluate for GERD, positional dyspnea or cough, SVC syndrome; heart failure symptoms.

Px: Vitals (orthostatic) volume status. airway – large tongue, hoarseness, goiter, radiation injury. Eyes for positioning. Respiratory - effusions, hypoventilation; CVS – hypovolemia, bradycardia, HTN, CHF. DTRs (reduced)

Investigations: CBC, lytes (SIADH, glucose), TSH, free T3/T4, ABG if respiratory depression; ECG (lowvoltage, long PR, QRS, QT, VT torsade's), CXR (effusions), ECHO (contractility, effusion) +/- CT (mediastinal mass)

Optimization: Delay elective case if symptomatic; Consult Endo +/- Cardio (risk of MI with CAD); Aspiration prophylaxis; Avoid pre-operative sedation; Supplemental O2 and ventilatory support as indicated; Drain symptomatic pleural effusions; Restore intravascular volume; Euthyroid prior to elective surgery - thyroxine PO titrated to achieve normal TSH over 6-8 weeks; Emergency Surgery - Pre-operative thyroid and glucocorticoid replacement (levothyroxine 400-500 ug IV load then 50-200ug/day, T3 has more rapid onset - liothyronine
0.15 – 0.3 ug/kg IV q6h, Hydrocortisone 100 mg IV then 25 mg IV q6h)

Options: Regional is acceptable option if CNS, ventilation, and cardiac status are appropriate

Room Setup: CAS+5lead, temperature; nerve stimulator; Art line; forced air warmer; PAC/TEE if indicated

Management: anticipate hypotension – consider ketamine; judicious NdMB – full reversal; consider ephedrine for hypotension – need some B agonist given cardiac dysfunction, may be refractory to catecholamines; multimodal analgesia (limit opioids); high risk for delayed emergence

Postop disposition: Dependent on degree of cardiorespiratory compromise. Low threshold for ventilation & HDU; monitor for fluid and electrolyte derangements

Perioperative Hypoxemia

1. **Low FIO2** – machine, circuit
2. **Airway** – obstruction, mal-positioned ETT
3. **Hypoventilation** – airway, Bronchospasm, **PTX**, **light anesthesia** / pain, dec. LOC (ventilator drive)
4. **V/Q mismatch** – pre-existing lung disease, palm edema (CHF), **atelectasis, aspiration**, infection, Cardiac arrest (dec. pulmonary perfusion), Obstruction (PE, VAE, AFE, FE)
5. **Anatomic Shunts** – Cardiac lesions (PFO, ASD, VSD, PDA)
6. **Low SvO2** – **Low CO**, anemia, hemorrhage, high VO2, hemoglobinopathies

Anesthetic Management

- Emergency - simultaneous diagnosis and management - Inform the surgeon and call for help
- Scan monitors: rate, rhythm, BP, $EtCO_2$, SaO_2, PIP
- Hand ventilates with 100% O_2 - increase PEEP, use larger volumes (recruitment maneuvers)
- **Check position of ETT:** pass suction catheter, FO bronchoscope (mucus plug, aspiration)
- Examine patient - cyanosis, rash, pulse, tracheal position, chest movement, B/L air entry, wheeze
- Support / Monitor Circulation
- Develop DDx and treat

Investigations: ABG (A-a gradient, Hemoglobin), CXR, ECG

Pediatric Hypoxemia

Aspiration (esp. FB), Laryngospasm, Post-obstructive pulmonary edema, Shunting (undiagnosed CHD), Endobronchial intubation (especially if small)

Obstetrical Hypoxemia/Dyspnea

AFE, PE, Aspiration, High spinal, Pulmonary edema (cardiomyopathy or valvopathy, autotx), Anemia

Trauma/Burns Hypoxemia

Airway obstruction, Airway disruption, Aspiration, PTX (simple or tension), CO toxicity, Pulmonary contusion, Hemothorax, Tamponade, Fat embolism, ARDS, Eschar around chest

OLV Hypoxemia

Mispositioning of ETT/DLT/blocker, Shunt through non-ventilated lung (inhibition of HPV), Atelectasis, PTX,low CO with potential RV failure

- **Management** – 100% FiO_2, confirm correct placement and lung isolation, PEEP dependant lung, CPAP operative side, Clamp PA

Massive Transfusion

TRALI, ABO incompatibility

Artifact

Poor peripheral perfusion, Hypothermia, Methemoglobinemia

Increased Airway Pressure

Definition: *an increase in PIP of more than 5 cm H2O; or a PIP greater than 40 cm H_2O*

DDx

1. Machine - stuck expiratory, inspiratory, APL, O2 flush valve, kinked scavenger, failed check valve
2. ETT - malposition, blocked (mucous, FB), kinked, cuff herniation, size
3. Increase airway resistance
   - **bronchospasm**
   - **light anesthesia**
   - **anaphylaxis**
   - foreign body
   - mucous/secretions
   - URTI
4. Decreased lung compliance
   - ALI / ARDS, **aspiration** / pulmonary edema
   - restrictive lung disease
5. Pleura – **PTX,** hemothorax, pleural effusion
6. Dec. chest wall compliance – kyphoscoliosis, muscle rigidity, MH
7. Increased abdominal pressures
   - abdominal compartment syndrome, obesity, insufflations, retractors, Trendelenburg

Management:

- Emergency which requires simultaneous diagnosis and management
- Increase. FiO2 to 1.0, inform the surgeon and call for help
- Initial Differential Dx:
  - Machine - Disconnect - assess lung compliance with ambo bag, patency of circuit
  - ETT - Check placement with laryngoscope and pass suction catheter to ensure patency
    - if marked obstruction: deflate cuff and recheck, extubate (consider exchange catheter), mask / LMA ventilate to increase SaO_2 then reintubate, consider FOB examination if difficulties

- If patient problem, initial management includes:
  - Deepen anesthetic with volatile (Sevoflurane) or IV (e.g., Lido or Ketamine)
  - Ensure paralysis
  - auscultate bilaterally for symmetry, breath sounds, wheezes, rales, crackles
    - Asymmetry
      - endobronchial tube - examine and reposition ETT
      - pneumothorax - assess BP, HR, palpate trachea, percuss chest
    - Wheezing or silence: bronchospasm – deepen, Ventolin, epinephrine
    - Crackles: pulmonary edema - PEEP, Lasix, morphine, NTG...
  - If hypoxemic or ↓ BP, initiate epinephrine (can bolus or put 1 mg in 1000 mls and run as an infusion)
- exclude other causes: MH, light anesthesia, inadequate muscle relaxation, opioids, surgical

<u>***Ethics/ Informed Consent***</u>

Principles of medical ethics:

- ***Autonomy****:* right to self-determination
- ***Non-maleficence***: Obligation to ‐do no harm‖ intentionally
- ***Beneficence****:* moral obligation to act for the benefit of others — do good‖
- ***Justice****:* obligation of fairness, entitlement to care & equity in its delivery
- ***Fidelity:*** right to confidentiality Informed Consent

Decision Making Capacity: *ability to make a particular decision at a specific time*

Voluntariness: Participate without coercion

Disclosure: The goal of disclosure is to provide information relevant to the decision-maker and the decision to be made (professional practice standard vs reasonable person standard vs subjective person standard (opera singer)

Recommendation: What the anaesthesiologist would recommend based on professional opinion.

Understanding: Patient needs to understand the risks and benefits of the proposed procedure

Decision: The patient should be encouraged to form a decision or be involved in the decision-making process

Autonomous authorization: To respect the patient's autonomy, the patient should give his/her consent for the procedure based on informed consent as an expression of the patient's self determination

Approaches to pediatric consent

Age	Decision-Making Capacity	Technique *
<6 years	None	Best interest's standard
6–12 years	Developing	Informed permission / Informed assent
12–18 years	Mostly developed	Informed assent / informed permission
Mature minor	Developed, as legally determined by ajudge	Informed consent
Emancipated minor	Developed, as determined by a situation	Informed consent

Assent
1. Helping the patient achieve a developmentally appropriate awareness of the nature of his or her condition
2. Telling the patient what he or she can expect with tests and treatment
3. Making a clinical assessment of the patient's understanding of the situation and the factors influencing how he orshe is responding, including whether there is inappropriate pressure to accept testing or therapy
4. Soliciting an expression of the patient's willingness to accept the proposed care

1. Decision Making Capacity: The ability to make a decision at a specific time which includes capacity to understand problems, proposed Rx, alternatives, options to refuse treatment, andforeseeable consequences, and express a preference based on rational, internally consistentreasoning.
2. Voluntariness – Pt participates willingly History /o coercion or manipulation

   Disclosure – To provide pt with info relevant to decision. (3) standards of disclosure: The professional practice standard, the reasonable (objective) person standard, and the subjective person standard (e.g., opera singer). Negligence related to informed consent is determined if Materiality‖ assesses whether the info given met the std of care, -Causation‖ then assesses whether sharing the omitted info would have caused the pt to choose a different option

3. Understanding – Patients need to understand the risks and benefits, distress does not seem to compromise the ability to recall risks, particularly among parturient. Recall and understandingare not correlated.

4. Recommendation – Anesthesiologists should offer an opinion

5. Decision – The Anesthesiologist should make substantial effort for to educate the patient prior to making a decision rather than to accept at face value the patient's refusal to be educated. If the patient chooses a technique which the anesthesiologist believes to be inappropriate, they are not ethically obligated to provide care in non-emergent situations.

6. Autonomous authority – Obtaining informed consent is how we acknowledge the responsibility to respect a patient 's right to self-determination.

Controversies:

1. **Emergencies**: Assume patient wants life-saving measures unless declared otherwise. Determine if intervention is reversible, if so, proceed. If irreversible make all attempts to clarify patient's wishes in advance.

2. **Moral Objections**: Anesthesiologist is not obligated to subjugate their Morales, however they must make a reasonable effort to find a competent and willing replacement. They should performcare in life-or-death circumstances.
3. **Confidentiality**: May disregard if a patient makes a credible threat to harm someone else.

Pediatric informed assent: -Informed assent‖ acknowledges that although most pediatric patients cannot legally consent to medical care, pediatric patients should share in decision making to the extent their development permits. Help the patient understand a developmentally appropriate awareness of the nature of her condition, what he/she should expect with proposed Rx, assess patients understanding, andsolicited an expression of the patient 's willingness to accept the proposed procedure. Generally, < 6 years don 't has decision making capacity > surrogate decision makers. 6-12 years DMC is developing, use informed assent, permission. 12-18 years, mostly developed DMC, Informed assent/permission. Mature Minor, developed as legally determined by judge -informed consent. ‖ Emancipated minor, developed as determined by situation
-informed consent‖

Informed Consent (7) Components

Indications: Anesthesia to entire extremity distal to tourniquet: limited to 60-90mins.

Contraindications: Usual + infection at site of needle insertion, coagulopathy (relative), pre-existing neuro deficits (relative), Raynaud 's or Scleroderma, Sickle Cell due to tourniquet, open wounds, obesity (may exceed capabilities of tourniquet), partial heart block (tourniquet release may precipitate. complete HB) i.e., RBBB/LBBB, bi-fascicular block).

Complications: Slow onset, may require 20 min, local anesthetic toxicity, inadequate block (better exsanguination = better block), hematoma (avoid multiple punctures), skin tears (minimize shear forces with Esmarch bandage, for fragile skin elevate arm for 3 mins prior to applying bandage + brachial artery compression. Post-operative pain, ecchymosis, nerve injury related to ischemia, usually transient.

Technique: Standard CAS monitors, 20-22g IV, Esmarch bandage, double-cuff pneumatic tourniquet. Exsanguinate arm for 1-3 mins (elevate, then apply Esmarch). Inflate tourniquet 100-150mmHg above SBP (at least 250mmHg). Remove Esmarch, confirm pallor and pulselessness. Then inject local.anesthetic.
Lidocaine 3mg/kg or 40 mL of 0.5%
Bupivacaine contraindicated due to CVS toxicity, Chloropropane contraindicated due to risk of thrombophlebitis.

Adjuvants: Guanethidine 10mg for 1st Rx, then 20mg for 2Nd U/E, 40mg for L/W
Reserpine 1-1.5mg (total)
NSAIDs for improved analgesia 20-60mg
Clonidine 1mcq/kg (not available in Canada)

Deflation: <20 mins = don 't
20-40 mins = deflate for 10s, inflate for 1 min, deflate (delays onset but not peak serum levels)
>40 min: deflate

For longer cases and tourniquet pain inflate distal cuff (over anesthetized area) then deflate proximal cuff.

For expected long cases, deflate after maximum time limit reached, allow limb to reperfusion x 5 mins, then repeat Bier Block with 50% original dose.

DDx Post-operative Jaundice

Prehepatic:

- Hemolysis, Hematoma, Blood transfusion

Intrahepatic:

- Drug induced: ETOH, Toxins
- Infectious: Hepatitis ABC
- Shocked Liver
- Sepsis
- TPN (acalculous cholecystitis)
- congenital conjugation defects
- Hypoxia

Post hepatic

- Gallstone, mechanical obstruction or acalculous cholecystitis

Tests: CBC/Lytes/Haptoglobin/Coombs/Smear/LFTs/Bili/GGT/Alk-P/Hepatic U/S / Hepatitis Serology/ Toxicology Screen (EtOH/Tylenol)

Considerations of fulminant hepatic failure: Considerations of maintaining hepatic perfusion pressure, correcting coagulopathy, avoiding toxins. Recognize increased risk of post-operative ventilation and encephalopathy and ICU. Consider altered PK/PDs.

Jehovah's Witness

Jehovah's Witnesses are an international religious organization that rejects much of modern mainstream Christianity *in favour of what they believe is a restored form of first-century Christianity.*

1. Risk of **perioperative morbidity and mortality secondary to massive blood loss** and patient refusal of allogenic blood products (RBCs, WBCs, platelets, plasma)
2. **Legal and ethical issues of consent** specifically regarding JW minors and in emergency scenarios
3. Considerations of pre-**operative optimization of hematocrit** (e.g., iron and Erythropoietin)
4. Considerations of **intra-operative blood conservation** techniques including hypotensive techniques, antifibrinolytics, hemodilution, cell saver

Specific obstetrical considerations

1. In cases of **mother vs. fetus**, courts have ruled in favour of blood transfusions when fetus considered viable
2. Consider (and discuss) **hysterectomy** for life-threatening hemorrhage
3. Epidural blood patches are generally accepted (Watchtower)

Anesthetic Goals/Conflicts:

- Maximize pre-operative HCT, minimize blood loss (antifibrinolytics, controlled hypotension, hemodilution), discuss cell salvage techniques (cell saver), factor VII!!
- Consider Regional Technique, tourniquets
- Document Refusal of Blood Products
- Conflicts: Parents vs. pediatric patient's incapable of giving consent (courts have uniformly intervened to deny the ability to refuse transfusion therapy), Pediatric patients nearing the age of consent

HX: Cardiopulmonary status, previous anemia, personal beliefs, cell-saver.

Optimization: If elective, delay surgery until hematocrit/red cell mass is optimized with iron +/- erythropoietin (300U/kg SC x 3 injections/week for 3 – 4 weeks). D/C Anticoagulants. Hematology Consultation, blood utilization program. JW Hospital Leeson. Legal counsel if dealing with minors. Consider pre-operative angiographic embolization. Venofer (IV iron sucrose 100mg iron) – Side effectsinclude hypotension, GI symptoms, muscle cramps, headaches

Intraoperative: Arterial line, minimize venipuncture, +- cell saver, controlled hypotension, regional,meticulous surgical technique, tourniquet, antifibrinolytics, avoid coagulopathy

Tranexamic acid – reversibly binds plasminogen. S/E: hypotension, N/V, abdominal cramps,thromboembolic, retinal degeneration with prolonged use.
E-aminocaproic acid – reversibly binds plasminogen, 6-10x less potent than TXA. Side effects include hypotension, sinus bradycardia, GI symptoms, CNS symptoms, anaphylactic reactions (paraben hypersensitivity), agranulocytosis, and rhabdomyolysis (rare)
Aprotinin - Inhibits many serine proteases including; trypsin, chymotrypsin, **plasmin (inhibition of fibrinolysis)**, and **kallikrein (inhibition of factor XIIa** – anaphylactic reactions.
Topical Collagen – causes platelet aggregation and initiates clotting cascade.

POST-OPERATIVE: Severe anemia > Consider sedation, ventilation, temperature control, iron supplementation.

L to R shunt

1. Consideration primary lesion ASD or VSD, or PDA (L –R shunt)
2. Consideration of Eisenmenger syndrome
   a. PTH
   b. RV dysfunction
3. Physiological interaction with pregnancy
   a. ↑ afterload Suring labour can ↑ L-R shunt and result in pHTN and RV failure
   b. dec. SVR → exacerbate the severity R-L shunt if pre-existing pHTN

Anesthetic Goals / Conflicts

- Hemodynamic Goals
  - Maintain Rate, Rhythm, preload, and contractility
  - Avoid extremes of afterload
  - Avoid air bubbles
- Pregnancy
  - Slowly titrated epidural (dec. SVR – reversal of shunt – hypoxia)
  - Assisted 2Nd stage – RV failure
  - Avoid increase. pHTN - hypoxemia, hypercapnia, acidemia, hypothermia, pain

Laryngotracheal Trauma

1. Emergency case
   a. Risk of aspiration

2. Trauma patient with associated injuries:
   a. c-spine
   b. CHI
   c. major vascular
   d. thoracic (PTX, pneumomediastinum)
   e. esophageal

3. Potential for airway obstruction:
   a. evolution of underlying process
   b. manipulation of tenuous airway (laryngoscopy, cricoid)
   c. PPV and neuromuscular blockade
   d. May require emergency surgical airway

Anesthetic Goals / Conflicts

- Identify the injury and evaluate extent
- Avoid PPV and neuromuscular blockade until airway controlled distal toinjury Identify associated injuries

Hx: high index of suspicion for occult injury – airway, vascular, pulmonary, esophageal (especially with penetrating neck injury); mechanism of injury

Px: 25% of patients have no external evidence of injury – neck trauma, subcutaneous air leaks & emphysema, dyspnea, hoarseness or voice change, hemoptysis, stridor, dysphagia, cervical pain, flattening of thyroid cartilage, ecchymosis in neck

Inv: CXR – pneumothorax, pneumomediastinum, subcutaneous air; c-spines – paravertebral air; CTneck – quantify disruption, associated injuries; Laryngoscopy / Bronchoscopy / esophagoscopy are mandatory; CTA or angiography to assess for vascular injury

Anesthetic Setup: If stable, transfer to OR; difficult airway equipment (FOB); equipment and personnel for immediate rigid bronchoscopy, tracheostomy

Airway management: if time, delineate injuries prior to airway instrumentation; consider AFOI (difficult topicalization); consider awake trach; if GA required – SV (inhalational, TIVA) vs. RSI (NO Cricoid or PPV); Confirmation of tracheal intubation – $EtCO_2$, CXR, FOB

LASERS (Light Amplification by Simulated Emission of Radiation)

1. **Patient safety and potential complications**: atmosphere contamination, perforation of a vessel or structure, embolism, inappropriate energy transfer.
   - **Atmospheric Contamination** (mean size 0.31um) small enough to reach alveoli. Note most surgical masks filter particles down to 3um. Potential mutagenic/carcinogenic biproducts.
   - **Tissue and Vessel Perforation**: Vessels > 5mm are not coagulable by laser, pneumothorax. With Nd: YAG laser perforation or bleeding may not be apparent until edema and necrosis become maximal several days post-operative
   - **Embolism**: Nd: YAG laser system associated with venous gas embolism due to the gas coolant
   - **Energy Tx** to inappropriate locations (reflected or transmitted through air)
2. **Operating room safety** and appropriate precautions (eyewear, appropriate masks, window covers and warning signs)
3. Prevention and possible emergency management of **airway fires** (low FiO_2, avoidance N_2O, specialized ETT, potential for jet ventilation, intermittent laser use).

Patient Safety: Eyes taped closed, cover with saline soaked gauze
OR staff Safety: Laser specific lenses, wraparound goggles, all windows covered and warning signs

ETT Tube Fires: Incidence 0.5-1.5% - Any hard carbon material (tissue/plastic/rubber) can ignite Puncturing cuff and O2 enriched gas increase chance of fire.
3 Preventative strategies: 1) Reduce flammability of ETT 2) Removal of flammable materials from airway using metallic venture jet ventilation cannula 3) Reduction of O_2 content of inhaled gas
Ease of ignition with Nd: YAG: PVC > Red Rubber > siliconeEase of initiation with CO_2: PVC > Silicone > red rubber
Options: Wrap ETT with reflective tape, protecting ETT cuff with laser resistant cuffs, saline filled cuffs with methylene blue for early detection, covering cuff with pledges, Metal ETTs (Laser Flex), Jet Ventilation, intermittent Apnea. Reduce FiO2 < 0.4. Avoid volatiles as they can form toxic compounds in the presence of an airway fire (not inherently flammable).

Airway Fire Protocol:
1) Remove source immediately
2) OR staff notified, call code
3) Flaming material extinguished in bucket of water/saline (keep available)
4) Ventilation resumed with 100% O2 once extinguished by mask
5) Direct laryngoscopy/Rigid bronchoscopy /FOB to assess damage +/- saline lavage
6) Reintubation if any airway damage
7) Tracheostomy if severe
8) Assess oropharynx for burns
9) CXR
10) Consider steroids?

Lithium Toxicity

Toxicity occurs with serum levels > 2mEq/L, with signs of skeletal muscle weakness, ataxia, sedation, widening of QRS.

1. Multisystem effects of toxicity:
    a. CNS: Sedation, decreased LOC, Seizures
    b. CVS: Wide QRS, AV block, hypotension
    c. Respiratory: potentiate NdMB
    d. Renal: Nephrogenic DI >> Fluid and electrolyte imbalance
2. Treatment:
    a. Medical emergency requiring Hemodialysis
    b. Diuresis – Loop or osmotic diuretics
        i. Thiazide diuretics increase lithium resorption in proximal tubule

Anesthetic Goals/Conflicts:

- Avoid NSAIDS and ACEi 's which decrease lithium excretion
- Supportive management, correct fluid and electrolyte abnormalities of DI

Liver Failure

1. Underlying etiology and associated concerns
    - Viral hepatitis, drugs (ETOH, Tylenol), Autoimmune, Hemochromatosis
2. End-organ Dysfunction
    - CNS – encephalopathy
    - CVS – hyperdynamic (increase.CO, dec. SVR), cardiomyopathy, portal hypertension
    - Respiratory – chronic hypoxemia (V/Q mismatch, intrapulmonary AV shunts), RLD (ascites)
    - Renal –hepatorenal syndrome, CRF
    - Hem – anemia, coagulopathy (thrombocytopenia, dec. clotting factors), immunodeficiency
    - Endo – hypoglycemia, hyponatremia, lactic acidosis
    - GI – esophageal varices
3. Altered pharmacology (increase Vd, dec. protein binding, dec. hepatic clearance)
4. TBW excess with dec. effective circulating volume (dec. albumin)

Anesthetic Goals/Conflicts:

- Identify and optimize multi-organ dysfunction
    - Delay elective cases until optimized
    - Correct hypovolemia, coagulopathy, acute hepatitis is a contraindication to surgery
- Universal precautions

Hx: determine etiology & associated comorbidities (hemochromatosis – restrictive cardiomyopathy, ETOH – dilated cardiomyopathy); Identify end-organ dysfunction – encephalopathy, varices, hepatopulmonary/renal syndromes, dyspnea, ascites/SBP; Ongoing treatment and response to date.

PE: Vitals, postural BP, GCS, temperature, volume status. Cardiopulmonary exam assessing for high output heart failure, aortopulmonary HTN, pleural effusions (supine vs upright sat can indicate hepatopulmonary syndrome), sigmate of chronic liver disease (caput, spider nevi, clubbing, asterixis, hepatosplenomegaly), icterus

Investigations: CBC (anemia, thrombocytopenia), lytes (hyponatremia), BUN, Cr (renal failure), coags, Ca, Mg, Cross Match, glucose, albumin, bilirubin (Child-Pugh), CXR (pleural effusions), ECG (pHTN), PFTs (restrictive), ECHO (PAP, EF, cardiomyopathy

Optimization: Consultation with GI/hepatologist – treat encephalopathy, evaluate for varices, Correct coagulopathies (vit K, FFP), electrolytes, **anemia**, volume deficit. Risks stratify with Child-Pugh, Aspiration prophylaxis, Optimize nutritional status. If RLD is severe, then thoracentesis or paracentesismay be required.

Anesthetic Options: local, GA, Regional – contraindicated with massive hemorrhage, increase. infectrisk – if required, single shot (coagulopathy may recur)

Room Setup: CAS + 5, temperature, nerve stim, pre-induction A-Line, Blood warmer, large IV accesswith rapid infuser, CVP, PAC/TEE rarely (if varices banded for the latter), ICP monitoring can be discussed in setting of fulminant hepatic failure, PRBC, pressors and infusions

Intraoperative Management: RSI vs. Hemodynamic instability, Anticipate altered pharmacokinetics – use propofol, fentanyl, remifentanil, cis-atracurium. Follow glucose, colloid for volume, follow U/O

Post-operative: High dependency unit. Low threshold for postop ventilation

Complications: Delayed emergence (encephalopathy, increase ICP, drugs), ARF, Hemorrhage (surgical vs. medical, variceal bleed – octreotide 25-50 ug/kg/hr, vasopressin, Blakemore tube), Sepsis, transfusion reactions, ETOH withdrawal

Liver Transplant

1. Urgent Case
2. Considerations of End Stage Liver Disease
   - Underlying etiology
   - Physiologic & metabolic derangement – encephalopathy, high output cardiac failure, pHTN, chronic hypoxia, coagulopathy, renal failure, varices
3. Risk of massive transfusion – Perioperative coagulopathy and management
4. Hemodynamic instability
   - Liver manipulation
   - IVC clamping
   - Post-reperfusion syndrome (acidosis, ↑ cardiac output, ↓ SVR, ↓ BP)
5. Risk of hypothermia
6. Postoperative disposition (ICU)

Anesthetic Goals/Conflicts:

1. Optimize end-organ dysfunction – volume resuscitate, correct coagulopathy
2. Preparation for major blood loss
   - Correct coagulopathy, Good IV access, cell-saver, fluid warmers, rapid infuser, Coordination with blood bank, consider antifibrinolytics
3. Preparation for 3 stages of liver transplantation and hemodynamic effects
   - Dissection, Anhepatic, Reperfusion/neohepatic

Hx: determine etiology & associated comorbidities (hemochromatosis – restrictive cardiomyopathy, ETOH – dilated cardiomyopathy); Identify end-organ dysfunction – encephalopathy, varices, hepatopulmonary/renal syndromes, dyspnea, ascites/SBP; Ongoing treatment and response to date.

PE: Vitals, postural BP, GCS, temperature, volume status. Cardiopulmonary exam assessing for highoutput heart failure, Porto pulmonary HTN, pleural effusions (supine vs upright sat can indicate hepatopulmonary syndrome), signs of chronic liver disease (caput, spider nevi, clubbing, asterixis, hepatosplenomegaly), icterus

Investigations: CBC, lytes (hyponatremia), BUN, Cr, coags, Ca, Mg, Cross Match, glucose, albumin, bile (Child-Pugh), CXR (pleural effusions), ECG (pHTN), PFTs (restrictive), ECHO (PAP, EF, cardiomyopathy)

Optimization: Consultation with GI/hepatologist – treat encephalopathy, evaluate for varices, Correct coagulopathies (vit K, FFP), electrolytes, **anemia**, volume deficit. Risks stratify with Child-Pugh, Aspiration prophylaxis, Optimize nutritional status. If RLD is severe, thoracentesis or paracentesis may be required.

Room Setup: CAS + 5, temperature, nerve stim, pre-induction A-Line, Blood warmer, 2-3 large IVs with rapid infuser, CVP, PAC/TEE rarely (if varices banded for the latter), ICP monitoring can be discussed in setting of fulminant hepatic failure, PRBC (10 units to start), pressors Calcium, and infusions

Intraoperative Management: Induction: RSI/ETT. Maintenance: Balanced anesthesia. Maintain relaxation with Cis (or atracurium). Minimize crystallize. Albumin 5% or, less optimally, PS/VV for fluid resuscitation. Monitor lytes

Stages: Dissection: Results in bleeding/hypovolemia – volume resuscitate and maintain renal perfusion

Anhepatic: Clamping results in dec. preload, dec. CO, dec. renal perfusion, dec. citrate clearance (with associated citrate toxicity), fibrinolysis – volume load, vasopressors, consider veno-veno bypass
Neohepatic/reperfusion: most unstable period, abrupt increased in K+, HISTORY +, dec. temperature, release of vasoactive substances. Postreperfusion syndrome – hypotension, bradycardia, arrhythmia – pre-emptive bicarb, Calcium, hyperventilation, insulin/glucose, vasopressors, free radical scavengers (methylene blue)

Post-operative: Conservative management involves transferring to ICU ventilated and weaning over 6-8 hours.

Local Anesthetic Toxicity

1. Prevent and recognize toxicity
    a. Toxic doses, monitoring, mild signs and symptoms (Analgesia, Light-headedness, Tinnitus, Numbness of tongue)

2. Emergency management of CNS toxicity
    a. seizures, coma and respiratory arrest
    b. airway management and hyperventilation

3. Emergency management of CVS toxicity
    a. arrhythmias, hypotension, and cardiac arrest
        i. ACLS, escalating doses of Epinephrine, Vasopressin
        ii. Intralipid therapy (1.5ml/kg may rpt q5 to max 3ml/kg followed by 0.25ml/kg/min)

Anesthetic Goals/Conflicts:

- Prevention of toxicity: aspiration, test doses, slow infusion
- Avoid exacerbating factors: acidosis, hypercarbia, hypoxia
- Prompt administration of possible antidote: Intralipid 20%

Presentation: initial sx of

CNS toxicity - tinnitus, visual disturbance/diplopia, light-headedness, metallic taste, circumoral numbness - Progression to myoclonus, grand mal seizures, coma & respiratory arrest

Cardiotoxicity usually follows neurotoxicity; ~10% may present with arrhythmias, hypotension and CVS collapse rather than seizures - Arrhythmias include conduction delay, BBB, prolonged PR interval, complete heart block, sinus arrest, or asystole - ventricular ectopy, and malignant arrhythmias such as ventricular tachycardia, torsade's de pointes, and ventricular fibrillation

Toxic doses: Chlorprocaine 12mg/kg, Cocaine 1.5-3mg/kg, Bupivacaine 2-3mg/kg, Lido 4.5-7mg/kg (History / epi), Ropivacaine 3mg/kg

Rates of Absorption: Arterial > venous > Tracheal > Intercostal > Caudal > Paracervical > Epidural > Brachial Plexus > Sciatic/Femoral > Subcutaneous > Topical

Prevention: Aspirate, give incremental doses, test doses with epinephrine (15mcg should increase HR by 10 bpm, SBP by 15mmHg, or lead to a 25% decrease in T-wave amplitude in lead II (peak in peds), wait 40-60 seconds, max BP response at 90 seconds. When using tissue depots, limit dose and use epinephrine

Optimization: Benzo 's raise seizure threshold, avoid hypoventilation

Management: Stop the injection / Maintain oxygenation and ventilation / avoid hypoxemia, hypercarbia, and acidosis –midazolam, prop for Sz – Mild CVS depression (brady, HTN) ephedrine, atropine - Profound CVS depression and malignant dysrhythmias, ACLS, escalating epi, vasopressin, intralipid – avoid Ca channel blockers

Note: Intralipid may cause pulmonary vasoconstriction, pancreatitis.

Long QTc Syndrome

1. Hemodynamic compromise / collapse from rapid polymorphic VT (Torsade de Pointes) and sudden cardiac death
2. Optimize QTc
    a. B-blockade, Lt stellate ganglion block
    b. Avoid
        i. Medications: Butyrophenones (Droperidol), Quinidine, TCAs, ketamine, Lidocaine
        ii. Electrolytes: Acute hypokalemia, hypomagnesemia, hypocalcaemia,
        iii. SNS activation: hypothermia, hypoxia, hypercarbia, acidosis, stress,anxiety,auditory stim
        iv. Valsalva
3. Consider underlying etiology
    a. Congenital (catecholamine dependant) vs. acquired (pause dependant)
4. Pacemaker / AICD

Anesthetic Goals/Conflicts:

- Recognize & optimize patients with prolonged QTc
- Avoid prolongation of QTc
    - SNS stimulation, physical stress, anxiety, auditory stimuli
    - bradycardia in acquired long QT
    - Medications
- Rapidly recognize and treat Torsade's de Point

Hx and PE: FMHx of sudden death, associated congenital abnormalities, syncope, arrhythmias

Investigations: Lytes (K, Ca, Mg); ECG (prolonged QTc (F >480 msec, M>470 msec)

Optimization: EP study; B-blockade; Left SGB if refractory to medical therapy or ER surgery; Correct Lytes (K^+, Mg^{2+}, Ca^{2+}); Continue antiarrhythmics; Cardioversion/defib pads on patient; Anxiolysis

Anesthetic Options: Local; GA; RA

Room Setup: Resus drugs (phenyl and ephedrine); esmolol; Mg^{2+}; ACLS drugs; DEFIB & CRASH CART

Intraoperative Management: Propofol shortens Q-T; Deep prior to airway instrumentation; TIVA optimal;Volatiles prolong QT but used safely; Avoid N_2O and abrupt rise in Des (SNS +); Consider deep extubation; Avoid reversal atropine, glycol & antiemetics (droperidol & ondansetron) they all prolong QTc;

Post-operative: Monitored bed; quiet atmosphere; Good pain control (Methadone prolongs QTc); consider Phenytoin in severe QTc prolongation (it shortens QTc)

Drugs: Prolongs QT: thiopental, ketamine, Iso, Sevoflurane, Succinyl , pancuronium, Sufentanil, Neostigmine, edrophonium, atropine, glycopyrrolate, Epinephrine, Norepinephrine, class I & III antiarrhythmics, haloperidol, droperidol, quetiapine, risperidone, SSRIs, Macrolide Abx, 5-HT agonists, cisapride

No QT prolongation: Propofol, etomidate, methohexital, Halothane, vecuronium, atracurium, alfentanil, fentanyl, midazolam, phenylephrine

Lower limb Revascularization

1. Considerations of a vasculopathy
    a. comorbidities: HTN, CAD, DM, renal insufficiency, CVA, COPD
    b. increased risk perioperative CV event (stroke, MI)
    c. increase HD monitoring/tight HD control
2. Type of anesthetic and suitability - GA vs regional
3. Etiology of occlusion/Urgency of surgery
    a. Acute (emergency case, risks limb viability)
    b. Chronic vascular atherosclerosis –high risk pt with time for optimization
4. Prevention and recognition of perioperative complications
    a. MI, CHF, HTN
    b. Mitigate stress response – adequate analgesia
    c. Graft patency - IV hydration, avoid hypothermia, spinal anesthetic
        i. Acute thrombosis and Graft dehiscence

Anesthetic Goals:

- Prevention of perioperative complications – ischemia, CHF, CVA, renal insufficiency
    - Optimization of oxygenation, perfusion of end organs
    - Adequate intra-operative, post-operative analgesia
    - HD control, volume status
- Promoting graft patency
    - Early recognition of postop graft thrombosis
    - Adequate hydration, perfusion, warm limb to avoid vasoconstriction

Hx & Px: Indication for surgery - claudication, ischemic rest pain or ulceration, gangrene; Etiology - acutearterial occlusion (embolic source? A-fib, recent MI, prosthetic valves, aneurysm, paradoxical embolus) vs. chronic vascular insufficiency/atherosclerosis; thorough assessment for comorbid disease; contraindications to regional

Inv: CBC, lytes Cr, BUN, Type and screen, coags, ECG +/- echo, PFT, baseline ABG, CXR as appropriate

Optimization: aspiration prophylaxis if emergent, diabetic, if elective consider need for cardiology/respiratory workup/optimization

Monitoring: 5 lead ECG with ST analysis, Artline, +/- CVC, large IV,

Anesthetic Plan: consult History / surgeon Re: length of case, expected blood loss, cell salvage, Spinal, Epidural, GA all reasonable, depends on procedure and patient's comorbidity

Intra-operative considerations: Intraoperative IV Heparin (Delay heparin 1 History after needle, Remove catheter 2-4 History after last heparin dose and patient 's coagulation status evaluated, Re-heparinize 1 History after catheter removal, Bloody/difficult tap may increase risk; no data to support mandatory delay, discuss with surgeon), Potential uncontrolled bleeding, HD swings – laryngoscopy, emergence, tunnelling for graft, Ischemic Reperfusion Syndrome (hypotension, hyperkalemia, acidosis, myoglobinuria - ATN

Complications: Optimize hemodynamics to prevent myocardial ischemia, ensure adequate analgesia, Monitor graft patency (Acute thrombosis – urgent take back, expect significant blood loss with thrombectomy, Graft dehiscence – massive bleeding, hypovolemic shock requiring resuscitation and urgent take back)

Lung Isolation

1. Indications
    - Relative vs. Absolute (see below)
2. Relative Contraindications
    - High aspiration risk
    - Severe hypoxemia (intolerant of brief periods of apnea)
    - Tracheal stenosis or obstruction
    - Difficult airway
3. Technique
    - DLT
    - Bronchial blocker
    - Endobronchial ETT
4. Complications
    - Trauma (laryngeal, tracheal laceration)
    - Tube malposition
    - Cuff herniation/obstruction

Anesthetic Goals/Conflicts:

- Rapid and accurate placement of lung isolation device
- Common conflicts: aspiration, difficult airway

Absolute Indications

A. Prevention of contamination
   1. Unilateral pulmonary hemorrhage 2. Unilateral infection (prevention of contamination)

B. Control of distribution of ventilation
   1. Giant unilateral bullae 4. Bronchopleural/broncho cutaneous fistula
   2. Tracheobronchial tree disruption 5. Surgical opening of major conducting airway
   3. Life-threatening hypoxemia d/t unilateral lung disease

C. Unilateral bronchopulmonary lavage (alveolar proteinosis)

Relative Indications

1. Surgical Exposure (high priority): thoracic aortic aneurysm, pneumonectomy, upper lobectomy, mediastinal exposure, thoracoscopy
2. Surgical Exposure (medium priority): middle / lower lobectomy, esophageal resection, procedures on thoracic spine
3. Post CPB status after removal of totally occluding chronic unilateral pulmonary emboli
4. Significant hypoxemia from unilateral lung disease

Predictors of low arterial oxygen saturation during OLV: 1) Side of Surgery (right side has 10% more blood flow than left) 2) Poor PaO_2 on Two Lung Ventilation 3) Pre-operative percentage of predicted FEV1 (inverse correlation) 4) Supine position

Management of hypoxemia on OLV Manual ventilation, FiO_2 1.0, notify surgeonCheck position of DLT/ blockerwith FOB
CPAP to non-dependent lung, PEEP to ventilated lung Insufflation of non-dependent lung with 1-2L/min oxygen
Intermittent 2 lung ventilation, Clamp operative lung PA to eliminate shunt

Lung Transplant Recipient

1. Assessment of graft function
    a. rule out chronic rejection (BAL, biopsy) & active infection (immunosuppressed)
2. Assessment of non-transplanted lung function
    a. differential lung compliance
    b. potential for pHTN, cor pulmonale, and RVF
3. Physiology of denervated lung
    a. impaired cough reflex and mucociliary function
    b. increase. risk of bronchoconstriction
4. Knowledge of anastomotic location, with placement of ETT under direct vision
5. Immunosuppression and resulting end-organ dysfunction
6. Considerations for the planned surgical procedure

Anesthetic Goals / Conflicts

- Minimize injury to allograft and native lung
    - meticulous aseptic technique
    - avoid instrumentation of lung
    - lung protective ventilation
    - avoid excessive intraoperative fluids
- prompt recovery of respiratory function (early extubation)

COMPLICATIONS OF LUNG TRANSPLANT

1. Primary Graft Failure (15-35%)
2. Pneumonia
3. Acute Graft Rejection (50%)
4. Bronchial Stenosis
5. Chronic Graft Rejection (aka Bronchiolitis obliterans)

History and Physical

- What surgery?
- Function of the allograft/SLTx vs DLTx
- Evidence of bronchial narrowing, other disease

Investigations

- Usual labs –especially CBC, kidney function
- CXR - evidence of rejection or infection (but may be normal in presence of both)
- Spirometry and ABG mandatory

Optimization: postpone if evidence of infection; stress steroids; prophylactic antibiotics

Anesthetic options: neuraxial/regional may be preferred if possible

GA: careful placement of ETT - avoid site of anastomosis

- Prone to infection, early extubation, judicious fluids, prone to bronchoconstrictor 'n
- If SLTx, consider different lung compliance in native vs transplanted lung

Complications: hypoxemia, trauma to native or transplanted lung

Malignant Hyperthermia

Anesthesia induced-hypermetabolic state characterized by rigidity, rhabdomyolysis, hyperkalemic arrest, ARF,DIC and cerebral edema

1. Recognize susceptible patients a provide a **trigger free anesthetic** (volatiles/Suxamethonium)
2. **Early recognition, declaration of emergency and continuous therapy** (dantrolene, cooling, ICU)

Anesthetic Goals/Conflicts:

- Avoid triggers (volatiles and Succinyl) in MH susceptible patient
- Early recognition and Rx: D/C triggering agents, correct hypoxemia / hypercarbia by hyperventilating on 100% O2 at >10L min, reverse hypermetabolic state with dantrolene, correctmetabolic acidosis with HCO3-, treat hyperkalemia, dysrhythmia control (avoid CCBs!), Cool patient until Core < 38 degrees.
- Continue management after acute episode to prevent secondary complications

Hx: Personal or Family History of MH, intolerance to caffeine containing foods, previous testing, hx of unexplained fevers or cramps. 3 associated disorders: CCD (Central Core Disease), King-Den borough syndrome, Evans's myopathy. Generally normal PE unless they have associated myopathy.

Investigations: Electrolytes, Crt, CK (70% of MH patients have elevated resting CK), urine for myoglobin, ECG may have ventricular dysrhythmias), Coagulations, ABG. Special: Caffeine-halothanecontracture test = gold standard, sensitivity 98-100%, specificity of 73-93%. Genetic testing has low sens ~25%.

Optimization: Dantrolene prophylaxis not recommended, avoid triggers

Room Setup: CAS monitors, central temperature monitor, 5 lead ECG, urinary catheter, large bore IV, consider arterial line. MH anesthetic machine or clean machine with 100% o2 at 10L/min for 10mins. Replace all disposable circuits, fresh gas outlet hoses, CO_2 absorbers. Remove Suxamethonium. Use ofexpired gas analyzer can help demonstrate that all volatiles have been removed. Dantrolene (~36 ampules = 720mg)

Intraoperative Management: N_2O considered safe, TIVA, MH may present after surgery

Post-operative: If uneventful anesthetic, patient can be discharged 4 hrs after surgery provided, they are accompanied by a responsible adult who has been educated about MH **Management of MH Crisis Initial Management:** 1) Declare emergency 2) Notify Surgeon to finish ASAP Call for MH Cart 4) D/C volatiles and succinyl 5) Hyperventilate with 100% O_2 at >10L/min **Dantrolene 2.5mg/kg IV q5-10mins** push, may req 10-30mg/kg, cont. until signs of MH resolved. Dissolve each bottle (20mg) in 60 cc sterile warm water. Each bottle has 20mg dantrolene + 0.3mg mannitol **Supportive Rx:** Establish IV Access, increase monitoring (temperature/ foley/art/CVC), Labs: ABG 's, lactate, CK, SVO2, CBC, Lytes, urine myoglobin, **sepsis workup, TSH,** coags, volume resuscitation. Cool patient to target core temperature of 38', ice packs to surface, gastric and urinary lavage, cold IV. $HCO3^-$ 2-4MEQ/kg for urine alk and acidosis, Treat Hyperkalemia (OK to use calcium with caution)

Dysrhythmias: Lido 1-1.5mg/kg, Procainamide 3-15mg/kg, forced diuresis with Lasix/Mannitol

Post-operative: Recrudescence in 25% in the first few hours, Dantrolene 1mg/kg q4-6hrs for at least36hrs. Measure CK q4-6hrs. Watch for DIC, renal failure. Refer patient and family for testing!

Marfan's Syndrome

Connective tissue disorder affecting cardiovascular, skeletal and ocular systems. Particular relevance with associated valvular defects, thoracic aneurysms, kyphoscoliosis and emphysema.

1. **Airway** - TMJ laxity with risk of dislocation / Potential C-spine (C1/ C2) laxity/ instability
2. Respiratory insufficiency
    - RLD/**pHTN**/cor pulmonale due to kyphoscoliosis, pectus carinatum/excavatum
    - Emphysema / bullous lung disease – increase. risk of **spontaneous pneumothorax**
3. Significant risk of CVS disease and perioperative complications
    - **Arrhythmias & conduction** defects
    - Aortic **aneurysm and dissection** (due to cystic medial necrosis) – minimize SNS
    - MI (due to dissection of coronary arterioles)
    - MVP, **MR, AR**
4. Technical difficulties with **positioning** and **neuraxial techniques**.

Pregnancy:

- Risk of 3rd. trimester aortic dissection due to estrogen mediated inhibition of collagen/elastin deposition in aorta.
- Screening TTE and pre-conception elective repair if aortic root > 4cm
- Beta blocker therapy during pregnancy, labour, and delivery – minimize sympathetic stimulation.
- Difficult epidurals (kyphoscoliosis) > GA and C-section may allow optimal hemodynamic control

Anesthetic Goals/Conflicts:

- Gestational HTN and risk of rupture, risk of pneumothorax with PPV

Hx: Focused history for CVS involvement, previous investigations, sx 's of AI/MR. Hx of restrictive lungdisease, spontaneous pneumothorax, pHTN. Functional capacity. Neurologic sx 's from cervical instability. Ocular sx 's (lens displacement).

PE: Focused cardiac exam. Murmurs of AR (-blowingll diastolic murmur LSB), MR holosystolic murmur at apex. Evidence of CHF. Skeletal abnormalities: pectus, scoliosis, reduced elbow extension, pes planus, joint hypermobility, high palate with dental crowding. Respiratory: Increased WOB, hyperinflation.

Investigations: Usual BW, CXR: cardiomegaly, dilated vessels, bullous disease. 12lead: conduction abnormalities / BBB. Echo – for root dilatation, valves, EF, PAP. Consider PFTs.

Optimization: cardiology / respiratory consult. Beta blockade, anxiolysis. Appropriate hemodynamic manipulation based on underlying lesions or ventricular dysfunction.

Anesthetic Options: GA/ Neuraxial (maybe difficult) / regional all appropriate if hemodynamic. goals achieved. Consider avoiding PPV due to risk of pneumo if hx of emphysema or bullous disease.

Room Setup: 5 leads +- invasive lines, +- TEE/PAC, Beta blockers, NTG/Nitrides/Inotropes, + Chest tube kit (32-40F)

Intraoperative Management: Avoid increase in SBP/catecholamine surges. Observe peak airway pressures. Ensure adequate analgesia on emergence and full NMB reversal.

Post-operative: May require monitored setting based on underlying cardiorespiratory reserve. Observe for perioperative pneumothoraxes, aortic dissection/rupture/tamponade/coronary artery dissection.
Worsening MR
/ MVP.

Massive Hemoptysis

1. Emergency procedure with no time to optimize (full stomach, resuscitation)
2. Difficult airway r/t hemorrhage with the need for immediate lung isolation
3. Shared airway and potential for airway obstruction, acute asphyxiation and aspiration
4. Potential for hemorrhagic shock requiring resuscitation and massive blood transfusion
5. Considerations of underlying disease/etiology
   - TB (infectious precautions); bronchiectasis (chronic infection = 90%)
   - Neoplasm (4 M 's)
   - Cardiovascular aetiologies (mitral stenosis, AV malformations, PE)
   - Coagulation
   - Trauma
   - Iatrogenic (PAC insertion, post-operative)

Anesthetic Goals/Conflicts:

- Mobilization of resources
- Efficient and rapid airway management with lung isolation
- Volume resuscitation
- Effective communication with surgeon and facilitation of surgical access for bronchoscopy

Hx: AMPLE; Dx, onset, progression, known location of bleed? Etiology (TB, Bronchiectasis, Neoplasia), recent procedure (iatrogenic), contraindications to surgery include inoperable pulmonary carcinoma, failure to localize site of hemorrhage, and presence of severe bilateral pulmonary disease

Px: VS, Stable or unstable, airway for ease of intubation/DLT/obstruction, volume status, IV access, LOC

Inv: CBC, lytes, Ur, Cr, PTT / INR, ABG & crossmatch, CXR, CT to localize, ECG (pHTN), baseline PFTs, rigid bronchoscopy (single most important technique to identify cause of active bleeding), FOB if not actively bleeding

Optimization: Avoid sedation, bronchial artery embolization (contraindicated if collaterals to spine),

Anesthetic Setup: Discuss plan with Surgeon, large bore IVs, Blood products immediately available, Vasopressors, High FiO2, suction, bleeding lung down (prevents contamination), early lung isolation (DLT, endobronchial SLT, blocker), Thoracic surgeon with rigid bronchoscopy, HFJV, fogarty catheter

Management of Anesthesia: bleeding lung dependant prior to isolation, then reverse after isolation; Acute airway obstruction or treatable cause - rigid bronchoscope (iced saline, vasoconstrictors, bronchial blocker, packing, Nd:YAG laser); not treatable with rigid bronchoscopy – rapid lung isolation (awake vs. asleep laryngoscopy; difficult topicalization; intubate in semi-fowlers; possible RSI with ketamine and succinyl/rocuronium; endobronchial SLT vs. blocker vs. DLT) SLT maneuvers include – advance endobronchial - ETT goes down bleeding bronchus (attempt to reposition ETT into nonbleeding bronchus - try ventilating alongside endobronchial ETT by inserting an additional small ETT through glottis -consider placing Fogarty catheter down ETT and occluding bronchus, then withdrawing ETT into trachea); ETT goes down nonbleeding bronchus (suction ETT to remove residual blood, ventilate with 100%, if oxygenation continues to be a problem, prepare to insert DLT

Complications: Can 't ventilate / high airway pressures: (Massive airway clot, Tension pneumothorax, light anesthesia), Aspiration, Hypoxemia, Hypotension, Cardiac arrest

Massive Transfusion

Replacement ≥ 1blood/24 hrs (~10 units PRBCs in adult), or 50% blood vol/3 hrs, or 4 units/1 hour with ongoing losses, or 6 units in 1 bleeding episode with on-going losses

1. Early recognition of potential for massive transfusion and mobilization of resources
   - Blood Bank, Lab, Hematopathology, Help for transfusion-related duties in OR/ER/LDR
2. Consider transfusion-sparing modalities — cell saver, antifibrinolytics, Factor VIIa
3. Monitor hemoglobin (>70), platelets >50 (>100 with ICH), INR <1.5, PTT within 1.5 of lab 's normal, fibrinogen >1, and replace appropriately. Octaplex to reverse Coumadin.
4. Monitor electrolytes including K^+, Ca^{++} and Mg^{++}
5. Avoid hypothermia
6. Obstetric patient – etiology (fetal demise, AFE, placental abruption) may contribute to DIC

Anesthetic Goals/Conflicts:

Acute phase resuscitation - Maintain hemodynamics - volume, crystalloids, pressors; Oxygenation - RBC transfusion; Hemostasis - factors, platelets, euthermia
Maintenance phase resuscitation: time to base resuscitation on labs - standard lab tests have poor correlation with in vivo coagulopathy.

Hx: Bleeding Hx, previous transfusion, inherited coagulopathy, medications (ASA, coumadin, etc.).
Obstetric Risk factors: Placenta Previa, Prior C-section, Multiple gestation, Chorioamnionitis, Placental Abruption, Abnormal fetal presentation

PE: Vitals + Temperature. Surgical bleeding, medical bleeding with dec. clot formation (nose, gums, IV sites

Investigations: CBC, INR, PTT, fibrinogen, Mg, Ca, Lytes, LFTs, Lactate, mixed venous

Optimization: Prevention - Pre-operative Fe ± EPO, position to dec. venous engorgement, normothermia, controlled hypotension, antifibrinolytics, tourniquet, cautery. RBC conservation - ANH, Hypervolemic hemodilution. Cell salvage (obstetric concern of fetal debris/AFE causing anaphylactoid Rx – use after delivery of fetoplacental unit. Inform Blood Bank & Laboratory

Anesthetic Options: GA for massive transfusion

Room Setup: CAS+5lead, A-line, CVL, temperature, large bore IV. 's, rapid infuser, warmers, Foley, pressors/ Inotropes

Intraoperative Management: **PRBC**: Hct 0.70 in 250mL, **FFP** – all coagulation factors, dec FV and FVIII (15-30%), Factors replaced if INR / PTT > 1.5x. **Cryo**– has fibrinogen, fibronectin, factor VIII, vWF and factor XIII (fibrinogen < 1.0 g/L), 1-unit FFP has 0.5g of Fibrinogen & 1u of cryo = 0.25g. **Platelets** For surgical hemostasis goal is PLT > 50 or > 100 for intracranial or neuraxial stuff. **Recombinant Factor VIIa** reduces the number of units transfused in cases of massive transfusion. **Octaplex** (prothrombin complex concentrate of F II, VII, IX, X) for rapid Coumadin reversal + Vit K.

Post-operative: ICU to monitor HD stability, coagulation abnormalities, electrolyte imbalance, acid-basestatus. ETT & PPV continue until temperature and HD goals are met and stabilized.
Complications: Infections, Hemolytic transfusion reactions Non-hemolytic (Febrile, Delayed transfusion reactions, Anaphylactic, TRALI / TACO, transfusion-associated Graft vs Host disease). Hyperkalemia; hypocalcaemia, Hypomagnesemia. Hypothermia, Coagulopathy: Diluted factors (< 30% activity) and plts with crystalloid, colloid and RBCs

Mediastinal Mass

1. Potential for catastrophic cardiopulmonary collapse on induction
   a. airway and CVS (RVOT) compression
   b. May require pre-induction CPB setup
2. SVC syndrome
   a. Upper airway edema, Lower extremity IV access
3. Comorbid disease
   a. Myasthenia gravis/Eaton-Lambert (Thymoma), Thyroid, Lymphoma
   b. Tumor 4 M 's (mass effect, metastasis, metabolic, medications)
4. +/- Considerations for mediastinoscopy – **relative contraindication to mediastinoscopy**
   a. Shared & difficult airway
   b. Complications (hemorrhage, inn. art. compression, PTX, TB injury, VAE)

Anesthetic Goals/Conflicts:

- Optimize – biopsy peripheral tissue or mediastinoscopy under local, steroids, radiation, chemo,
- Maintain airway patency
  - Awake FOI with armoured ETT, spontaneous ventilation until ETT distal toobstruction, gentle PPV, judicious use of muscle relaxants
  - Assisted <u>expiration</u> may be lifesaving in complete obstruction (pulmonary tamponade)
- Maintain hemodynamics
  - careful positioning - lateral decubitus or prone if cardiovascular collapse
  - **maintain preload** (RV may be volume dependent)
- Preparation for urgent resuscitation - rigid bronchoscopy, VVBP, positional changes, epinephrine, Heliox

Hx:

Airway compression (positional dyspnea, cough, stridor, hoarseness),

SVC Syndrome (HISTORY /A, upper body edema/plethora, cough, dyspnea),

Right Heart Compression (positional syncope/dyspnea, hepatosplenomegaly).

Comorbid Disease based on DDx (thyroid, thymoma, MG/ELS, lymphoma (especially adolescents), neuroblastoma in children)

PE: Vitals (hypoxemia, postural HTN), HISTORY &N (edema/plethora, tracheal deviation, masses), CVS (syncope with Valsalva, quite HS/JVD for pericardial effusion, pulsus paradoxus), RESPIRATORY (WOB, stridor, **supine dyspnea**) **Investigations:** Labs, CXR, CT scan (>50% tracheal comp ↑risk), +/-ECHO, PFTs not useful

Optimization: Consider pre-operative steroids, chemo, radiation to decrease mass depending on diagnosis if too high risk (recognizing that this may impair definitive diagnosis), check for extra thoracic LN sites for biopsy especially if lymphoma, treat pulmonary infections, consider pre-operative Airway / SVC stents

Anesthetic Options: Always consider local/sedation first, otherwise GETA

Room Setup: CAS + 5L ECG, arterial line, vasoactive drugs, lower extremity IV if SVC syndrome, consider having rigid bronchoscopy & CPB available.

Intraoperative Management: If asymptomatic with no radiologic evidence of heart/airway compression proceed with routine induction and maintenance. If positional symptoms/compression, consider awake FOI with positioning of ETT distal to obstruction with ENT/rigid bronchoscope/CPB backup. Maintain SV during induction and carefully transition to PPV & muscle relaxation. Consider inhalational vs slow TIVA for uncooperative patients or kids.

Post-operative: Needs intensive monitoring in HDU to monitor for airway obs (mass or if resected, tracheomalacia) and airway edema.

Special: Intraoperative emergencies - Acute airway compression or inability to ventilate (reposition, return to SV, rigid bronchoscopy, CPB, consider dynamic hyperinflation), Cardiovascular collapse (reposition, SV, fluids, inotropes, CPB)

Mediastinoscopy

1. Limited intra-operative access to the airway
2. Significant intra- and post-operative complications relating to
   a. compression or trauma to important structures - stroke – innominate artery compression; tracheobronchial compression or laceration; hemorrhage – aorta, SVC, PA; RLN injury
   b. pneumothorax
   c. venous air embolism
3. Short procedure requiring still patient
4. Comorbid conditions
   a. COPD / RLN
   b. Myasthenia gravis/Eaton-Lambert (Thymoma), Thyroid, Lymphoma
   c. CAD
   d. Smoking

Anesthetic Goals/Conflicts:

- Hemodynamically stable induction of anesthesia with airway securement
  - AFOI, SV induction, standard
- Optimal surgical conditions (still patient)
- Minimize potential for complications (e.g., stroke from innominate artery compression)

Indications: tissue dx for mediastinal nodes – NOT for AMM tumors (ant. Mediastinotomy)

Contra: previous mediastinoscopy, radiation, Relative – SVC syndrome, tracheal deviation, CVD, TAA

Hx and Px: S/S of AW obstruction (stridor, hoarseness, wheezing); Positional Sx (SOB, Stridor, cough) SVC syndrome (edema, venous congestion of airway & N and UE, altered mental status (high ICP); Hypotension; Hypoxia; Myasthenic (Eaton-Lambert) syndrome in patients with oat-cell carcinoma; Stroke;Underlying diagnoses and investigations/therapy (chemo and end-organ effects, radiation); evaluate for co-morbidities (EtOH, smoking/COPD, CAD, CVD, 4MS)

Investigations: CBC, E7, Cross Match; ECG – RV strain; CT- distortion/compression; PFTs; Echo - if indicated

Optimization: Anti-sialagogue (glycopyrrolate); position patient to minimize airway obstruction; Avoid sedation

Anesthetic Options: Local Anesthetic – depending on patient 's comorbidity (AMM, CVD, limited pulmonary reserve) GA with muscle relaxation and PPV - preferable, still patient, more control, more flexible surgical manipulation, dec. risk of VAE

Room Setup: CAS and 5 lead EKG; difficult airway cart; large bore IV's (above and below diaphragm); A-line or SaO_2 monitor on R side (innominate artery compression) & NIBP on L side; +/- CVP/PAP/precordial doper; PNS with ELS; Blood in room; Rigid bronchoscope, Armored ETT

Intraoperative Management: tailor induction to suit specific airway needs (AFOI vs. SV induction vs. RSI vs. surgeon with rigid bronchoscopy in OR prior to induction); topicalize airway to minimize coughing strain at emergence short-acting NMB (consider TIVA with remifentanil); head-up position may minimize venous engorgement and improve surg conditions, but increased risk of VAE; minimal need for post-operative opioids; extubate in OR

Complications: Hemorrhage (Aorta, PA, SVC – surgical tamponade, Lung Isolation, resuscitate below the diaphragm, Rt thoracotomy); Tracheobronchial compression (reposition scope); PTX (usually post-operative); bradycardia (Vagal); VAE; Stroke (compression of innominate); RLN paralysis (usually Lt, airway if Bilateral)

Metabolic Acidosis

1) Underlying etiology (AG vs non-AG)
2) Other associated metabolic derangements
3) Related multiorgan dysfunction
    - malignant arrhythmias
    - impaired myocardial function
    - altered seizure threshold
4) Altered pharmacology
    - Augments / prolongs NdMB
    - Respiratory acidosis inhibits neostigmine reversal of NdMB

Anesthetic Goals/Conflicts:

- Treatment of underlying etiology
- Treat associated metabolic abnormalities
- Anticipate/manage physiologic sequelae of metabolic derangement
- Patient with severe metabolic acidosis with limited respiratory reserve
    - bicarb administration when minute ventilation is already near patient 's maximum

Hx: Identify etiology - Organ hypoperfusion and shock (Obtundation, dyspnea, angina, abdominal pain)Toxidrome (altered LOC, visual/balance disturbances, CNS irritability, N&V, palpitations, muscle weakness)

PE: Vitals + temperature, volume status, focused neuro (GCS, cranial nerves), peripheral perfusion (peripheral pulses), hyperventilation (fatigue may herald rapid deterioration), Kussmaul 's breathing, abdominal exam

Investigations: ABG, Lytes, BUN, Cr, Ca, Mg, Glucose. CBC. Urinalysis. osmolality. specific toxins.

Optimization: Identify and treat cause prior to an anesthetic. Bicarb (1 mEq/kg) or Tris-Hydroxymethyl Amino-Methane (1.1 x base deficit x body weight = cc required) if significant physiologic derangement. Dialysis for acidosis refractory to medical management or acidosis with significant physiologic derangement

Anesthetic Options: GA. Regional likely not tolerated 2'to physiologic derangement

Room Setup: CAS + 5. Art line (for serial sampling), Warming blanket, Nerve stimulator (impact on NdMR)

Intraoperative Management: Agents used for maintenance/induction dependent on etiology of acidosis. Anticipate exaggerated response to induction agents. Ventilation should aim for pH > 7.2 to optimize enzyme function.

Post-operative: Low threshold for high dependency unit.

Causes of AG metabolic acidosis: MUDPILES CART = Methanol, Uremia, DKA, Paraldehyde/Phenformin, Iron/Isoniazid, Lactate, Ethylene glycol, Salicylate, Cyanide, Arsenic, Rhabdomyolysis, Toluene

Causes of Non-AG metabolic acidosis: GI losses, pancreatic fistulae, renal bicarb loss, renal dysfunction, hypoaldosteronism, hyperventilation, ingestion (ammonium chloride, acetazolamide, hyperalimentation, ketoacidosis while on insulin)
Other key points: AG = Na – Cl-HCO_3. Normal is 12 with range of 8-16.
Adjustment of AG for hypoalbuminemia -> (Normal Albumin – Observed albumin) X 0.2 (some sources used 0.25 = Actual anion gap

Osmolar gap = 2 X [Na] + glucose/18 + BUN/2.8

Micro laryngoscopy

1. Potential difficult airway with risk of perioperative airway obstruction
2. Shared airway with possible jet ventilation
    a. barotrauma, TIVA, gas exchange
    b. need for vocal cord paralysis
3. Unprotected airway with risk of loss of airway and aspiration
    a. debris, blood, gastric contents
4. Laser complications
    a. Airway fire, ocular/cutaneous burns, VAE, air contamination
5. High risk for perioperative myocardial ischemia / infraction

Anesthetic Goals/Conflicts:

- Safe induction and airway management
    - AFOI, awake look, spontaneous vent, ENT laryngoscopy
- Maintain adequate oxygenation and ventilation
- Prevention of barotrauma and Laser related complication
- Unobstructed, motionless surgical field

Hx: extent of lesion, location, and airway obstruction – hoarseness, dysphonia, stridor, dyspnea, dynamic obstruction; etiology – previous anesthetics; contraindications to jet ventilation (airway obstruction, restrictive lung disease - obese, ped, bullous lung disease, aspiration risk); coexisting diseases - CAD

PE: careful airway exam, positional changes if airway obstruction, standard PE

Investigations: imaging (CT), nasopharyngoscopy, CXR, PFTs, blood work and further tests dictated by comorbidities – -safell small ETT with regular PPV, jet ventilation via suspension -ventilating laryngoscopell, jet ventilation via bronchoscope (for sub-glottic masses), apneic technique with alternating ETT or BMV, high frequency PPV via a catheter

Room Setup: Laser precautions (goggles, masks, notice on doors, smoke evacuator, eye protection, saline bucket, Laser Shield ETT with Methylene blue for cuff); Jet ventilator – rigid bronchoscope; TIVA; Standard monitors
+/- art line

Intraoperative Management: If difficult airway – awake DL, AFOI, SV induction (inhalational vs. TIVA); if no airway concerns – IV induction, Succinyl TIVA; DL prior to handing patient over to surgeon; succinyl boluses (bradycardia). Limit FiO_2, communication with surgeon is crucial

Post-operative: head-up to decrease edema, Dex, monitor for PTX

Complications: airway obstruction – rigid bronchoscope, cricothyroidotomy; Dec. chest excursion – suction, check for PTX, airway fire: 4 E 's = extract, eliminate, extinguish, evaluate – reintubate and observe; Barotrauma, VAE, hemorrhage, HTN / tachycardia

Mitral Regurgitation

MR can be acute or chronic and results in volume overload and decreased forward cardiac output. In acute MR, no compensatory hypertrophy and lack of compliance results in CHF / cardiogenic shock.

1. Increased risk of perioperative cardiovascular complications including CHF and MI
2. The pathological hemodynamic changes of mitral regurgitation:
   - **Chronic** – **LA volume overload** and decreased forward cardiac output / **LV dysfunction** / atrial **arrhythmias** due to LA dilatation / **pulmonary hypertension** and RV dysfunction
   - **Acute** – sudden LA and LV overload without compensatory hypertrophy leads to reduced forward cardiac output and simultaneous pulmonary congestion
     - may require emergent surgical / anesthetic management
3. Associated co-morbidities including:
   - Other valvular pathology (MS, AR) / Endocarditis / Connective tissue disease
4. Underlying Etiology: (1) Leaflets/commissures: Rheumatic, endocarditis, MVP (2) Tensor apparatus: rupture papillary muscle (ischemia), dysfunction (fibrosis) (3) LV cavity or annulus: LV enlargement (myocarditis/cardiomyopathy), calcified mitral ring, marfans
5. Medical therapy (ACEI, BB, digoxin, CCBs), anticoagulants for A-fib

<u>Anesthetic Goals/Conflicts:</u>

Fast, full, and forward

- Maintain forward flow: Adequate preload, high N HR~90bpm, NSR, slight reduction of afterload, maintain or increase contractility.

Hx: Onset, severity of disease. **NYHA class** (1=no limitation History / ordinary activity, 2=mild limitation of activity, comfortable at rest or mild exertion, 3=marked limitation, comfortable only at rest, 4= confined to chair, sx 's at rest) signs of CHF: orthopnea/PND. Comorbid illness: CAD, Mitral Stenosis, pHTN, **A-fib**,

PE: Elevated JVP, edema, rales. Displaced LV apical impulse (chronic), holosystolic apical murmur radiating to axillae. S3 / S4. If associated MS, may have diastolic murmur. Findings of pHTN.

Investigations: Usual BW, troponins, blood cultures (if endo), **ECG**: dysrhythmias, LVH +- RVH/ strain, **CXR**: pulmonary vascularity and congestion, **ECHO**: EF, severity, LV + atrial size, thrombus. +- angiogram.

Optimization: Cardiology consult, consider MVR/replacement>> Class 1 indications include: Acute symptomatic MR, NYHA II-IV sx 's with N EF, Symptomatic or asymptomatic with mild LV dysfunction (EF 0.5-0.6) and dilatation / optimize CHF

Anesthetic Options: GA, neuraxial (as long as hemodynamic goals met) early epidural in pregnancy

Room Setup: 5 lead, Art, +/- TEE/PAC / +/- IABP/Perfusion services, Inotropes (milrinone/dobutamine), NTG/Nitrides, AChs for brady, NO for pHTN.

Intraoperative Management: Observe hemodynamic goals, consider mitral stenosis if rheumatic heart disease. Avoid hypercapnia/hypoxia and pain on emergence (increase PVR). May require inotropic support post MVR/replacement.

Post-operative:

MVP: empty LV causes increase. MVP and acute MR /
RV failure: Avoid precipitants of pHTN /
SAM: increase. SVR, volume expansion and decreased contractility /
Ischemia: CAD vs. hypotension /
Arrhythmia: cardioversion vs. IV drugs /
Hypotension: preload vs. afterload vs. contractility /
Air embolism: keep lines free of air bubbles
Pregnancy and MR: MR with NYHA 1-2 and N LVEF are low risk for mom and baby. NYHA III-IV sx 's, MR with pHTN or LV dysfunction considered high risk. Maintain specific hemodynamic goals, early epidural, art line, ACEi contraindicated due to adverse effects, hydralazine ok.

Mitral Stenosis

1. Identify severity of disease
    a. mod. area 1-1.5cm2 (symptomatic), critical area <1cm2 (CHF, pHTN, RVF)
2. Hemodynamic complications of Mitral Stenosis - CHF (increase. LA pressure with underfilled LV), atrial arrhythmias, pHTN with RVF, systemic embolization (TIA 's/CVA 's)
3. Precipitants of decompensation – increase. CO and dec. diastolic time
    a. Pregnancy, thyrotoxicosis, sepsis, A-fib, fever
4. Co-existing disease: Associated valvular disease (Ao valve, TR), rheumatic fever
5. Medications: anticoagulation, diuretics, BBs, digoxin

Pregnancy: moderate to severe MS usually increase NYHA status by 1 or 2 classes
Invasive monitoring +- PAC (for unexplained hypotension) / Judicious fluid management, BB for Tachycardia / Early titrated epidural / Avoid pushing (low forceps) / C-section of obstetric indications /Management of autotransfusion – intubation & PPV / oxytocin, methylergonovine, and hemabate (PF2-alpha) all increase. PVR

Anesthetic Goals/Conflicts:

- Hemodynamic goals: Slow HR 60-80 bpm, Strict NSR, maintain preload and contractility, avoid drops in afterload.
- Avoid precipitants of pHTN: hypoxia/acidosis/hypothermia/pain/N2O

Hx: Hx of dyspnea, CHF, PND, orthopnea, functional capacity, hemoptysis, arrhythmias, anticoagulation, risk of thrombosis. Hx of pHTN (dyspnea, fatigue, angina), Hoarseness d/t compression of L recurrent LN, CNS sx 's of stroke/TIA.

PE: Irregular pulses, prominent S2 and a diastolic murmur, decreased pulse pressure, loud S1 (highclosing pressure across MV) +- opening snap. Sx 's of pHTN. Tachypnea, crackles, wheezes, hepatomegaly, pedal edema.

Investigations: ECG – A-fib common, p mitral, RVH, CXR: Enlarged LA, pulmonary edema. Echo: Thickened MV, MVA, gradient, presence of thrombus. ? head CT. INR, PTT if on anticoagulants, LFTs.

Optimization: Cardiology consult, consider MVR or percutaneous valvulotomy prior to surgical procedures: Class I indications for valvotomy include: NYHA II-IV symptoms, asymptomatic patients with PAS > 50 mm Hg at rest or 60mm Hg with exercise. Class I for MVR: NYHA III-IV when PMBV is not an option. Mod-Severe MR. Medical management: Beta blockers, digoxin, diuretics, anticoagulation.

Anesthetic Options: Narcotic based GA +- regional, controlled epidural, avoid spinal. Strict NSR, slow HR avoid exacerbation of pHTN.

Room Setup: 5 lead ECG, A line, consider TEE>PAC, prepare for cardioversion, vasoactive meds.

Intraoperative Management: Observe hemodynamic goals, control sympathetic outflow, avoid tachy/pain on emergence. BB for tachycardia, early cardioversion, Consider NO if pHTN.

Post-operative: Monitored setting, observe for hypotension, MI, ischemia, CHF. If MVR
Note post CPB these patients often have depressed myocardial fnx despite N LVEF. Anticipate, augment preload, reduce SVR, inotropic support.

Mucopolysaccharidosis (hurlers and hunter's)

1. Potential Difficult airway: Macroglossia, infiltration of tissues, short neck
2. Potential unstable C-spine - AAI
3. Developmental delay, growth retardation
4. End-organ dysfunction
   a. Cardiomyopathy, valvular disease
   b. Hepatic dysfunction, Neurologic dysfunction
   c. Hemorrhagic diathesis due to platelet's dysfunction
5. Perioperative risk of hypoglycemia (glycogen cannot be hydrolyzed in hepatocytes)
6. Metabolic acidosis d/t inability to convert lactic acid to glycogen (avoid ringer 's)

Anesthetic Goals/Conflicts:

- Perioperative monitoring of serum glucose, minimization of fasting times when possible
- Pre-operative identification and optimization of cardiac system
- Safe establishment of airway
- Avoid respiratory-depressants

Multiple Sclerosis

Autoimmune, demyelinating CNS disease with multisystem effects

1. Demyelination results in:
   - Increased risk of **aspiration**
   - **Respiratory failure**
   - **Autonomic dysfunction** - hemodynamic instability
2. **Altered response to neuromuscular blockers**
   - Hyperkalemia with Succinylcholine if symptomatic
   - May be sensitive to NdMR or resistant (b/c upregulation of NAchR)
3. Potential for **exacerbation of MS**
   - Surgical stress
   - Neuraxial technique (spinal > epidural) – unknown why
   - Hyperthermia
4. **Immunosuppressive medications** (steroids, interferon, MTX)

Anesthetic Goals/Conflicts:

- Prevent exacerbations - Avoid hyperthermia and neuraxial anesthetics
- Minimize aspiration risk - Aspiration prophylaxis
- Maximize respiratory muscle strength
- Maintain hemodynamic stability
- Conflicts – RSI vs. Hemodynamic stability, Neuraxial for labour or C/S

Hx: Functional capacity, respiratory insufficiency, hemodynamic / autonomic instability, bulbar dysfunction. Course of disease, medical therapy.

PE: Focussed cardiorespiratory exam, cough, resting tachycardia, neurologic exam.

Investigations: Usual bloodwork, PFTs / ABG, CXR.

Optimization: Delay elective surgery for symptomatic disease, consider neurology consultation, aspiration prophylaxis, stress dose steroids.

Anesthetic Options: Avoid spinal and high doses of LA, epidural is not associated with exacerbation. GA and PNB 's Ok.

Room Setup: CAS monitors, 5 lead ECG, PNS, consider arterial line, temperature monitor (avoidhyperthermia), assistant for crinoids, vasopressors for hypotension.

Intraoperative Management: Consider RSI vs hemodynamically stable induction. Judicious NDMR. Ensure reversal. Avoid emotional stress / pain.

Post-operative: Monitoring for post-operative respiratory insufficiency and or neurologic dysfunction.

Special: Presents with ascending spastic paresis (Legs>arms), optic neuritis, gait disturbances, limb parasethesias, L 'hermette 's sign F>M, non-smokers, Caucasians. Relapses in 3rd. trimester with exacerbation 1-3 months post-delivery. Most common neuro-demyelinating disease 1:1000. Dx by IgG in CSF, MRI. Rx = Steroids = mainstay, Interferon B for RRMS, Glatiramer acetate = myelin mimic protein that blocks myelin destruction, Azathioprine: decreases rate of exacerbations but not course, others: MTX.

Muscular Dystrophy

Hereditary disease (x-linked recessive) of painless degeneration and atrophy of skeletal muscles with preserved innervation, often accompanied by developmental delay

1. Aspiration Risk – dec. gut motility, laryngeal muscle weakness
2. Coexisting disease
    a. Respiratory - Pre/post-operative respiratory insufficiency, RLD (d/t scoliosis) – pHTN & RVF, OSA, recurrent pneumonia
    b. Cardiac – Cardiomyopathy (sensitivity to myocardial depression), MR (MVP), Arrhythmias
3. Altered pharmacology
    a. Susceptibility to Anesthetic-induced Myodystrophy (Succinyl/Volatiles)
        i. Hyperkalemia (rhabdomyolysis)
    b. Sensitivity to NdMR (usual dose but prolonged action)
4. +- Considerations of a pediatric patient

Anesthetic Goals/Conflicts:

- Minimize risk of aspiration
- Minimize risk of cardiopulmonary insufficiency / failure
- Trigger free Anesthesia - Avoid succinylcholine + volatile anesthetics
- Conflicts: RSI (NdMB) vs titrated induction

Hx: Personal or Family History of MH/Rhabdo, Cardiac - functional capacity, CHF, orthopnea, PND; Respiratory - home O2, recurrent lung infections, chronic aspiration, OSA, Bi-pap, nocturnal ventilation, hospitalizations

PE: Vitals + BMI; Airway - Macroglossia, Respiratory – Adequate cough, kyphoscoliosis; Cardiac – CHF: crackles, JVP, S3, PHTN: loud P2, RV heave, TR, JVP; Assess for difficult IV access.

Investigations: Usual bloodwork, Lytes to assess K, CXR (chronic aspiration) ECG (tachy, short PR, tall R in V1, and deep q's in limb leads), Echo (fxn & valves), PFTs (FVC <35% poor outcomes, >45% unlikely to req post-operative ventilation), ABG, CK 30-300x N even in female carriers.

Optimization: Delay elective Sx to optimize cardiopulmonary status (Tx infection, optimize CHF) Avoidsedation (aspiration), aspiration prophylaxis, consider cardiology consult (CHF, arrhythmias, pacemaker)

Anesthetic Options: Trigger free anesthetic; consider local/regional technique (Muscle biopsy underlocal), GA - TIVA with low dose NdMB, possible post-operative ventilation

Room Setup: CAS +5 lead, temperature, foley, invasive monitoring as needed, dantrolene in room, drugs to treat hyperkalemia, PNS for NdMB

Intraoperative Management: Non-triggering RSI (NdMB, remi), avoid SUX/Volatiles, avoid myocardial depression with cardiomyopathy, ensure adequate reversal

Post-operative: Possible post-operative ventilation, Adequate post-operative monitoring for 24-48hrs -delayed Respiratory distress up to 36hrs, Telemetry for arrhythmia

Special: Presents in boys 3-5 years, with Gowers's sign, proximal weakness. Wheelchair by 8-11years.

Treatment of MH: Hyperventilate, change machines, circuit and CO2 absorber, Dantrolene 2.5mg/kg (20 mg in 50 mg sterile water), rpt as needed, max 10mg/kg. 2-4 mq/kg HCO3-, Cool, management ofhyperkalemia. Management of dysrhythmias, avoid Ca+ blockers due to myocardial depression and hyperkalemia when used with Dantrolene. ABGs.

Myasthenia Gravis

Autoimmune disorder- Ab against nAch-R à decrease in functional Ach-R at NMJ

1. Pseudobulbar dysfunction and increased risk for aspiration
2. Increased risk of perioperative respiratory complications and post-operative ventilation
   - risk factors: diagnosis > 6 years, daily pyridostigmine dose > 750mg/day, Hx of COPD, VC < 2.9L
3. Association with thymoma and considerations of an anterior mediastinal mass, thyroiditis, RA, cardiac myocarditis, cardiomyopathies, A-fib, heart block
4. Altered response to NMB – resistance to succinylcholine and increased sensitivity to NdMR
5. Perioperative management of medications
   - Steroids, anticholinesterases, immunosuppressants
6. Risk of myasthenic or cholinergic crisis

Anesthetic Goals/Conflicts:

- Optimize neuromuscular function
- Prevent or minimize complications: aspiration, respiratory failure, myasthenic crisis, cholinergic crisis
- Minimize exacerbation of perioperative weakness.
- Conflicts: RSI vs NMB, RSI vs cardiac involvement, RSI vs. ant. mediastinal mass

Hx: Symptoms of muscle groups involved, bulbar dysfunction, respiratory embarrassment, exercise tolerance, stability of symptoms, medical treatment. Associated comorbidities, thyroid/cardiac, arrhythmias. Presence of mediastinal mass.

PE: Focused cardiorespiratory exam, airway examination, dynamic symptoms due to AMM.

Investigations: Usual bloodwork, spirometry, Echo if suspect myocarditis / cardiomyopathy, CXR forAMM, if RA lateral neck films)

Optimization: Postpone elective cases for symptomatic patients. If acute myasthenic crisis, patient will need IVIG, plasmapheresis, and high dose steroids. Continue pyridostigmine perioperatively. ASPIRATION prophylaxis (sodium citrate, ranitidine, maxeran)
Anesthetic options: Regional or local preferred. Epidural for pregnant patient. GA. Discuss risk of POV.

Room Setup: Assistant for RSI, consider invasive monitoring for AMM / difficult airway

Intraoperative Management: Stress dose steroids, IV induction with remi preferred. May need 2mg/kg Suxamethonium or 10% of NDMR dose.

Post-operative: Respiratory failure: Myasthenia crisis Cholinergic crisis: 2ry to excessive anticholinesterases (also bradycardic, salivation, miosis (SLUDGE) –distinguish by giving edrophonium (Tensilon Test = 1 to 2 mg and titrate up 3mg, 5mg to max of 10mg) which improves symptoms if myasthenic crisis, worsens symptoms if cholinergic crisis)
Residual anesthetic drugs: muscle relaxants
Hypothermia; Hypokalemia; antiarrhythmics; Mg; antibiotics; psychotropics;
Special: Dx: Tensilon (Edrophonium), RMG, RIA against Ab RX: Pyridostigmine, IVIG / Plasmapheresis for Myasthenic crisis, Steroids/ Immunosuppressants. Surgery (Thymectomy improves 85%). Rule of 1/3's in pregnancy (get better/same/worse)

Myasthenic Syndrome

1. Association with Small Cell Cancer
2. Sensitive to Succinylcholine and Non depolarizing relaxants
3. Respiratory weakness/RLD
4. Risk of Aspiration
5. Medications: Anticholinesterase's don 't work well, IVIG, Plasmapheresis, 3-4di-aminopyridine.

Myotonic Dystrophy

Myotonia is the delayed relaxation of skeletal muscle after voluntary contraction, electrical stimulation or mechanical stimulation. As disease progresses, weakness and atrophy become more prominent and loss of DT Reflexes (distal muscles before proximal!!!)

1. Risk of **aspiration** secondary to bulbar weakness
2. **Respiratory insufficiency**, restrictive lung disease and **PHTN**, **central sleep apnea**
3. Cardiovascular involvement and **conduction abnormalities**: 1st degree heart block, atrial and **ventricular arrhythmias**, **cardiomyopathy** and MVP (20%) but rarely sx.
4. Endocrine abnormalities: DM, hypothyroid, hypogonadism, Addison 's
5. Sensitive to CNS and respiratory depressants, Avoid **Suxamethonium** - Hyperkalemia, Association with **MH** – trigger free
6. Risk of **Myotonic Crisis** with cautery, mechanical stimulation, succinylcholine and cholinesterase inhibitors, post-operative shivering. (Rx: Lido 0.5% infiltration, mb stabilizers, phenytoin)

Anesthetic Goals/Conflicts:

- Avoid aspiration and triggers of myotonic crisis, and post-operative shivering
- Treat Myotonia if it interferes with ventilation, be prepared for post-operative ventilation
- Conflict: RSI with avoidance of Succinylcholine or cholinesterase inhibitor vs cardiac induction for cardiac co-morbidities
- Avoid long-acting opioids due to risk of central sleep apnea

Hx: Functional history. Elucidate respiratory sx 's, central sleep apnea, restrictive disease. Elucidate cardiac involvement, symptomatic heart disease or evidence of cardiomyopathy/rhythm disturbance. Inquire about endocrine disease. Bulbar symptoms, dysphagia. AMPLE hx.

PE: Chest excursion, ability to cough, myotonic hand grip (unable to release), Cardiac examination for MVP (systolic apical click +/- late systolic murmur), arrhythmias, RVH (loud P2), failure. Developmental delay, frontal balding, expressionless facial weakness, dysarthria, SCM wasting.

Investigations: Usual BW / ECG / +-ECHO / +- Spirometry / tSH / Electrolytes / CK = N to slight high

Optimization: Aspiration prophylaxis, avoid sedation (CSA) / CPAP / Keep Warm /? Stress dose steroids

Room Setup: CAS / 5lead ECG / TEMPERATURE / Lido 0.5% / Mexilitine / Pheyntoin and Procainamide 18mg/kg over 20 – 30 mins IV / Quinine 300-600 mg IV

Anesthetic options: Theoretical risk of MH > trigger free preferred. Avoid Sux, Regional / Neuraxial for pain preferred. Avoid long-acting opioids for CSA.

Intraoperative Management: Avoid myocardial depression. Judicious use of NDMRs to avoid reversal agents. Although Neostigmine is usually ok. IV or propofol may precipitate contracture >> EMLA / lido.

Complications / treatment of a Myotonic Crisis:

muscle infiltration with dilute 0.5% lidocaine
phenytoin 18 mg/kg IV over 20-30 mins
procainamide 18 mg/kg IV over 20-30 mins
quinine 300 – 600 mg IV, phenytoin, mexiletine and tocainide depress Na+ influx, decreasing spread of action potentials.

Necrotizing Enterocolitis (NEC)

1. Considerations of Prematurity
2. Increased risk of aspiration
   - Bowel obstruction, dilated bowel loops, pneumatosis intestinalis
   - Full stomach
3. Associated multisystem derangements
   - Hypoxia
   - Sepsis / Hypovolemia
   - DIC, thrombocytopenia
   - Metabolic acidosis
4. Associated conditions
   - Birth asphyxia, hypotension, RDS, PDA, recurrent apnea, intestinal ischemia, UV cannulation, systemic infections, early feedings

Anesthetic Goals/Conflicts:

- Optimize multisystem abnormalities of prematurity
- Prevent aspiration (consider RSI)
  - Conflict with sepsis/hypovolemia and hemodynamic stability
- Anticipate and optimize fluid / electrolyte / glucose derangements
- Ensure good IV access (or central line above the diaphragm)
- Ensure continuous temperature monitoring and maintain normothermia
- Correction of coagulopathy

Hx: Obstetrical hx, PCA/prematurity and complications of prematurity (BPD, RDS, PDA, IVH, ROP), NEC hx: abdominal distension, vomiting, bloody or mucoid diarrhea, occult blood loss in stool, lethargy, irritability

PE: Vitals, weight (volume loss), focus on volume assessment (IV access, u/o); Respiratory – intubated, WOB, FiO2; CVS – perfusion, cap refill, murmurs; abdominal exam

Investigations: CBC (anemia, thrombocytopenia), lytes/Cr (hypovolemia), glucose, coagulation profile, G & S, ABG, ECHO if indicated, AXR (pneumatosis, intestinalis, dilated loops, free air)

Optimization: Unless intestinal necrosis/perforation, initial management in medical – decompress stomach,NPO, Abx, Fluid/TPN; Volume resuscitation – Crystalloid, blood, FFP, Plts; good IV access +/-CVP

Anesthetic Options: GA – caution d/t hypovolemia/sepsis, RSI for aspiration

Room Setup: Warm room/warming devices, resuscitation drugs (epi) drawn up, extra personel, neonatalcircuit

Monitors: CAS, +/- arterial line, temperature probe, foley

Intraoperative Management: muscle relaxant/opioid +/- ketamine, Volatiles may be poorly tolerated,avoid N2O (distends bowel), FiO_2 to maintain Sats ~90%

Post-operative: NICU, post-operative ventilation, +/- inotropes

Complications: hypothermia, hypovolemic shock, metabolic acidosis, coagulopathy

Special: Operative indications – Absolute: pneumoperitoneum, gangrene; Relative: clinical deterioration, portal vein gas, erythema abdominal wall, fixed abdominal mass, persistently dilated loop. Non-indications are severe GI hemorrhage, abdominal tenderness, intestinal obstruction, gasless abdominal with ascites

Neuraxial Opioid Monitoring

1. Identify risk factors for respiratory depression
    - Sleep apnea
    - Advanced age
    - Co-existing disease (diabetes, obesity, unstable medical condition)
    - High dose opioid, repeated neuraxial doses, concomitant enteral or parenteralopioids and sedatives
2. Select appropriate opioid and dose
    - Lipophilic vs hydrophilic
3. Select appropriate monitoring and disposition for the patient

    (Based on patient factors, opiate choice and neuraxial technique)

Anesthetic Goals

- All patients should be monitored for adequacy of VENTILATION, OXYGENATION andLEVEL OF CONSCIOUSNESS after receiving neuraxial opioids
- Single shot of hydrophobic (i.e., fentanyl or sufentanil) = continuous for 20min then q1h x 2h
- Single shot of hydrophilic (morphine) = q1h x 12 hr, then q2h x 12 hrs
- Continuous infusion: continuous x 20min then q1h x 12 hrs, q2h x 12 hrs, q4h until infusion stopped
- Sustained/Extended-release epidural morphine: q1h x 12hrs, then q2h x12hrs, then q4h after 48hrs

Intensify monitoring in the presence of risk factors – Continuous pulse oximetry

Hx: OSA Sx 's, concomitant Opioid/CNS depressant use (benzo, EtOH)

Pathophysiology: Neuraxial opioids mechanisms of respiratory depression:

1. Vascular uptake by epidural/subarachnoid venous plexuses & circulation to brainstem respiratory center
2. Arachnoid penetration and movement into the spinal cord
3. Rostral spread via the aqueous CSF to the brain stem or via direct peri-medullary vascular channels

Investigations: BUN/Creatinine for renal insufficiency

Drug Effects: Lipophilicity (fentanyl) rapid onset of effect & dec. duration of action. In single doses of 10-30ug, has rapid onset (10-20min) and short duration (4-6hrs) with minimal cephalad spread, making it least likely to cause delayed respiratory depression. May cause **early** (0-1hr) respiratory depression. Hydrophilicity (i.e., morphine) increase. duration of action and dec. onset time. Slow onset (30-60min), dose related duration (13-33hrs) and potential for both early and **delayed respiratory depression**. Delayed depression is primarily assoc with hydrophilic opioids because of cephalad spread andtypically occurs within 12hrs post-injection (up to 24hrs, with a **peak at 6hrs**).

Treatment:

Supplemental Oxygen - available, administered if dec. LOC or respiratory depression, routine use may increase. the duration of apneic episodes and hinder diagnosis of hypotension.

Reversal Agents – available, IV access mandatory, administered if respiratory depression develops, ABC approach, infusion will likely be required (2-10mg/24hrs).

NIPPV – may be considered to improve ventilator status.

Neurofibromatosis

Definition: *multi-system, AD disorder effecting neural crest cells during development causing a tendency to form multiple soft tumours (neurofibromas) in the skin and CNS*

1. Potential **difficult airway:** pharyngeal tumor, laryngeal stenosis, limitation of c-spine ROM
2. Potential **restrictive lung disease** (kyphoscoliosis 30% or pulmonary fibrosis from parenchymal infiltration of tumor)
3. Cardiovascular involvement: **essential hypertension**, Pheochromocytoma 1% increaseidence, renal artery stenosis, may have **idiopathic hypertrophic cardiomyopathy**, dysrhythmias
4. Altered response to NB 's: **Sensitive to Suxamethonium**, **unpredictable respiratoryonse to NdMR**
5. Potential **contraindication to neuraxial technique** due to spread of tumor, and potential raised ICP from intracranial tumours, seizures.

Background:

- Three subtypes: NFI, NF2, Segmental, hallmark café au lait spots >1.5cms, > 6
- Autosomal dominant but 50% are new mutations. Often worsens in pregnancy
- NF1: Classic, multisystem neurofibromatosis. 1:3000 early dx, increasereases severity with age
- F2: More localized dx(Café spots and neurofibromas ↓common). Bilateral acoustic neuromas. Also have abn growth of other cell types, i.e. schwannomas, meningiomas, gliomas, cataracts.
- Segmental: Mosaic form of disorders with neurofibromas in some areas and other areas unaffected.

Hx: Airway issues, hoarseness, previous hx of difficult intubation. Respiratory sx 's, functional capacity, history of restrictive lung disease, cor pulmonale. Cardiac involvement: HTN, pheo, RAS, RV outflow obstruction. Hx of headaches, seizures, raised ICP, visual symptoms. Endo- pituitary involvement, pancreatic tumors, thyroid tumors.

PE: Airway exam (hoarseness, dysphonia, stridor), focused cardiopulmonary exam, kyphoscoliosis, fine crackles, clubbing, BP(HTN/perspiration), neurological exam for ICP, visual defects, papilledema decreased LOC + neuro exam for regional technique

Investigations: Usual BW +- imaging related to symptoms, MRI if planning regional technique. CXR in severe kyphoscoliosis, consider PFTs or ABG. 24-hour urine collection for creatinine, total catecholamines, vanillylmandelic acid, and metanephrines.

Optimization: Consider endocrine consult, MRI if planning regional technique, BP control, respiratoryconsult if restrictive lung disease?

Anesthetic Options: GA preferred or MRI prior to regional / neuraxial technique. May avoid LMA from laryngeal obstruction by tumor. Consider raised ICP.

Room Setup: Entirely dependent on manifestations of disease, consider difficult airway equipment, antihypertensives, alpha blockade (phentolamine). PNS for unpredictable respiratoryonse to NMB.

Post-operative: Seizures, residual NMBs

Neuroleptic Malignant Syndrome

1. Potentially life-threatening emergency with high mortality (4-20%)
   - Altered LOC: Coma which may mandate airway management
   - Autonomic instability: tachycardia, hypertension, cardiac dysrhythmias (most likely cause of death)
   - Hypermetabolic State: fever, rhabdomyolysis, DIC, volume depletion, renal failure and acidosis
   - Tachypnea and potential respiratory insufficiency from hypoventilation/rigidity
2. DDx: MH, infection, drug toxicity/withdrawal, Serotonin Syndrome, heat stroke, status epilepticus, malignant catatonia, thyrotoxicosis, pheochromocytoma
3. Underlying psychiatric condition

Anesthetic Goals/Conflicts:

- Resuscitation and ICU monitoring following trigger
  - Stop offending agents (? Suxamethonium, antidopinergics), supportive treatment, cooling, treat acidosis and electrolyte abnormalities, hemodynamic support
  - Pharmacologic: bromocriptine, dantrolene, benzodiazepines
  - ECT
- Rule out high risk conditions on differential diagnosis
- Trigger freell anesthetic in patients with history of NMS (controversial)

Hx: AMPLE + recent neuroleptic drugs started or increase dosage, psych hx, most common drugs: haloperidol, phenothiazines, butyrophenones, thioxanthines. Withdrawal of anti-Parkinson meds (dopamine agonists; Symptoms – Mental status changes (confusion, stupor, delirium) motor rigidity, akinesia, bradykinesia, dystonia, mutism, dysarthria, involuntary mov 'ts.

PE: Vitals (orthostatic, temperature): autonomic dysfunction, CVS: tachycardia, diaphoresis, arrhythmias; MSK: rigidity that resolves with NdMB (unlike MH); Respiratory failure (WOB, cyanosis, hypercarbia), CNS: altered LOC, hyperthermia

Investigations: CBC (+/- increased WBC), ABG (Met acidosis), CK (rhabdo – correlates with disease severity), coags (risk of DIC), increased LFTs, electrolyte abN (hypo PO4, Ca, Mg; hyper Na, K), pan-culture to r/o sepsis, tox screen, renal function, myoglobinuria. ECG, CXR (aspiration, infection), CT Head

Optimization: Delay elective surgery. D/C any offending meds (Haldol, loxapine, maxeran, perphenazine, droperidol), **rehydrate**, maintain U/O (rhabdo), cool, r/o Ddx, ICU consult, +/- intubation for dLOC, Bromocryptine (2.5-20mg PO TID), muscle relaxants, dantrolene (reduced rigidity and heat production), ECT.

Room Setup: Trigger-free anesthetic to be conservative, inotropes available, avoid the above-mentioned drugs (most anti-emetics), CAS + invasive monitors, temperature probe, Suxamethonium controversial if these pts need ECT. Crash cart available.

Intraoperative Management: As above: trigger free. Use NdMBs to aid rigidity.

Post-operative: Likely need ICU post-operative.

Special: Complications: hyper/hypotension, hyperthermia, hypermetabolic, volume deplete, renal failure, MH, thromboembolism, residual catatonia.

Non-obstetrical surgery for the Parturient

1. Parturient
   a. Risk of aspiration, difficult airway, rapid desaturation, aortocaval compression, 2 patients
2. Maintenance uteroplacental perfusion
   a. Avoid hypoxemia, hypotension, acidosis and hyperventilation
   b. FHR and uterus monitoring
3. Risk of preterm labour
   a. Obstetrical consultation, tocolytics, Steroids if viable and < 37 wks.
4. Surgical considerations of a gravid uterus
5. Appropriate timing related to gestational age
   a. Exposure to potential teratogenic drugs

Anesthetic Goals/Conflicts:

- Ensure obstetrical involvement and FHR monitoring when possible
- Avoid Teratogens
- Maintain uteroplacental perfusion
  - maintain oxygenation,
  - maternal MAP
  - prevent acidosis, normocapnia

Hx: Gestational age, Obstetrical history, underlying medical condition, adverse pregnancy associated features(PIH/HELLP/hyperemesis/Gestational Diabetes), CVS status, Preterm labor.

PE: Volume status, CVS exam, detailed airway examination, uterine tone/contractions.

Investigations: Review fetal U/S, usual bloodwork, +- PIH bloodwork +- Echo depending on CVS exam

Optimization: Delay elective surgery, essential surgery in early 2Nd trimester, aspiration prophylaxis, consider steroids for fetal lung maturation (Betamethasone 6mg q 24hrs x 2days for infants < 37wks), consider tocolytic therapy (Nifedipine/terbutaline (s/e 's tachycardia, hypokalemia, hyperglycemia)/MgSo4/Indomethacin (high risk of ductus closure). OBS consult!

Room Setup: Airway adjuncts, fetal heart rate monitor after 20-24 wks./vaginal probe/consider arterial line for CO_2 insufflation. Left uterine displacement, calf compressors, temperature. Avoid laparoscopic procedures after end of 2Nd trimester

Intraoperative Management: GA or regional acceptable, avoid N_2O (controversial). Maintain oxygenation, uteroplacental perfusion, avoid hypocarbia (aim 30-35mmHg) and acidosis

Specific Procedures: Laparoscopy – open trochar placement, low insufflations pressures 8-12mmHg; ECT – OB Consult, intubate beyond 1st trimester (aspiration prophylaxis for all), monitor FHR, not a risk factor for SA; Trauma - Early fetal U/S and FHR, All diagnostic modalities required (primacy of mother), C/S (stable mother, a viable fetus in distress, traumatic uterine rupture, unsalvageable mother with viable fetus, If fetus is pre-viable or dead, optimize mother (i.e. do not go for c-section, vaginal delivery can be performed later)

Post-operative: Monitor FHR and uterine contractions, Risk of DVT

Complications: Most serious fetal risk associated with surgery is due to intrauterine asphyxia: Maintainmaternal oxygenation, oxygen tension and carrying capacity, uteroplacental perfusion.
The most common causes of maternal hypotension: deep GA, sympathectomy with high spinal or epidural, aortocaval compression, hemorrhage, and hypovolemia

Obesity: BMI >30, Morbid Obesity: BMI>40 kg/m²

1. Physiologic Changes of Obesity:
    a) Airway – potential **difficult BMV / Intubation / Cricothyroidotomy**
    b) Respiratory – **Restrictive lung defect** (decrease. FRC/ERV/VC), assoc. **OSA**, risk of post-operative hypoxemia / ventilation. Potential **pHTN** related to OSA.
    c) CVS – Increased demand with limited reserve, increaser. blood volume, CO, LVH, wall stress
    d) GI – Increased risk of **aspiration**
    e) Heme – **Hypercoagulability** (2x risk of DVT)
2. Co-morbid disease: OSA, Obesity hypoventilation, HTN, IHD, CAD, CHF, Type 2 DM,
3. Altered Pharmacokinetics and Pharmacodynamics:
    a) Increased LBW, altered drug dosing, increased pseudocholinesterase
    b) **Sensitivity to opioids**
    c) **Reduced LA requirements** 20-30% for NA techniques
4. Potential technical difficulties: (positioning, monitoring, IV access)

Anesthetic Goals/Conflicts:

- Evaluate and optimize the physiologic impact of obesity: OSA, pHTN, DM, CAD
- Safely secure airway, avoiding aspiration and long-acting agents: minimize post-operative respiratory complications
- Avoid thrombotic complications and peripheral nerve injury
- Consider regional technique, post-operative pain management vs respiratory depression

Hx: Hx of difficult airway, OSA, CPAP, HTN, DM, hypothyroid, CAD, CHF, functional capacity, pHTN,Stroke, Renal failure, GERD, Meds.

PE: Detailed airway exam for ease of laryngoscopy and BMV, CVS: BP, Cardiomegaly: displaced PMI, CHF S3/S4, basilar crackles. pHTN: JVD, R parasternal heave, loud P2, Murmur of TR, hepatomegaly, edema). Respiratory: Focus on restrictive dysfunction (rapid RR, shallow respiration, ruddy color, OSA (ruddy color, thick neck). Gastro – hepatic dysfunction (hepatomegaly, ascites, spider angiomas, jaundice).

Investigations: CBC: Polycythemia, Lytes, Cr, BUN, glucose – if HTN, DM or on diuretics LFTs, PT, PTT if hepatic dysfunction. ABG if hypoxemia. ECG: Typically shows low voltage, LVH, strain: LA abnormalities. If pHTN: RVH, RBBB, P Pulmonale. Echo / Consider PFTs if severe (not costeffective in asymptomatic obese patients nor utility in optimizing the postoperative management.
Polysomnography: 10 sec or more cessation of flow **(apnea) (5/hr)** or 50% reduction in flow or decrease in sat >4% **15/hr (hypopnea)** is diagnostic of OSA. Apnea/Hypopnea index **>30 = severe**

Optimization: Aspiration prophylaxis, avoid pre-operative sedation, anti- sialagogue for AFI, DVT prophylaxis (SC heparin / compression stockings), Optimize co-existing diseases. CPAP.

Room Setup: Difficult airway equipment, glucometer, remainder depends on co-morbid disease. OR tables designed for 120-140kg patients. Position and pad carefully.

Intraoperative Management: Local/Regional/GA. Avoid long-acting agents. Do not use LMA 's in morbid obesity. Difficult spinal/epidural, use 20-30% less dose due to increased spread. Doses based on lean body weight esp. NMDs. Use PPV / PEEP, extubate awake.

Post-operative: Respiratory insufficiency, consider OSA protocol, overnight oximetry, semi – recumbent positioning, CPAP / BiPAP.

Obstetrical Hemorrhage

1. Emergency Situation with high maternal and fetal morbidity & Mortality
   - o requiring immediate resuscitation
2. Etiology & Risk factors
   - o APH: Abruption, placenta previa, uterine rupture, vasa previa, other
   - o PPH: Tone, tissue, thrombin, trauma, turnout Antepartum
3. Hemorrhagic Shock
4. Potential for DIC & massive transfusion
5. Pregnant Patient

Anesthetic goals:

- Intrauterine Resuscitation
  - o Optimize uteroplacental perfusion
- Maintain adequate circulating blood volume and coagulation factors
- Facilitate safe and timely delivery
- Clear lines of communications regarding ongoing HD & coagulation status
- Mobilize resources early

Conflicts:

- Need for oxytocin in a increasingly hypovolemic patient
- Risk of preterm delivery vs risk of delaying delivery in compromised mother
- Regional in hypovolemic patient (i.e., hypovolemic, unstable patient with difficult airway)
- Bleeding patient with contraindications to many uterotonics (e.g., Pulmonary HTN, severe asthma…)

Differentials: **APH** - placenta previa (Multipara, Uterine scar, Risk of placenta accrete); Abruption (HTN, cocaine use, trauma, PROM); Uterine rupture (Uterine scarring, Tumultuous or prolonged labor, Trauma, iatrogenic); Vasa Previa (Severe fetal distress)

PPH – Uterine atony (Uterine overdistension, Augmented labour, retained placenta, Operative delivery); Retained product; Genital trauma; Placenta accrete; Uterine inversion; Coagulopathy

History: **S**AMPLE, Obstetrician Hx, fetal distress, ongoing blood loss, maternal compromise, coagulopathy
P/E: Vitals, airway, classification of stage of shock

Investigations: CBC, G&S, DIC screen, repeat…US

Optimization: Intrauterine resuscitation, large bore IV access, Volume resuscitation, Aspiration prophylaxis

Anesthetic options: Directed by - Fetal distress, Airway, Coagulopathy, Hypovolemia
GA/RSI unless airway difficult. Regional contraindicated related to volume status / coagulopathy / prolonged procedure. FOB if difficult airway. Consider TIVA

Setup: CAS monitors, temperature, Artline, +/- CVP, rapid transfuser, Emergency drugs

Specific management of OB hemorrhage:
Volume, blood components, uterotonics (oxy, hemabate 250 mcg IM/IU, misoprostol 600-800 pr/po/pb, ergot 0.25 mg by slow IV infusion, vasopressin 20 U in 100 cc injected diffusely into uterus), surgical measures (B-Lynch, vascular clamping/ligation, emergency hysterectomy, packing, massage), interventional radiology, Factor VII

Postop disposition: Following massive transfusion a critical care bed is appropriate or at least a monitored bed with invasive monitoring

Obstructive Sleep Apnea

1. Potential difficult intubation/BMV
2. Increased incidence of peri-operative pulmonary complications
   a. Increased susceptibility to obstruction with sedatives/respiratory depressants
      - Need for post-operative monitoring
3. Cardiopulmonary alterations:
   a. Hypoxia, hypercarbia, polycythemia, systemic/pHTN, RV dysfunction
4. Co-morbid diseases including:
   a. Obesity (60-90%), diabetes, CAD, HTN and congenital syndromes in children

Anesthetic Goals/Conflicts:

- Identify patients at risk
- Anticipate potential for failed intubation/ventilation
- Avoid long-acting opioids, sedatives or other respiratory depressants
  - o NSAIDs, acetaminophen, regional/local techniques to minimize pain (i.e., opioid sparing techniques)
- Monitoring to decrease morbidity associated with apnea post-operatively

Hx: snoring, daytime somnolence, apneic periods during sleep, morning HISTORY /A, functional reserve, BiPAP, Home O2, congenital syndrome, history of difficult intubation/ventilation. Hx of Etoh, hypothyroid, sleep meds.

Risk Factors: Male, middle aged, BMI > 30, Alcohol (evening), drug induced sleep, down 's syndrome, acromegaly

PE: Room air sat, BMI > 30, neck circumference >17‖ M (16‖ F), airway for ease of intubation/BMV, signs of CHF (JVP, S3/S4), signs of RVF (JVD, right sided S3/S4, systolic murmur of TR, hepatomegaly, signs of PHN [loud P2])

Investigations: CBC (polycythemia), ABG (baseline PaCO2, PaO2), +/- Echo (cor pulmonale), TSH, GHif acromegaly. Overnight oximetry (at home). Gold standard is polysomnography (5 or more apneic events per hour or 15 or more hypopnea events per hour during a 7-hr sleep study. Apnea Hypopnea index: Mild AHI 6-20, Moderate 20-40, Severe = >40.

Optimization: Weight loss, CPAP pre-operative, smoking cessation, CAD/HTN optimization

Room Setup: Difficult airway cart, art line for repeat ABGs, CPAP in PAR

Intraoperative Management: Local>Regional>Neuraxial (opioids-free), GA – ETT > LMA Avoid long-acting respiratory. depressants, adjuvant analgesia (local, NSAIDS)

Post-operative: CPAP, step-down unit, continuous sat monitoring until saturation >90% sleeping. At VGH it 's a minimum of 3H in PAR. Consider 24H of monitoring if patient demonstrates apneic episodes <90% or severe pre-existing OSA (AHI > 30) or requiring complicated pain management. Patient d/c'd toward should continue intensive monitoring (RR/SS Q1H x 48h, then Q4h).

Open Eye

1. Surgical Emergency
   - Further expulsion of eye contents risks blindness
2. Full stomach/risk of aspiration
3. Trauma & other associated injuries
4. Considerations for Eye Surgery
   - Shared airway
   - Immobile patient
   - Oculo-cardiac reflex
   - Smooth emergence with minimal coughing

Anesthetic Goals/Conflicts:

1. Minimize risk of aspiration (prophylaxis, RSI)
2. Minimize increase in IOP
   - Avoid coughing, straining and hypertensive response to laryngoscopy
   - Avoid hypercarbia
   - Use deep anesthesia, barbiturates
   - Consider avoiding succinylcholine

Hx: Mechanism of injury, associated trauma, last meal (full stomach), PMHx (may be elderly)

PE: Airway examination

Investigations: As directed by Hx & PE

Optimization: For pediatric patient for which an inhalational induction is necessary, may consider delaying until fasted but generally cannot delay; aspiration prophylaxis

Anesthetic Options: GETA only option

Room Setup: CAS monitors, atropine available (OC reflex)

Intraoperative Management: Deep anesthesia and muscle relaxation needed to prevent coughing or movement.

Post-operative: Extubate awake with minimal coughing or straining (balance risk of aspiration with smooth emergence)

Pacemakers

1. Indication for implantation
    a. PM – SSS, AV block
    b. AICD – VT, V-fib, cardiomyopathy EF < 35%
2. Minimize risk of and prepare for potential for pacemaker / AICD interference & failure
    a. Magnet
    b. Pacer clinic interrogation perioperative
        i. **Disable anti-tachycardia functions**
    c. Alternate pacing strategies
        i. Sympathomimetics
        ii. Transvenous pacemaker or pacing PAC
        iii. External defib device
3. Co-existing disease
    a. Associated CAD / Cardiomyopathy EF<35%
    b. HTN / CRF / DM
    c. Medications

Anesthetic Goals/Issues:

1. Identify & optimize underlying cardiac status
2. Anticipate and prevent failure or interference
    a. Avoid inappropriate inhibition or triggering of pacemaker by electrocautery
    b. Avoid inadvertent activation of AICD leading to life-threatening rhythm
3. Prevent damage to device

Hx: Indication for pacemaker, pacemaker dependency, last interrogation, type of pace maker, responseto magnet, symptoms of pacemaker malfunctioning (CHF/Syncope etc.), ICD frequency. Coexisting illnesses, cardiac disease. Type of OR, cautery being used, location of surgery.

PE: Pulse, Location of generator, Rhythm, CHF >> **Investigations:** Lytes/EKG/CXR for type of pacemaker, lead location.

Optimization: Underlying disease, pre-operative interrogation if elective, **disable ICD/tachyarrhythmiasensing**, reprogram to demand mode, call manufacturer.

Room Setup:5 lead ECG (disable ‗artifact filter ', consider Artline for hemodynamic capture, Magnet (avoid in ICD unless necessary >> can disable permanently), Pacing pads (AP positioning, away from generator), Defibrillator, chronotropic meds (Atropine, Isoproterenol (2-10mcq/min), Epinephrine, Dopamine), consider telemetric programmer present if interference expected/hemodynamic instability.

Intraoperative: Bipolar, short bursts, avoid generator between cautery and ground. (With magnet 60%go to 60-100bpm asynchronized, 25% go to asynchronized at program rate, 15% brief 60-100 beats pacing event, some may produce no change)

Post-operative: Reprogramming and interrogation by pacemaker clinic prior to discharge to ward

Special: Pacemaker Mediated Tachycardia (PMT): Dual Chamber pacemaker History / magnet defaults to demand mode >> retrograde p waves which are then ‐trackedǁ after magnet removal. Tx: Reapply and remove magnet.

- 1 – Chamber Paced 2- Sensed 3- Response (T/I/D/0) 4- Rate Modulation 5 –Arrhythmia Treatment (Paced / Shocked / Dual)
- AICD: I = Shock Chamber, II = Anti-tachycardia pacing chamber A/V/D, III = Tachycardia detection Electrogram vs Hemodynamic, IV = Anti-bradycardia pacingchamber A/V/D

Pain

1. Emergency situation requiring immediate management and Dx
2. Classification of the pain
   - nociceptive
   - neuropathic
   - malignant or non-malignant
3. Develop DDx whiling ruling out a medical or surgical emergency
   - Compartment syndrome, nerve compression & ischemia
   - Metastases, infection, inflammation, fracture, visceral (GI, vascular, renal)
4. Develop a comprehensive management plan
   - biopsychosocial assessment (depression, suicide)
   - multidisciplinary resources
5. Specific Management Strategies - **Multimodal approach**
   - Biological - Disease-specific treatment, Physical (Exercise, stretching, heat, massage), Pharmacologic (symptom-related): PO, IV, SC, epidural, intrathecal,regional blocks, Neurostimulation (TENS, SCS), Neurorestorative (Chemical, thermal, surgical)
   - Psychological/Social

Red Flags - thoracic pain, fever, weight loss, bladder/bowel dysfunction, history Ca, gait problems, saddle anesthesia, age <20 or >55

Yellow Flags - negative attitude that back pain is harmful or severely disabling, fear-avoidance behavior, expectation that passive rather than active treatments is beneficial, depression, low morale, social withdrawal, social or financial problems, litigation

Differential Diagnosis for Lower Back Pain:

Mechanical:

- Discs: annular tears, internal disc disruption or herniation
- Sciatica (either referred mechanical or nerve root compression)
- ligaments, periosteum
- spondylosis, spondylolisthesis
- pinalstenosisnon- mechanical:

Spinal

- Neoplasia: metastatic (breast, prostate, lymphoma; primary spinal cord; retroperitoneal tumours
- Infection: osteomyelitis; septic discitis; paraspinal or epidural abscess; HZ
- Inflammatory arthritis: AS, IBD; Reiter's syndrome; Psoriatic Spondylitis
- Trauma(fracture)Visceral
- Pelvic organs: prostates; endometriosis; PID
- Renal: nephrolithiasis; pyelonephritis; perinephric abscess
- Vascular: AAA
- GI: pancreatitis; cholecystitis; perforated bowel

WHO Relief Ladder/Algorithm for Cancer Pain

1. 3-step -ladder‖ for cancer pain relief
   a. correct drug, correct dose, at the correct time → 80-90% effective
2. If pain occurs→ prompt oral administration of drugs in following order:
   a. Nonopioids (NSAIDs and Acetaminophen) +/- adjuvants
   b. Mild opioids (i.e., Codeine, oxycodone) +/- adjuvants
   c. Strong opioids (i.e., Morphine, hydromorphone) +/- adjuvants

Adjuvants also used to calm fears and anxiety.
To maintain freedom from pain: give regularly (q3-6h) and not -prn‖

Surgical intervention on appropriate nerves may provide further pain relief if drugs are not wholly effective

Anesthetic Goals/Conflicts:

1. Common chronic neuropathic, non-malignant pain - distinct from stump pain
2. Difficult to treat, warranting multidisciplinary involvement including physio, heat, and psychiatry
3. Multi-modal analgesia
   a. aggressive pre-operative pain management
   b. avoidance of aggravating factors, including cold, stress, stump irritation
   c. liberal use of regional anesthesia, anti-neuropathic agents, simple analgesics, opioids

Parkinson's Disease

Central dopamine deficiency leading to rigidity, tremors and late dementia.

1. Potential **difficult airway** due to cervical TMJ rigidity
2. Increased risk of **aspiration** secondary to bulbar dysfunction, gastroparesis, esophageal dysfunction.
3. **Autonomic instability**, NE depletion (med), increased risk of hypotension on induction + regional
4. restrictive lung disease secondary to chest wall rigidity
5. Increased risk of perioperative **airway obstruction, Respiratory. failure, exacerbation of Neurologic symptoms** (maxeran droperidol, nozinan)**, and delirium**
6. Interactions with **medical therapy**: continue current therapy, MAOi 's (type B) and Demerol (seizures rigidity and hypertension), Levodopa (can deplete NE stores).
7. Elderly patient

Anesthetic Goals/Conflicts:

- Safely manage patient 's airway: RSI vs. hemodynamic lability, difficult airway.
- Continue anti-Parkinsonism medications perioperatively, avoid anti-dopaminergic meds
- Maximize respiratory function

Hx: Onset and severity of disease, medications, previous anesthetic history.

PE: Particular attention to airway, orthostatic symptoms, neuro exam (pill-rolling tremor, rigidity etc), volume status.

Investigations: Nothing specific

Optimization: Continue anti-parkinsonism medications (L-dopa only oral, absorbed proximal SB) >> NG for long surgery, immediately post-operative. Aspiration prophylaxis.

Anesthetic Options:

Room Setup: Appropriate airway equipment, direct acting agents for hypotension, consider arterial line

Intraoperative Management: Volatiles or TIVA, be aware of narcotic induced rigidity

Post-operative: Increased risk for hypoventilation, respiratory compromise, and post-operative delirium >> use atypical antipsychotics, if necessary (Olanzapine/Quetiapine/Risperidone), worsening Parkinson 's >> restart meds ASAP.

1. Physiologic changes:
    a. Altered airway anatomy
    b. higher risk of laryngospasm
    c. rapid desaturation on induction or apnea
    d. Dec. Cardiovascular Reserve
        - increased vagal tone
    e. altered pharmacokinetics
        - higher MAC, higher TBW
2. Limited or no cooperation
3. Need to communicate with and manage parents

Respiratory Rates	
Age	***Rate***
Neonate	40-60
1yr old	24
18yr old	12

Normal Heart Rates			
Age	***Awake***	***Mean***	***Sleeping***
0 to 3mo	85-205	140	80-160
3mo to 2yr	100-190	130	75-160
2yr to 10yr	60-140	80	60-90
> 10yr	60-100	75	50-90

Normal BP		
Age	***Systolic***	***Diastolic***
Birth (12h, < 1000g)	39-59	16-36
Birth (12h, 3kg)	50-70	25-45
Neonate (96h)	60-90	20-60
Infant (6mo)	87-105	53-66
Toddler (2yr)	95-105	53-66
School Age (7yr)	97-112	57-71
Adolescent (15yr)	112-128	66-80

Pediatric Stridor

1. Emergency
    - Increase. risk of aspiration, Limited time for optimization and investigation
2. Airway compromise
    - Potential for catastrophic loss of the airway, hypoxemia, respiratory acidosis, cardiac arrest, negative pressure pulmonary edema
    a. Mobilization of resources and collaboration with other specialties: ENT, ICU, ER
3. Pediatric patient

DDx

- **Congenital** (generally chronic symptoms) – Nose (Choanal atresia, Septum deformities, Turbinate hypertrophy), Pharynx (Craniofacial anomalies – Crouzon 's, Pierre-Robin, Alpert 's syndromes; Tongue – macroglossia and glossoptosis), Larynx (Laryngomalacia, webs, cysts, hemangioma, stenosis), Trachea (stenosis, vascular rings & slings, tracheomalacia)
- **Infections** – epiglottitis, tracheitis, peritonsillar and retropharyngeal abscess, croup (parainfluenza), RSV, Influenza A and B, Mycoplasma
- **Tumors** – Omphalocele, Teratoma, Lymphoma, Granuloma, Fibroma, Papilloma, Neuroblastoma, Hemangioma, Rhabdomyosarcoma, Cystic hygroma
- **Trauma** – RLN palsy (post PDA repair, thyroid surgery), Post extubation (Croup/ edema, Vocal cord injury or paralysis, Subglottic stenosis), Caustic injury, Inhalational injury, Facial trauma or burn
- **Allergic** – Anaphylaxis, hereditary angioneurotic edema
- **Miscellaneous** – Hypocalcaemia, Foreign bodies (airway or esophageal), Spasmodiccroup, Exercise, GERD, Juvenile RA with cricoarytenoid involvement

HISTORY AND PHYSICAL MAY BE ABBREVIATED DUE TO URGENCY

Hx: SAMPLE; onset of symptoms (acute, subacute vs chronic); circumstances (related to feeding);associated symptoms (constitutional, drooling, dysphagia, vocal changes/muffling, hoarseness); previousepisodes (chronic or recurrent episodes – congenital, tumor or vocal cord dysfunction); OSA (suggests pharyngeal cause: tonsils or adenoids); PMHx – intubation, PDA/necl Sx, immunization Hx

Px: VS; general (Toxemia, Fever, Hypotension, tachycardia) weight; airway exam (size of tongue and mandible, craniofacial anatomy, neck edema); Respiratory (WOB/ accessory muscle use, nasal flaring, retraction, Cyanosis, Clubbing: underlying CHD or bronchiectasis, stridor may be heard in inspiration, expiration or during the entire respiratory cycle); Hemangiomas, café au lait spots; Anaphylaxis: rash, hypotension

Inv: CBC: leukocytosis, Blood Cross match; **Imaging:** unstable: skip radiology and evaluate their airway in the OR with ENT; accompany to radiology suite with airway equipment; Neck radiographs – generally nonspecific; CXR – Mediastinal masses, Vascular rings, R aortic arch, FB; Airway fluoroscopy; CT scan; nasopharyngoscopy **Options:** Compromised airways should be evaluated and secured with direct visualization in the OR with ENT present under spontaneous ventilation; **FB:** SV with rigid bronchoscope

Anesthetic Setup: difficult airway cart, ENT surgeon, skilled help, Rigid bronchoscope, cricothyroidotomy (age >6)

Monitors: CAS, consider transcutaneous CO2 monitoring for rigid bronchoscope

Drugs: Succinylcholine, Atropine, vasoactive agents if suspicion of severe sepsis, TIVA vs Inhalational

Management:

Moribund: awake DL;

Stable child: SV GA, IH – 4% ET sevoflurane, TIVA – Propofol infusion at 200 u/k/m, Remi 0.1 u/k/m; DL when unresponsive (may take ~10min); ETT placed (use 0.5-1.0 size smaller); Topicalize airway prior to rigid bronchoscopy (lido 3mg/kg)

Emergence: PICU, FB removal: consider intubating and extubating awake (aspiration & laryngospasm risk)

Post extubation Stridor: Typically, 1-4yrs, max in 4hr, resolution in 24h; DDx; humidified oxygen; Neb epi 0.5 ml/kg –watch for rebound; Dex: 4-8mg IV; Emotional support; Heliox; Admission

Pharyngeal Abscess

1. Urgent/Emergent Procedure with Risk of Aspiration and acute airway obstruction
2. Difficult airway management
   a. Distorted Anatomy, trismus, difficult topicalization
   b. Risk of abscess rupture and lung soilage
   c. Shared airway
3. Life Threatening Complications
   a. AW obstruction, abscess rupture & aspiration, sepsis/toxic shock syndrome, mediastinitis
4. Risk Factors / Co-morbidities
   a. Pediatric, DM, IVDU. HIV, ETOH, ENT malignancy

Anesthetic Goals/Conflicts:

1. Efficiently + Safely secure airway recognizing *evolving obstruction*
   - Consider pre-operative abscess needle drainage
   - Prevent abscess rupture and lung soilage
2. Fluid resuscitation and appropriate Abx
3. Potential conflicts:
   - uncooperative patient (peds) vs. difficult airway
   - full stomach vs. potential inhalational induction
   - deep plane of anesthesia vs. potential hypotension from sepsis/ dehydration
   - awake FOB does not visualize ETT passing abscess (potential for rupture by ETT)

Hx: Abscess time course, associated symptoms (drooling, dysphagia, stridor, dysphonia, hoarseness); presence of sepsis; establish risk of comorbidities - DM, IVDU, HIV, underlying head & neck malignancy, alcoholism

PE: Vitals (respiratory distress, sepsis); detailed airway examination (mouth opening/trismus - pterygoid muscle spasm, edema, submandibular edema, tracheal deviation, Torticollis / dec neck ROM, Horner 's syndrome & cranial nerve palsies); respiratory exam for infection/empyema; CVS exam for hypovolemia/sepsis

Investigations: Limited impact on management; CBC, Blood Cross match, CXR, neck Xray, **CT head & neck**

Optimization: Aspiration prophylaxis, Anti-sialagogue, fluid resuscitation, antibiotics, needle aspiration and decompression by surgeon

Anesthetic Options: SV induction (peds); awake FOI (may be difficult to topicalize); tracheostomy underlocal (maybe difficult anatomy); blind techniques not recommended. Use slow, gentle technique to minimize risk of abscess rupture.

Room Setup: Difficult airway cart, skilled assistants, ENT surgeon present

Intraoperative Management: Discuss plan with surgeon (shared airway); dexamethasone to decrease edema

Post-operative: Consider postop ventilation/ICU or extubation over tube exchanger depending on severity

Complications: Airway obstruction, aspiration of abscess contents, laryngospasm, sepsis, post-obstructive pulmonary edema, abscess spread (meninges, lung, epidural space, etc.), vascular injury/ hemorrhage

Pheochromocytoma

1. Prevention and Management of hemodynamic instability:
   - Pre-operative optimization, Avoidance of SNS stimulation, histamine release, & unopposed alpha
   - Intra-operative monitoring and management of HTN, tachycardia, arrhythmias
2. Relative intravascular volume depletion
3. End-organ dysfunction
   - Hypertrophic or dilated cardiomyopathy, IHD, CVA, Hyperglycemia
4. Associated endocrinopathies:
   - Hyper parathyroid (MEN2a)
   - Medullary thyroid CA (MEN 2a & 2b)
   - Neurofibromatosis (Von Recklinghausen's)
   - von Hippel-Lindau disease (cerebellar hemangioblastoma, RCC)
5. Post-operative complications:
   - HTN or hypotension, Hypoglycemia, Adrenal insufficiency

Anesthetic Goals/Conflicts:

- Prevent, recognize and be prepared to treat pheochromocytoma crisis:
  - Adequate pre-operative optimization - Alpha blockade; Volume resuscitation; Anxiolysis
  - Tight hemodynamic control
    - Avoid SNS surges (anxiolysis, deep induction, Epidural)
    - Avoid histamine releasing drugs (catecholamine release from tumor)

Hx: Triad of diaphoresis, tachycardia in HTN patient; flushing; orthostatic hypotension; end-organ dysfunction (CHF; IHD), endocrinopathies; 5Ps – Pressure (HTN); Perspiration; Pallor; Pain Palpitations (associated with tremor, weight loss, fever)

PE: Vitals (including postural), CHF Signs; volume status; caution with abdominal exam

Investigations: CBC (polycythemia), Lytes, BUN, Cr, Glucose (hyperglycemia), Ca^{++} (Men 2), CXR, ECG (LVH, ischemia, prolonged QTc, abnormal R waves, ECHO (hypertrophic or dilated cardiomyopathy), MIBI (CAD), PET/CT to localized non-adrenal masses

Optimization: Endo consult; 10-14 days required; correct hypovolemia; Phenoxybenzamine 10-20 mg po bid or Prazosin 1 mg tid or qid until Hct drops by 5%, no BP>165/90 in hospital x 48hrs (1hr continuous in PACU), orthostatic hypotension (not below 80/45), ECG normalization, <1 PVC q5min (Roizen criteria). B-Block for tumours that secrete epi, or reflex tachycardia (after effective alpha blockade); Steroid replacement for bilateral adrenalectomies, CCB & Mg for refractory HTN; Preg - <24 weeks remove, >24 treat – epidural, C/S

Anesthetic Options: GETA +/- Epidural; no data that RA is better than GA

Room Setup: CAS + 5 Lead; Aline; Foley; CVP; (PAC, TEE); Temperature; Glucometer; ER Drugs (use rapid acting titratable meds, particularly during high-risk times like intubation (remi, lido), tumour manipulation (phentolamine, NTP) and ligation of venous drainage (fluid, phenylephrine)

Intraoperative Management: communicate with surgeon throughout; Deep plane of anesthesia prior to stimulation (lido, remi); avoid (ketamine, ephedrine, pancuronium, histamine releasing agents, desflurane);
Pre-removal: HTN, Tachycardia, arrhythmia (Phentolamine 1-5mg IV, SNP 1-2ug/kg IV bolus, NTG, labetalol, lido, Mg);
Post-removal HTN (fluids, phenyl, dopamine, decrease anesthetic)

Postoperative: HDU; Monitor HDs and glucose may still be HTN post-operative (cleared over 7-10days)

Complications: Hypertension; Hypotension; Hypoglycemia; Adrenal insufficiency (if bilateral)

Pneumonectomy

1. **Postresection pulmonary function** (suitability for procedure)
   - o Mechanics (ppo FEV1>40%) / Lung Function (ppo DLCO>40%) /Cardiopulmonary interaction (ppo VO_2 max>15ml/kg/min)
2. Perioperative **respiratory and cardiac complications**
   - o Hypoxemia, hypercapnia, atelectasis, pneumonia, ALI, respiratory failure
   - o pHTN with RV failure, Ischemia, Arrythmias (A-fib)
3. Co-morbid disease
   - o Malignancy 4 Ms (Mass, Metastases, Metabolic derangement, Medications), Smoker, COPD, CAD, PVD
4. Considerations of OLV
   - o DLETT placement / Physiologic changes - hypoxia
5. Postoperative pain and monitoring for complications
   - o Respiratory failure, Arrhythmia, BPF, Herniation

Anesthetic Goals/Conflicts:

- Optimize respiratory function pre-operatively
- Optimize oxygenation during OLV and plan for immediate extubation
- Optimize respiratory mechanics post-operatively
  - o pain management, fluid management
- Minimize modifiable complication risks
- hypothermia, arrhythmias, ischemia

Hx: assess RF for difficult EBT; RESPIRATORY: dyspnea, exercise tolerance, cough, wheeze, positional aw aggravation; pneumonia; CVS: functional status, RV dysfunction; Hx of underlying respiratory disease; Malignancy → 4 M 's

PE: VS; Distress; AW; RESPIRATORY (COPD, tracheal compression); CVS (CAD, arrhythmias, pHTN, SVC syndrome)

Investigations: CBC, coags, lytes, ABG, X-match; CXR, ECG, CT, +/- ECHO; PFTs, V/Q scan
Slinger's 3-legged Stool: Respiratory Mechanics (ppo FEV1 < 40%) Gas exchange (ppo DLCO < 40%) Cardiopulmonary interaction (ppo VO_2max <15ml/kg/min) Other factors: RV/TLC ratio > 50%; < 2 flights stairs; 6 min walk < 2000ft; Exercise SpO2 <4%; ppoVo2 max < 10 ml/kg/min may be an absolute contraindication to pulmonary resection

Optimization: Smoking cessation; COPD optimization; CAD optimization; +/- antiarrhythmicprophylaxis

Anesthetic Options: GA +/- TEA; lung isolation → R or L DLT; Bronchial blocker; Mainstem Bronchusintubation with single lumen tube or 2 single lumen tubes

Room Setup: Drugs (inotropes, vasopressors & antiarrhythmics); CAS monitors, 5 lead ECG, pre-A-line; CVP; +/- TEE & PAC; Difficult AW cart; FOB; different size DLT & bronchial blocker; DLT size based on tracheal width (mm)
→ 18 = 41; 16 = 39; 15 = 37, 14 = 35

Intraoperative Management: Volatiles inhibit HPV (halothane worst), consider TIVA; epidural LA / narcotics; maintain 2 lung ventilation as long as possible; avoid N2O; FiO2 0.5-1.0, VT 5-8ml/kg, PEEP dependant Lung, permissive hypercapnia; may need intermittent 2-lung ventilation, intermittent recruitment maneuvers, CPAP or O2 insufflation to nondependent lung; minimize peri-operative IV fluids; Extubate early to ↓ risk of barotrauma / pulmonary infection; for ppo FEV1 >40%, normal extubation criteria; for ppo FEV1 <30% + poor exercise tolerance, staged weaning from mechanical ventilation is best.

Post-operative: HDU/PAR; Pain control; supplemental O2

Complications: Hypoxia with OLV; ↑ airway pressures; herniated heart; ruptured bronchus; RLN injury, RV overload; torsion of lobe on operative side; post-pneumonectomy ALI.

Special→ **Predictors of Hypoxemia during OLV:** Side (R>L); Hypoxemia on 2 lung ventilation; Supine; Normal PFT

Popliteal Nerve Block L4-S3

Note: US techniques use high frequency 10-15MHz probe.

Indications: Ankle and foot surgery

Anatomy: Sciatic nerve at the level of popliteal fossa, superficial and lateral to popl. Art.Common peroneal gives off sup. and deep peroneal nerves and lateral sural nerve. Tibial gives of medialand lateral plantar nerves and medial sural nerve.

Contraindications: Post-operative neurological monitoring, risk of post-operative compartment syndrome, previous popliteal artery bypass (relative)

Risks: Infection, hematoma, nerve injury, LA toxicity

Approach: Inter-tendinous (Classic): Prone, Landmarks: popliteal. Crease, tendons of semitendinosus and semimembranosus medially and biceps femoris laterally. Insert 10cm 22g needle 7cm above the crease, and 1 cm lateral to the midway point bw the tendons. Goal 0.2-0.5mA, 0.7mA if peripheral neuropathy!
Aim: Plantar flexion or inversion indicative of tibial nerve stimulation which is more reliable than CP (dorsiflexion and eversion).

Lateral: Supine, landmarks are popliteal crease, vastus lateralis (superior) and biceps femoris (inferior). With palpating hand on biceps femoris muscle, insert needle (10cm) perpendicular to skin at point marked 7cm above popliteal crease, midway between tendons. Contact Femur, then withdraw to skin and redirect
30 degrees inferiorly.
35-40mL LA, slow onset 10-25mins

Saphenous NB: *for tourniquet, or supplement popliteal block*

Inject 7-10ml LA subcutaneously from the Tibial Tuberosity, medially.

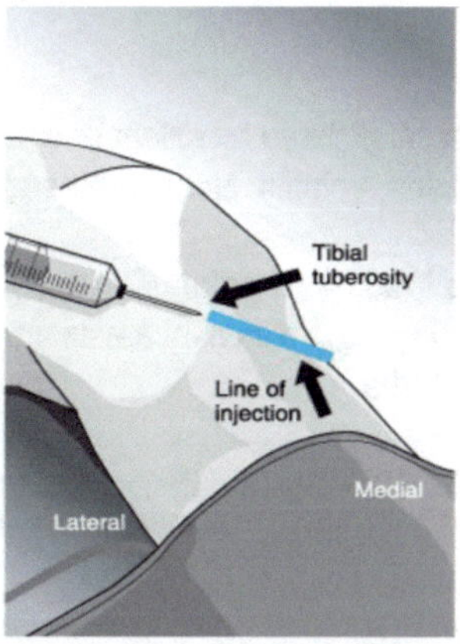

Porphyria

1. Risk of Porphyric Crisis
   a. Avoidance of pharmacologic and physiologic triggers
2. Neurologic dysfunction

Autonomic - **Hypertension, Tachycardia**, Abd pain, Vomiting, diarrhea,
   a. orthostatic hypotension
   b. Cranial - Bulbar dysfunction (**Aspiration Risk**)
   c. Peripheral - **Respiratory weakness**, peripheral neuropathies, quadriplegia
   d. Anxiety, confusion, hysteria, **seizures**, coma
3. CRF with severe **volume depletion** and electrolyte abnormalities Hypokalemia, hyponatremia (SIADH), hypomagnesemia

Anesthetic Goals/Conflicts:

1. Adequate optimization
   a. Avoid prolonged fast (dehydration), correct anemia, manage pain/anxiety
2. Avoid triggers:
   a. Barbiturates, etomidate, steroids, diazepam,
   b. Fasting, progesterone, estrogen, infection, anemia
   c. Smoking, ETOH, marijuana, ecstasy, amphetamines, cocaine
3. Be prepared to treat an acute crisis
   a. Fluids, glucose, hematin, cimetidine, somatostatin, plasmapheresis
   b. Manage Sz with midazolam/propofol – avoid diazepam, STP, phenytoin

Hx: Determine type of porphyria (acute/inducible), family history, known triggers, current symptoms - focus on CNS (Sz, confusion, neuropathy), bulbar dysfunction, tachycardia, palpitations, CHF, respiratoryfailure.

PE: Vitals + postural, volume status, GCS, neuro exam, CVS (HTN / hypotension, tachycardia, CHF)

Investigations: CBC, lytes, BUN, Cr, Glucose, LFTs (if any suspicion of hepatic dysfunction), Mg, Calcium, Coags, ECG (LVH), CXR, +/-PFTs, ABGs

Optimization: Hematology consult, Correct anemia, avoid prolonged fast (IV glucose), aspiration prophylaxis, Correct metabolic abnormalities and volume status, Anxiolysis with midazolam

Room Setup: CAS + 5, art line, aggressive multimodal (regional only if you have a good pre-operative neuro exam)

Anesthetic options: Local, Regional (Pre-operative neuro exam, respiratory function, bupivacaine), or GA (trigger free)

Intraoperative management: Management dictated by extent of cardiorespiratory dysfunction. Generally – Propofol, Succinyl, Rocuronium, Opioids, Volatile, Neostigmine/glycopyrrolate

Acute Porphyria crisis: IV glucose load, fluid bolus (D10NS), Beta-blocker (ifhypertensive/ tachycardic), Hematin (3-4 mg/kg), octreotide, plasmapheresis (may reduce pain), midazolam/ propofol for Sz, Manage electrolyte disturbances

Unsafe Drugs: barbiturates, etomidate, NSAIDs (diclofenac, ketorolac), ACE-I, CCB, Diazepam, Steroids (estrogen, progesterone…), Cephalosporins, Phenytoin, ergotamine

Disputed: Lidocaine, Maxeran, other NSAIDs

Posterior Fossa Surgery

1. Risk of increase. ICP / obstructive hydrocephalus
2. Intra –operative Complications
   - Injury to vital brainstem structures (CNs IV-XII, CVS/Respiratory centers)
   - VAE and paradoxical air embolism
   - Hemodynamic instability during brainstem manipulation (arrhythmias, hypotension)
   - Hemorrhage
   - Hypothermia
3. Neurophysiologic monitoring
4. Intraoperative considerations
   - sitting position
   - Shared airway
   - Prolonged surgical time

Anesthetic Goals/Conflicts:

- Maintain CPP
- Vigilant monitoring of hemodynamics for early signs brainstem injury
- Provide brain relaxation to facilitate surgical exposure
- Prevent and manage complications related to positioning (VAE, hemodynamic instability,tension pneumocephalus, macroglossia, quadriplegia, peripheral nerve injury)

Hx: Establish pre-operative neurologic dysfunction – increase. ICP (a.m. headache, N/V), cranial nerve deficits (airway obstruction, aspiration). Contraindications to sitting position - absolute (Ventricular-atrial shunt; RAP>PCWP; PFO; Cerebral ischemia when upright & awake) & relative (extremes of age; uncontrolled HTN; COPD)

PE: Vitals including GCS, postural BP; Cardiopulmonary for instability & aspiration; Neurological exam for ↑ICP, Cranial Nerve, cerebellar & bulbar dysfunction.
Investigations: CBC, Lytes, BUN, Creatinine, X-match, Osmolality (Mannitol). Imaging – ECHO to screen PFO; CT head for mass effects/↑ICP/herniation/obstructive hydrocephalus.

Optimization: pre-operative dexamethasone for tumor edema, ICP management, volume loading to mitigate positioning hemodynamics, Aspiration prophylaxis

Anesthetic Options: GETA – balanced technique with volatile or TIVA if neurophysiological monitoring (BAER, EMG facial nerve)

Room Setup: CAS with 5 lead (dysrhythmias with brainstem compression), temperature probe, Art line transducer on arm (appreciate that Cerebral circulation is above in sitting position), CVP/Bunegin multi-orifice catheter 2 cm below SVC/RA junction (confirmed with TEE/CXR), Precordial Doppler (3rd-6th Right sternal ICS).
Vasopressors/vasodilators (post-operative HTN), mannitol, atropine +/-TCP for bradycardia (if in brainstem)

Intraoperative Management: Sitting position: SCD 's/ G-suit minimizes venous pooling, two finger breadths between sternum and chin to ↓potential for macroglossia and cervical cord ischemia, avoid excessive hip flexion (sciatic/ peroneal nerve injury), confirm ETT position with neck flexion;

Post-operative: possible **ventilation** d/t airway edema, CN dysfunction, Cardiopulmonary dysfunction, dec. LOC;HDU to monitor for CVS, respiratory, neurologic deterioration – increase. ICP, dysrhythmia, central apnea, aspiration

Complications: VAE, brain stem dysfunction (ECG changes are sensitive), tension pneumocephalus(CSF replaced with air – HISTORY /A, Sz, confusion, dec. LOC – CT, burr hole), quadriplegia (ischemia d/tcervical flexion)

Preeclampsia and HELLP Syndrome

1. Pregnancy
2. Difficult airway
   - Airway edema of pregnancy exaggerated
3. Complications and organ dysfunction
   - ICH, seizures, cerebral edema
   - Compensated hypovolemia, LV dysfunction, HTN crisis, HD instability and shock
   - Noncardiogenic pulmonary edema (dec. oncotic pressure)
   - Renal dysfunction, Thrombocytopenia, coagulopathy, infrequently DIC
   - HELLP syndrome (Hemolysis, Elevated Liver enzymes, Low Platelets)
4. Considerations of antihypertensive / anticonvulsant therapy
5. Risk of fetal distress and need for operative delivery
6. Decreased UPP, IUGR, abruptio placentae, premature labor and delivery

Anesthetic Goals/Conflicts:

- Control maternal HD - prevent HTN crisis & ICH
- Prevent & manage eclampsia – MgSO4
- Optimize intravascular volume & avoid pulmonary edema
- Optimize end organ perfusion and oxygen delivery, including UPP

DDx: Pain, Cushing 's, hypoxia/hypercarbia, cocaine, withdrawal, NMS, serotonin syndrome, essential hypertension, pheochromocytoma, thyrotoxicosis, carcinoid

Hx: Rule out other causes, evaluate for end organ dysfunction (evaluation of CNS, cardiorespiratory, coagulation, GI, renal all important); Risk factors – Chronic HTN, Previous Hx, multiples, Age, Race, Obesity

PE: airway; VS, volume status, heart failure, bruising

Investigations: serial CBCs, G&S, lytes, BUN, Cr, Uric Acid, U/A for protein, LFTs, CXR, 12 lead, ECHO

Optimization: Asp. prophylaxis, close communication with OB & NICU, early IV access/bloodwork, serial CBCs, early labour epidural, Mg SO4 for Seizures prophylaxis (6 g IV bolus over 15 minutes, then 1 – 2 g/hr / monitor for toxicity / respiratory depression, decrease reflexes / Calcium Gluconate 1 amp, potentiates NMB), antihypertensive therapy (Labetalol 5 mg IVP, doubling q5min max 300 mg, Hydralazine 5 – 10 mg IV q10 minutes, NTG 50 – 100 μg IVP, nitroprusside, Nifedipine, Esmolol 1.5 mg/kg to blunt ↑ BP associated with laryngoscopy); platelets (count <50), steroids?

Room Setup: CAS +5 lead +/-art line +/-CVP for CHF, IV x2; difficult airway cart; Consider blood warmer, immediate access to PRBC, FFP, Plts; Draw up additional induction agent +/- remi, esmolol;Peds and OB

Intraoperative Management: Regional if no contraindications (coags, thrombocytopenia, increase. ICP) – volume load with colloid prior to regional (no fluid with GA – aim for 80ml/kg), tight hemodynamic control; GA requires deep induction – Thiopentone 4mg/kg, lido 1.5mg/kg, remi 1-2u/kg (or +/- esmolol 1.5mg/kg), succinyl 1.5mg/kg; treat hypotension. If bleeding secondary to uterine atony, TIVA is reasonable

Post-operative: HDU for 24-48 hrs post-operative (hypertension may peak post-partum)

Complications: DIC, PPH, pulmonary edema, Seizures, ICH, ARF

Classifications: Chronic HTN: before 20wks; Preeclampsia: HTN > 20 weeks SBP>140 or DBP >90 AND proteinuria of >0.3g/24h; Severe preeclampsia: SBP>160 or DBP>110; proteinuria >5g/24h or >3+; CNS dysfunction: blurred vision, altered mental status, severe headache; Liver capsule distension: RUQ or epigastric pain; ↑ transaminases of 2X normal; Thrombocytopenia < 100,000; Oliguria < 500 mls in 24 hours; IUGR; Pulmonary edema or cyanosis; CVA; Eclampsia: above plus seizures

Prematurity

1. Altered airway anatomy
2. Impaired temperature and glucose regulation
3. Other physiologic derangements of prematurity
   - o Respiratory – RDS, BPD, rapid desaturation, post-operative apnea, persistent pHTN
   - o CVS – HR/preload dependant CO, Transitional circulation/PDA, bradycardia, CHD
   - o CNS - IVH, seizures, ROP
   - o GI – GERD, NEC
   - o Heme - Anemia, thrombocytopenia
   - o Altered pharmacology – increase. Vd, opioid sensitivity, dec. clearance, protein binding,metabolism, dec. MAC
4. Difficult IV access and monitoring

Uncuffed ETT size
2.5 for < 1000g or 28 weeks
3.0 for 1000-2000g or 28-34 weeks
3.5 for 2000-3000g or 34-38 weeks
3.5-4.0 for larger / older neonates

<u>Anesthetic Goals/Conflicts:</u>

1. Ensure optimization of multisystem derangements including respiratory, cardiovascular, hepatic, renal, hematological
2. Anticipate fluid / electrolyte / glucose derangements and optimize pre-operatively
3. Ensure continuous temperature monitoring and maintain normothermia

Hx: PCA, Obstetrical hx, PMHx since birth and assess for complications (IVH, retinopathy, PPHTN/PDA, CHD, RDS/BPD, hx apnea, GERD, NEC, hypoglycemia, anemia, thrombocytopenia, etc.), meds

PE: Vitals, weight, ins/outs, IV access, ventilator parameters, CVS (cap refill, fontanel, perfusion, murmurs, CHF), RESPIRATORY (WOB, retractions, wheeze, crackles)

Investigations: CBC, lytes, Cr, coags, bilirubin, glucose, ABG, CXR, AXR, head U/S, ECHO

Optimization: Optimize volume status (especially if CHF), glucose, acidosis, coagulopathy, transfuse (Hb>100 if cardiorespiratory disease), NPO (2hrs clear fluid, 4hrs breast milk), pre- treat with atropine/glycopyrrolate, Vit K (1mg)

Anesthetic Options: GA – muscle relaxant + opioid may be tolerated best.

Room Setup: Warm room/forced air warmer, consider NICU ventilator, epinephrine/resuscitation drugs drawn up to exact doses, pre & post-ductal SpO2, appropriately sized ETT (leak at 20cm H_2O, circuit

Intraoperative Management: Depends on case, avoid SNS stim (risk of IVH), muscle relaxant/narcotic vs. desflurane/remifentanil for rapid emergence; be aware of impaired metabolism/excretion of drugs, FiO2 to maintain SaO2 88-92%

Complications: PTX, hypoglycemia, paradoxical air embolism

Post-operative: Apnea monitoring if PCA < 50-60 weeks (risk factors: prematurity, PCA, HCT <30%, hx apnea, chronic respiratory disease e.g., BPD, neurological disease)

Pulmonary Hypertension

Mean PAP > 25mmHg at rest or 30mmHG during exercise

1. Potential for acute perioperative RV dysfunction and hemodynamic collapse
2. Optimize pulmonary pressures and right heart function
    - o Avoid hypoxia, hypercarbia, acidosis, hypothermia, sympathetic stimulation(pain), high/ low lung volumes
    - o Cautious fluid administration
    - o Maintain RV perfusion
3. Associated Conditions
    - o COPD, obesity, OSA, CHD, valvular disease (MR), CHF, CTD, HIV, recurrent thromboembolic disease
4. Medication
    - o Anticoagulation / CCBs / Vasodilators (e.g., sildenafil) / Prostacyclin analogs (e.g., Epoprostenol/Flolan) / Endothelin antagonists (e.g., Bosantan) / Diuretics
5. Need for invasive monitoring, optimized analgesia & post-operative disposition

<u>*Anesthetic Goals/Conflicts:*</u>

- Ensure patient is OPTIMIZED – Respiratory, Cardio, alternatives to OR (medical management etc.)
- Avoid increase in PVR (minimize pain, sympathetic stimulation, hypoxia, hypercarbia,acidosis, optimize airway pressures - **Conflict with hypoxia/hypercarbia vs. PPV**
- Optimize RV function (careful fluid administration, maintain RV perfusion (afterload)
- Be mindful of ventricular interdependence

Hx: Fatigue, functional capacity, ischemia, RHF, presyncope/syncope, orthopnea/PND, cyanosis, hemoptysis. Underlying etiology, medications, investigations/ECHO.

PE: pHTN: large A wave, Loud P2, RV heave, TR (high pitched pansystolic murmur at 4th intercostalspace in the parasternal region), dec. CO, S3/S4, JVD, hepatomegaly, ascites, dependent edema

Investigations: CBC (polycythemia), elect, coags if on AC 's, ABG, ECG – RVH R/S ratio in V1 and V2 of 1 and S waves >than 3mm in V5 or V6, P pulmonale > 2.5mm II/III/AVF. CXR – globular heart, prom. or engorged pulmonary. vasculature, chronic lung dx. ECHO-TR/PAP, EF, cardiac size, fnx. VQ scan if thromboembolic disease, PFTs, R sided Angio= gold standard, can trial nitric oxide and assessrespiratory.

Optimization: Respiratory consult: Rx respiratory infections, Rx bronchospasm (bronchodilators, mucolytics, steroids), Inotropes for RVF (dobutamine/milrinone) consider neb 5mg. Ensure optimal preload. Rx: pHTN, heparinize patient if indicated, continue pHTN meds. Must cont. PGI2 infusion (shorthalf-life)3-5 mins, can get rebound HTN. Start or cont. chronic therapy for pHTN: Nifedipine 30-240mg PO OD, Diltiazem 120-900mg PO OD, Epoprostenol (PGI2) 2-150ng/kg/min IV or inhaled (60mcg aerosolized?), Sildenafil 50mg PO BID, Bosentan (a dual endothelin receptor antagonist) 125mg bid - S/E: anemia/fluid retention. Home O2, phlebotomy if HCT >50%

Anesthetic Options: Regional preferred (sympathectomy), avoid ketamine (↑PVR), IV anesthetics aresafe

Room Setup: Pulmonary vasodilators: NO, NTG, Nirpride, Hydral, Inhaled NO (SE: inhibit plt agg, - inotrope, methHgb), CCB: Nifedipine/Diltiazem, PGE1, prostacyclin (PGI2), Adenosine, Ach, Inotropes:Dobutamine (0.1-10mcg/kg/min)/Milrinone/Vasopressin if needing increase. SVR History /o PVR increaserease.
CAS/Invasive lines/PAC/TEE (note PAC risks arrythmia/rupture)

Intraoperative Management: Risk of hTN/CVS collapse, avoid ketamine, hyperventilate, ↑ or ↓ TVHistory / PEEP ↑PVR. Any tech. is ok, as long as hemodynamic goals me, consider TIVA.

Post-operative: HDU, consider RVAD for RHF or ECMO if awaiting Tx.

Pyloric Stenosis

1. Medical, not surgical, emergency
2. High risk for aspiration
3. Metabolic derangement
    a. Hypochloremia metabolic Alkalosis
    b. Hyponatremia & hypokalemia
4. Severe dehydration
5. Risk of post-operative apnea
    a. Persistent metabolic alkalosis
    b. Considerations of neonate/infant

Anesthetic Goals/Conflicts:

1. Optimize fluid and acid-base deficits prior to anesthesia
    a. (Na^+>130; K^+>3.0; Cl^->90; HCO3<27; U/O 1 cc/kg/hr; normal HR/BP/RR)
2. Prevent aspiration – OG suction prior to induction
3. Ensure adequate postoperative monitoring
4. Conflict being difficult airway and RSI

Initial Goal is to determine the degree of dehydration: <5% - 50cc/kg 5-10% - 100cc/kg >10% -150cc/kg

Hx: 1st born M; 2^{Nd} – 6th week; projectile nonbilious vomiting (Hx), feeds; Vol. status (tears, diapers, lethargy)

PE: VS; Weight; MM; Ant fontanelle; Sunken eyes; Cap refill; Skin Turgor; Activity (lethargy; olive sign

Investigations: CBC, electrolytes, BUN, Cr, glucose, ABG, bilirubin unconjugated, U/A; Classic abn: hypocalcaemia, hyponatremia; hypokalemia metabolic alkalosis; Hypokalemia (2'hyperaldosteronism); If severe volume depletion, can have metabolic acidosis (metabolic abn less common now because of earlier presentation); US to confirm Dx.

Optimization: May take 12 to 72 Hrs to correct volume and metabolic abn: IV; Use NS in 20 cc/kg boluses to replace deficit and titrate to clinical criteria outlined above and U/O of 1 cc/kg/hr Maintenance of D5NS + KCl 20-40 mEq/L at 1 to 1.5x maintenance requirement of 4 cc/kg/hr Prevention of aspiration: 14F NG suctioned with child in various positions (does not ensure empty stomach); pre-operative acetaminophen 20-30 mg/kg rectally.

Anesthetic Options: Generally, GA vs neuraxial anesthesia (SAB: 0.8 mg/kg of bupivacaine 0.5% vs Caudal: Large doses of 1.6 mL/kg (4 mg/kg) of 0.25% bupivacaine)

Room Setup: Routine + ER meds (atropine, Suxamethonium); CAS + T° probe; Neonatal setup (neonatal circuit, warm room, warming blanket and lights).

Intraoperative Management: RSI (P 4-6; Suxamethonium 2; or Remi 2-4); Continue Maintenance IV; Maintain on Volatile or TIVA; Avoid hyperventilation (worsens respiratory alkalosis); LA to wound.

Post-operative: Monitored bed for apneas for 12-24 hrs (increase. risk with metabolic alkalosis); Analgesia: Caudal; Tylenol; Local anesthetic infiltration by surgeon; Postop narcotics are not required

Complications: Fluid, electrolyte & metabolic imbalance uncorrected; Aspiration; Apnea postoperative

Restrictive Lung Disease

1. Increased risk of **perioperative respiratory failure, pneumonia, PTX**
   - o Cancel elective procedures if there is an acute + reversible processes
   - **o higher risk if VC < 15 ml/kg, FVC<50% or 500cc, or pCO_2>45**

2. Potential **difficult BMV** and **rapid desaturation** - dec. compliance, lower SaO_2, dec. FRC

3. Respiratory physiologic changes
   - **o Hypoxemia** (V/Q mismatch)
   - **o Decreased compliance** - Increase. Pk Pressures - **barotrauma**
   - **o pHTN** and RV dysfunction / cor pulmonale-AVOID INCREASE PVR

4. **Etiology / Co-morbid** disease states
   - o CTD/ autoimmune disease, IPF, ARDS, Obesity, Neuromuscular, kyphoscoliosis

5. Medications
   - **o steroids**, immunosuppressives, **bleomycin**, amiodarone, oxygen
   - o May be very sensitive to CNS depressants (opioids)
     - degree depends on etiology / increase. dead space ventilation

Anesthetic Goals/Conflicts:

- Pre-operative optimization of pulmonary function
- Either minimally invasive (LA or regional) or maximally supportive (slow wean)
- Lung protective ventilation
  - o Low VT, increase. RR, inverse ratio, pressure control, PEEP
- Avoid precipitants of pHTN
- Optimal postoperative pain management
- Encourage postoperative mobilization

Hx: Etiology of RLD; Severity of RLD and treatments; Dyspnea, exercise tolerance, recent infections,hemoptysis, cough, meds (bleomycin), (home O_2); Smoking; CVS: Angina, CHF, orthopnea, PND; Supine symptoms (mediastinal mass)

PE: AW; SVC syndrome (facial swelling)**;** ↑WOB**;** cyanosis (SpO2<80%, PaO2 <50mmHg), clubbingAE: crackles (fine vs coarse) wheezing**;** *pHTN* - Loud, fixed, widely split S2, palpable P2**;** *RVH* - RV heave, S4**;** *RV failure* - JVD, S3, hepatomegaly, ascites, dependent edema; skeletal abnormalities, obesity, abdominal distension causing restrictive lung pattern

Investigations: CBC, lytes, CXR, ABG, EKG (RAE, RVH), PFT (dec VC, TLC, normal FEV1/FVC), consider echo

Optimization: Respiratory consult, treat infection, drain pleural effusion and ascites, diuretics if fluid overloaded, NG to decompress distended abdomen

Room Setup: pHTN drug, spirometry, difficult airway cart b/c risk of difficult BMV

Intraoperative Management: Minimize drugs that depress ventilation; Consider epidural; Avoid N2O(PTX); May need stress dose steroids; PCV – keep PAP < 30 mmHg, inverse ratio, permissive hypercapnia

Post-operative: Risk of Postoperative pulmonary complications /ventilation; Increaseentive spirometry; Early ambulation

Special: FiO_2 to goal O_2 sat = 88-92% if history of bleomycin

Rheumatoid Arthritis

1) Potential for difficult airway (AAI, limited neck ROM, unstable C-spine)
2) Multisystem disease including cardiac, pulmonary, renal, hematologic involvement
   - CVS: pancarditis, AI, pericardial effusions, conduction system defects
   - Respiratory: RLD, interstitial fibrosis, pHTN, pleural effusions, nodules
   - Renal: CRF
   - Chronic anemia
3) Co-existing Diseases
   - SLE, amyloid, IHD, cancer, DM, osteoporosis, PUD, infections
4) Medications
   - Corticosteroids, Immunosuppressives: cyclosporine, cyclophosphamide, MTX, NSAIDs, Chronic pain meds
5) Technical difficulties with access. patient positioning, & fragile skin

Anesthetic Goals/Conflicts:

- Assume unstable c-spine unless radiographic evidence to the contrary
- Difficult AW should be anticipated
- Careful positioning and documentation of pre-existing neurologic symptoms
- Multimodal analgesia

Hx: Duration of illness (RFs for AA subluxation include male gender, severe arthropathy and longstanding disease, neck symptoms, rheum factor positive), airway – cricoarytenoid arthritis, evidence of AAI (occipital HISTORY /A, dysphagia, dysphonia, diplopia, neck/arm pain, dizziness, U/E numbness); functional capacity, dyspnea, cough, chest pain; joints/systems involved; meds/side effects, bruising/bleeding, fatigue; peripheral neuropathies

PE: airway, neck ROM, mobility of airway structures, CVS exam (LV dysfunction, effusions, pHTN, valvular Dz); Respiratory (pulmonary fibrosis, effusions) Neurologic dysfunction; restricted mobility; accessoptions.

Investigations: CBC, Lytes, BUN, Cr, Coags, ECG, CXR (if significant pulmonary involvement), ABG +/-PFTs, C-spine Flex/Ex views (Atlanto-dental interval > 3-4mm is abnormal), MRI of C-spine; ECHO

Optimization: Consider Spine consult, ENT for cricoarytenoid arthritis (awake trach) stress dose steroids, Iron
+/-EPO pre-operative, blood conservation

Anesthetic Options: GA or regional may be used. Awake FOB is recommended but any technique thatminimizes neck flexion may be appropriate; LMA may be difficult. Neuraxial OK (relative sparing of TL spine).

Intraoperative Management: AFOB, smaller ETT; Exaggerated hemodynamic responses; Careful positioning; eye drops (Sicca); Aggressive multimodal analgesia. Extubate awake, warm, comfortable, reversed.

Post-operative: Dictated by degree of cardiorespiratory compromise; Ventilation may be required d/t RLD

Complications: neurologic deficits, post intubation edema or cricoarytenoid dislocation (stridor)

Other manifestations of disease: Peripheral neuropathies, anemia, thrombocytopenia, bruising/bleeding, renal dysfunction secondary to vasculitis/GN/infiltrative disorders, pleural effusions, interstitial fibrosis, pulmonary nodules, pulmonary hypertension, heart failure (may be ischemic or infiltrative), pericarditis, pericardial effusions, coronary arteritis, heart block, aortitis, airway involvement(with involvement of cricoarytenoids), and many other multisystem manifestations

Rigid Bronchoscopy

1. Shared / unprotected airway
    a. need for good communication with surgeon
    b. risk of aspiration
2. Anticipated complications
    a. airway obstruction (supra or infra-glottic), injury, or edema
    b. pneumothorax
3. Considerations of jet ventilation
    a. Barotrauma
    b. Pulmonary tamponade
4. Comorbidities
    a. Underlying condition – acute/chronic pulmonary problems, cancer – 4M 's
    b. cardiac disease, smoker, EtOH, elderly
5. Need for deep plain of anesthesia/muscle relaxation

Anesthetic Goals/Conflicts:

- Good pre-oxygenation
- Excellent muscle relaxation
- Maintain adequate oxygenation and ventilation
- SV with insufflation vs. paralysis and jet ventilation
    a. Depends on ease of airway access, intraluminal vs. extraluminal compression

Hx: Standard history with focus on respiratory, airway concerns, functional capacity; Eaton-lamberassociated with lung ca; Positional dyspnea associated with airway cancers

PE: Standard cardiopulmonary exam. Careful airway exam assessing for upper airway obstruction

Investigations: CBC, ABGs, CXR +/- CT chest, PFTs (don 't necessarily need all these tests but see ifavailable in chart)

Optimization: Pre-operative respiratory function (inhalers/nebs is appropriate), +/- anti-sialagogue

Room Setup: Standard monitors, prepare for TIVA, have ETT and appropriate airway equipment ready,jet ventilation

Intraoperative Management: Good pre-oxygenation, TIVA, SV for FB removal / difficult airway access, muscle relaxation (succinyl vs. NdMB), good communication with surgeon, timed ventilation with procedure. Hyperventilate in preparation for periods of apnea.

Post-operative: Emergence may be stormy with coughing up of secretions or blood. Usually, post-operative pain is minimal so only use short-acting opioids during the case.

Potential complications:
Hypoxemia, Hypercapnia, hemorrhage, Tacheo-bronchial injury, airway obstruction (bronchospasm, bleeding, tissue, FB), aspiration, dental damage, pneumothorax

Cerebral Aneurysm & Subarachnoid Hemorrhage

1) Emergency case
    - o unprotected airway/decreased GCS
    - o unsecured aneurysm with risk of rupture
2) Increased ICP with the need to maintain CPP while minimizing transmural pressure
    - o Maintain high/normal MAP to prevent critical reductions in CBF
    - o Avoid / manage increase. ICP (avoiding transmural pressure)
3) Identify and manage Complications
    - o Surgical: Rebleeding, vasospasm, hydrocephalus, seizures
    - o Medical: LV dysfunction, neurogenic pulmonary edema, SIADH, cerebral salt wasting
4) Facilitate surgical exposure - Brain relaxation after Dura is opened

Anesthetic Goals/Conflicts:

- Optimize O_2 delivery & CPP while avoiding intracranial transmural pressure (HTN, rapid dec. in ICP)
    - o With increase. ICP, conflict between minimizing transmural pressure (deep induction) and maintaining CPP (hemodynamic support)
- Avoid secondary injury - hyperglycemia, hyponatremia, hyperthermia, elevated HOB
- Prevention of rebleeding (early surgical management) & vasospasm (nimodipine, pravastatin)
- Facilitate rapid postoperative neurological assessment

Grade I – Asymptomatic or minimal headache/ slight nuchal rigidity;

Grade II – Mod – severe headache, nuchal rigidity, cranial nerve palsies but not other deficits;

Grade III – Drowsiness, mild confusion or mild focal deficit;

Grade IV – Stupor, mod-severe hemiparesis, possible early decerebrate rigidity, vegetative; disturbances;

Grade V – Deep coma, decerebrate rigidity, moribund appearance

Hx: Focused. Evidence of cardiopulmonary compromise. Timeline of events (rebleed most common inthe first 6-12 Hours). Mechanism (suspicion of aspiration, possible C-spine injury), co-existing aneurysms, co-morbidities that might alter targets for CPP or otherwise complicate management

PE: Vitals including temperature, GCS, airway for ease of intubation, continuous monitoring (arrhythmias), assess extent of increase. ICP, Cardiopulmonary assessment looking for evidence of ventricular dysfunction (S3, S4), pulmonary edema, or suspected aspiration. Focused neuro exam.

Investigations: CBC, Lytes (hyponatremia), BUN, Cr, glucose, G&S, ABG, ECG (ST changes, canon T waves, prolonged QT, U waves), inotropes if suspected ischemic changes, CXR, ECHO if suspicious for LV dysfunction

Optimization: Aspiration prophylaxis, Goal CPP is 60mmHg (ischemia <50, ARDS >70), euvolemic, minimize increase. ICP (caution dropping ICP if unprotected aneurysms) Nimodipine, Pravastatin

Room Setup: CAS + 5 lead, Art (don 't delay if severe increase. ICP) CVP (triple H therapy - volume status, vasoactive agents), Temperature, glucometer, foley, ICP control (mannitol, Lasix), titratable vasoactive agents (? Ups, downs, adenosine). Consider STP for burst suppression if rupture, Lumbar drain may be considered. Possible neurophysiologic monitoring (SSEP/EEG)

Intraoperative Management: Imperative to prevent rupture or rebleed during induction. Minimize transmural pressure during stimulating parts of procedure (lido/prop/remi for intubation) TIVA for maintenance (brain relaxation), consider increase. MAP by 15% during temporary clipping, Crisp emergence – avoid coughing

Complications: Hypertension +/- bradycardia = rebleed/rupture – therapeutic hypotension (dec. bleedingto allow surgical exposure and control of aneurysm) burst suppression (cerebral ischemia due to clips– reduce CMR), increase. MAP once aneurysm controlled, hydrocephalus, herniation, vasospasm

Post-operative: BP control (labetalol, hydralazine, ACE-I), ICU post-operative, triple-H therapy (hypertensive, hypervolemic, hemodilution – may result in pulmonary edema and myocardial ischemia), Dx for delayed awakening = anesthetic, ictal/post-ictal, bleeding, ischemia, metabolic (hypercarbia, hyponatremia, hypoglycemia). CT early.

Sub-Arachnoid Block Contraindications

1. Contraindications (see below)
2. Level of block needed for surgery
3. Complications of technique
4. Physiological consequences of sympathectomy and ability to tolerate given co-morbid conditions
5. Anesthetic of choice and pharmacological actions

Contraindications:

	Miller	Barash	Chestnut	Toronto notes
Absolute	-Patient refusal -Raised ICP -Inability to remain still	Patient refusal	No definitive list – very surprising and frustrating	-Patient refusal - Lack of proper equipment - Lack of IV access - Overlying infection -Hypovolemia -Coagulopathy - Raised ICP - Lack of trained personnel
Relative	-Coagulopathy -Overlying Infection -Severe Hypovolemia	Hypovolemia/Shock -Increased ICP -Coagulopathy -Sepsis -Overlying Infection		Unstable psychiatric disease or emotional instability
Other considerations	- Pre-existing neurological disease			

Sarcoidosis

Systemic granulomatous disorder that involves many tissues but has a predilection for intrathoracic lymph nodes and lungs

1. Multisystem granulomatous disease:
    a. CNS: Ocular sarcoidosis may produce uveitis, unilateral facial palsy.
    b. CVS: Conduction defects, dysrhythmias
    c. Respiratory: Endobronchial sarcoid, laryngeal sarcoidosis/stenosis, pulmonary fibrosis, pHTN and cor-pulmonale.
2. Metabolic derangement: Hypercalcemia
3. Medications
    a. Corticosteroids are administered to suppress the manifestation of sarcoid and totreat hypercalcemia – Stress dose steroids.

Subacute Endocarditis Pophylaxis (SBE)

TABLE 3. Cardiac Conditions Associated With the Highest Risk of Adverse Outcome From Endocarditis for Which Prophylaxis With Dental Procedures Is Recommended

Prosthetic cardiac valve

Previous IE

Congenital heart disease (CHD)*

Unrepaired cyanotic CHD, including palliative shunts and conduits

Completely repaired congenital heart defect with prosthetic material or device, whether placed by surgery or by catheter intervention, during the first 6 months after the procedure†

Repaired CHD with residual defects at the site or adjacent to the site of a prosthetic patch or prosthetic device (which inhibit endothelialization)

Cardiac transplantation recipients who develop cardiac valvulopathy

*Except for the conditions listed above, antibiotic prophylaxis is no longer recommended for any other form of CHD.

†Prophylaxis is recommended because endothelialization of prosthetic material occurs within 6 months after the procedure.

TABLE 5. Regimens for a Dental Procedure

		Regimen: Single Dose 30 to 60 min Before Procedure	
Situation	Agent	Adults	Children
Oral	Amoxicillin	2 g	50 mg/kg
Unable to take oral medication	Ampicillin	2 g IM or IV	50 mg/kg IM or IV
	OR		
	Cefazolin or ceftriaxone	1 g IM or IV	50 mg/kg IM or IV
Allergic to penicillins or ampicillin—oral	Cephalexin*†	2 g	50 mg/kg
	OR		
	Clindamycin	600 mg	20 mg/kg
	OR		
	Azithromycin or clarithromycin	500 mg	15 mg/kg
Allergic to penicillins or ampicillin and unable to take oral medication	Cefazolin or ceftriaxone†	1 g IM or IV	50 mg/kg IM or IV
	OR		
	Clindamycin	600 mg IM or IV	20 mg/kg IM or IV

IM indicates intramuscular; IV, intravenous.

*Or other first- or second-generation oral cephalosporin in equivalent adult or pediatric dosage.

†Cephalosporins should not be used in an individual with a history of anaphylaxis, angioedema, or urticaria with penicillins or ampicillin.

Scleroderma

1. **Difficult airway** (microstomia, ↓ neck mobility, bleeding from nasal & oral telangiectasia) and high risk of **aspiration** (esophageal dysmotility with ↓ LES tone)
2. Multi-organ Dysfunction (d/t fibrosis):
   - CVS: pancarditis, LV failure, pericardial fluid, conduction disease, HTN, ischemia
   - Respiratory: RLD (pulmonary fibrosis), pHTN, cor pulmonale and RVF
   - Renal failure & -renal crisis‖: accelerated HTN, ARF, hemolytic anemia; ensure ACEi
   - Hypothyroidism
3. Peripheral vasoconstriction with hypovolemia
   - Avoid hypothermia
4. Difficult vascular access / positioning / monitoring (dermal thickening, calcification, contractures)
5. Myopathy (sensitivity to NMBs)
6. Medications: immunosuppressives, steroids, vasodilators (ACEi), pulmonary vasodilators

Anesthetic Goals/Conflicts:

- Anticipate difficult airway and prevent aspiration
  - Difficult airway vs aspiration risk
  - RSI in patient with limited reserve
- Avoid increase in PVR
  - Difficult ventilation (RLD) vs. need to avoid increase. PVR
- Prevention of hemodynamic instability with volume resuscitation and titrated anesthetic
- Prevention of vasoconstriction episodes by avoiding hypothermia and other precipitants
- Possible CI to radial art line in patient with significant cardiorespiratory disease

Hx: Functional capacity. Symptoms of reflux, swallowing problems, biventricular failure (edema, coagulopathies, RUQ pain, PND, orthopnea...), arrhythmias (syncope, palpitations...); Dyspnea, no- productive cough neuropathy; Prior anesthetic history with focus on airway (nose bleeds), access. Medications including steroids last 6 months, cyclosporine (renal tox), cyclophosphamide (lung/renal tox)

PE: Vitals, with postural BP, volume status; Airway, access, extent of contractures, Reynaud's, cardiorespiratory exam (looking for evidence again of restrictive lung disease, CHF, pHTN and cor pulmonale - peripheral edema, hepatomegaly, ↑ JVP, +ve HJR, HSM, loud P2, RV heave, pericarditis –rubs, pulsus paradoxus)

Investigations: CBC, Lytes, Bun, Cr, LFTs, Coags (malabsorption), ABG, CXR (failure), ECG (conduction Dz, RVF, pHTN, pericarditis), PFTs, ECHO

Optimization: Consult Rheum, Respiratory (possibly pHTN specialist), Cardio, Nephro. Trial pulmonary vasodilators. Treat reversible pulmonary disease (eg pulmonary edema, infection…). Aspiration prophylaxis

Anesthetic Options: Regional preferred if possible – epi free local, avoid respiratory muscle block, assess coagulation. If GA then RSI vs FOB, avoid nasal d/t bleeding, difficult surgical airway

Room Setup: Dependent on extent of organ dysfunction. CAS monitors + 5 lead. Consideration of pre- induction A line despite risks. CVP, PAC, TEE depending on extent of pHTN, RV dysfunction; Pulmonaryvasodilators and wide selective of resuscitative drugs should be available (including vasopressors and inotropes). If inhaled nitric oxide or Flolan are considered then specialized equipment will be required.
Difficult airway cart. Consider ICU ventilator; Warm room (21'C) & fluid

Intraoperative Management: Need to identify goals (avoid increase. pHTN); Volume resuscitates; caution with NdMB; Aggressive multimodal analgesia (may be sensitive to CNS and respiratory depressants). May require post-operative vent.

Post-operative: Determined by cardiopulmonary involvement - HDU

Complications: Difficult airway, hypoxemia, Hemodynamic collapse on induction (hypovolemia, cardiac dysfunction)

1. Etiology: idiopathic vs. non-idiopathic (neuromuscular Dz, congenital abnormalities)
2. Restrictive Lung Disease:
    a. pHTN with cor pulmonale; postop respiratory failure; prolonged ventilation
3. Cardiovascular abnormalities:
    a. CHD; cardiac conditions associated with NM disease etc.
4. Surgical Consideration:
    a. blood loss; hypothermia; AW edema; Prone/Lat; OLV if Thoracic approach
    b. Spinal cord integrity: wake-up test / SSEP / MEP 's
5. Post-operative pain control – clonidine, gabapentin, ketamine, opioids

Anesthetic Goals/Conflicts:

- Avoid exacerbations of pHTN (hypoxemia, hypercarbia, acidosis, hypothermia, lightanesthesia & pain)
- Balance perfusion pressure to spinal cord vs. need for mild hypotension to minimize blood loss
- Manage anesthetic agents to allow adequate monitoring of spinal cord integrity (SSEPs / MEPs)
- Vigilance for life threatening complications of VAE or major vascular injury (aortic, vena caval oriliac vessel)
- Optimize for postoperative wean from ventilation

Hx: Scoliosis hx (extent of disease, etiology): functional capacity, recurrent infections; CHD, NM disease, CTD, pre-existing CNS deficits; NutritionalJ status; Surgical Plan – Approach & monitoring tobe employed.

PE: Vitals, airway, **CV/Respiratory exam**, RVH & cor pulmonale (increased JVP, peripheral edema, hepatomegaly,
+HJR, RV heave, loud P2, wide split S2, unexpected murmurs, cyanosis, clubbing), Neuro deficits, scoliosis.

Investigations: CBC, G&S, Coags, ABGs if RLD, CXR for chronic lung disease, spinal Xray, ECG, +/- echo if applicable, PFTs.

Optimization: Pre-operative Hgb optimization, Respiratory health optimal, Pre-operative Clonidine (3ug/kg) and Gabapentin (10mg/kg).

Room Setup: CAS monitors, 5 lead ECG, A-line, good IV access, fluid warmers, forced air warmer, emergency drugs, TIVA infusions, TXA, SLETT vs DLETT, monitor for VAE (Doppler, TEE).

Intraoperative Management: Induction with hemodynamic goals in mind, short-acting NdMBs, Maintenance MEPs→no muscle relaxation, SSEP→ TIVA or low-dose volatile, prepared for prone or lateral position, TXA (100mg/kg bolus and 10mg/kg/hr) adequate analgesia.

Post-operative: Possible ICU, post-operative vent – depends on pre-operative cardiorespiratory reserve, intra-operative events, length of procedure, adequacy of analgesia, temperature, airway edema, etc.: pulmonary function is expected to worsen in first 7-10 days.

Special: Complications: intra-operative blood loss, neuro deficit (stop surgery, ensure adequate oxygenation/ ventilation, raise BP to above pre-operative, check Hg, r/o surgical causes), VAE, vascularinjury, post-operative respiratory failure (RF: VC <40%)

Scoliosis

Paroxysmal discharges from abnormally excited neuronal foci, which can be generally classified as: PARTIAL (simple vs. complex) or GENERALIZED (convulsive vs non-convulsive)

1. **Underlying etiology of Seizure**: Drugs, Infection, Metabolic, Structural - Raised ICP, Trauma: (hypoglycemia/hyponatremia/hypocalcaemia/hypomagnesemia), Withdrawal
2. Perioperative management of medications / interactions:
   - **Continue anti-epileptic medications** peri-operative
   - **NdMB resistance** due to enzyme inducers (phenytoin, carbamazepine, phenobarbital), p450 upregulation.
3. **Risk of perioperative seizures**: Avoid medications that exacerbate/precipitate seizure (Methohexital, ketamine, Cis/atracurium, enflurane, Demerol)
4. Risk of **Aspiration** with Seizure

Anesthetic Goals/Conflicts:

- Maintain a physiological pharmacologic and metabolic milieu to minimize risk of perioperative risk of seizure

Hx: AMPLE, seizure history, etiology, type, Hz, duration, medications / doses / side effects, recent serum levels. Etiology: DIMS

PE: Vitals, gingival hyperplasia (dilating), airway exam, LOC if recent seizure, neuro exam, signs of liver failure, bruising etc., evidence of aspiration pneumonia.

Investigations: Usual blood tests, toxicology screen, glucose, TSH, consider antiepileptic serum levels, CT-head, CXR for aspiration.

Optimization: Neurology consult for uncontrolled or new onset seizures, ensure patient continues anti-epileptic medications perioperatively. Correct metabolic derangements. Consider benzodiazepine pre- medication.

Anesthetic options: Regional or GA, possibly lower seizure threshold with LA toxicity, avoid ketamine, cisatracurium/atracurium/enflurane/meperidine etc. Avoid regional in post-ictal.

Room Setup: Usual setup

Intraoperative Management: Ideally Propofol or STP induction, consider benzo, may require higher doses of NMDR due to increased metabolism. Emergence = highest time for seizure.

Complications: Seizure Management: ABC, 100% O_2, BM ventilation, Vitals, Rapid glucometer, lorazepam 0.1mg/kg or midazolam in 0.5-1mg doses, STP 25-50mg, Propofol 25-50mg doses. If sz does not break >> GA doses, Phenytoin 20mg/kg IV load slowly, Phenobarbital 20mg/kg IV, intubate, treat underlying cause. Consider ICP management!! Hyperventilate, Mannitol/Decadron/elevate HOB,

Special: Phenobarbitone – Agranulocytosis, Hepatic Toxicity, SJS. Phenytoin – Gingival hyperplasia, ataxia, anemia, SJS, hepatotoxicity. Carbamazepine – Neutropenia, agranulocytosis, hepatotoxicity. Clonazepam-Thrombocytopenia, Valproic Acid – Agranulocytosis, hepatotoxicity, pancreatitis.

Seizures: Emergency

DDx

- Hypoxemia / Hypercapnia
- Drugs
- Infections
  - o Encephalitis, Meningitis, abscess, Sepsis
- Metabolic
  - o Hypoxia / hypercarbia, **Hypo/hyperglycemia**, myxedema coma, adrenal insufficiency, Electrolytes (hypo/hypernatremia, hypercalcemia), Toxins (Uremia, hepatic encephalopathy)
- Structural
  - o TBI, CVA, ICH, Tumor
- Pyrexia

Obstetrical Seizure

- Eclampsia, Drug withdrawal/intoxication (cocaine), ICH (hypertension), Epilepsy

Pediatric Seizure

- Febrile/meningitis/infection, Ingestion, Hypoxemia, Epilepsy, TBI (trauma/abuse), Metabolic (DKA, hypoglycemia)

Seizure during Regional

- Hypoxia/hypercapnia, LA toxicity (intravascular injection), High spinal, Epilepsy

Management

- Emergency Situation – Prevent injury, call for help and inform surgeon
- Scan monitors for HR, Rhythm, EtCO2, SaO2, and cycle BP
- Hand ventilates with 100% O_2 - DO NOT hyperventilate→ ↓ seizure threshold
- Anticonvulsants
  - o Propofol 20-30mg (Thiopental 25-50mg) titrated to effect
  - o Midazolam 0.5mg titrated to effect
- If no resolution and difficult ventilation
  - o NdMR
  - o Higher doses of sedatives
  - o Anticonvulsants
    - Phenytoin 10mg/kg IV load - slowly
    - Phenobarbital 1-2mg/kg
  - o Investigate etiology
    - Blood glucose, Electrolytes, Toxicology screen
    - Focused neurological exam
    - Infection, trauma, ↑ ICP, drug reaction
- Consult Neurology
- Pregnancy - $MgSO_4$ 6 g IV bolus over 15 minutes, then 1 – 2 g/hr
- ↑ ICP
  - o Maintain low normal pCO_2, Mannitol 1g/kg bolus, Dexamethasone 10-20mg bolus, Lasix 10-20mg bolus, HOB > 30°

Septic Shock

1. Critically ill patient with high mortality
2. Distributive shock with severe relative hypovolemia
   - Early goal directed therapy
   - Potential for cardiovascular collapse on induction of anesthesia
   - Need for critical care monitoring/ICU post-operatively
3. Multi-organ failure
   - ARDS, ARF, DIC
4. Systemic Infection
   - Early treatment with antibiotics, source control

Anesthetic Goals/Conflicts

1. Early goal-directed therapy
   - **Early Abx** – meropenem / Vancomycin
   - Fluid resuscitation and inotropes/vasopressors titrated to MAP > 65, CVP > 8-12 & SvO2 > 70
   - Peds – fluid titrated as 20ml/kg, monitor cap refill, BP less useful monitor, dopamine is 1st line
   - Parturient – FHR as resuscitative end point
2. **Urgent source control**
3. Parturient Conflicts – HD instability vs. fetal distress/Stat GA, neuraxial vs. bacteremia/HD instability

SIRS: Two or more of the following – **Temperature** <36, >38; **HR** > 90; **RR** > 20; **WBC** >12, <4, or 10% bands

Hx & Px: Confirm Diagnosis– distributive vs. cardiogenic vs. hypovolemic; R/O other etiology – Pancreatitis, anaphylaxis, drug ingestions, transfusion Rx, myxedema coma, adrenal crisis; Source of Sepsis – CNS (GCS, pupils, focal findings, meningismus), Respiratory (WOB, Sputum, auscultation), CVS (murmurs, CVLs, endocarditis – Septic emboli), Abd (jaundice, acute tenderness, ischemic gut), GU (flank pain, dec U/O, positive U/A, foley) Derma (cellulitis, abscess), Pregnancy (Chorioamnionitis, PROM) ; Identify end-organ dysfunction – LOC, respiratory failure, decreased peripheral perfusion, ARF; Vitals with postural & temperature; assess volume status; IV access

Inv: CBC + diff, platelets, electrolytes, Ur, Cr, Glu; INR/PTT; Blood cultures; group & screen; ABG,lactate, LFTs, amylase; CXR; sputum; ECG; +/-ECHO (TTE vs TEE)

Optimization: Consult ICU; Goal directed therapy – Monitored bed, Adequate IV access, Arterial Line, CVC (IJ or SC); O_2 +/- ETT with PPV (dec. WOB / VO2); fluid to keep CVP 8-12; Vasopressors to keep MAP > 65; SvO2 >70% - PRBC to Hct >30%, Dobutamine 2.5ug/kg/min; Early Abx (Meropenem 1gm IV q8h, Vancomycin 1g IV q12h); Surgery for source control (minimal delay); Consider Steroids if refractory shock; APC if APACHE >24 (stop 2 hrs pre-operative, re-start 12 hrs post); Glycemic control; Early enteral feeding; DVT & stress ulcer prophylaxis

Options: GA; neuraxial relatively contraindicated (infection, unfavorable hemodynamics, altered coagulation)

Setup: CAS 5 lead +temperature, A-line, CVC; adequate IV access; inotropes, infusions; blood products

Management: Aspiration risk; avoid Succinyl with prolonged immobility / intra-abdominal sepsis; HD stable induction (titrated, ketamine, minimize propofol, avoid etomidate); lung protective vent (Vt 6 mls, Ppl <30, permissive hypercapnia, PEEP titrated to PaO2 >60), Remember goals of resuscitation

Disposition: leave intubated; transport to ICU

Serotonin Syndrome

A potentially life-threatening adverse drug reaction with typical symptoms including agitation, delirium, autonomic hyperactivity, hyperreflexia, clonus, and hyperthermia.

1. Multisystem effects of serotonin excess:
   - CNS: seizure, altered LOC; CVS: Tachycardia and HTN, autonomic instability, arrhythmia; MSK: rigidity, rhabdomyolysis, hyperkalemia and renal failure; Hyperthermia; DIC
2. Avoid drugs that will precipitate Serotonin Syndrome in patients taking MAO inhibitors
   - Demerol, Fentanyl, Ondansetron, Metoclopramide, SSRI 's & TCA 's
3. Management strategies:
   - Cyproheptadine (5-HT antagonist), Benzodiazepines for rigidity
   - Hemodynamic support - may be altered and exaggerated responses to indirectacting sympathomimetics (avoid ephedrine and dopamine)
4. Psychiatric Patient – Co-operation, Informed consent / Substitute Decision Maker

Anesthetic Goals/Conflicts:

- Stop offending medications and provide supportive care
  - Aggressive cooling, antipyretics, NdMBs or benzodiazepines for rigidity
  - 5-HT receptor antagonists (b-blockers, cyproheptadine)
- Avoid drugs which may exacerbate serotonin syndrome: meperidine, fentanyl, ondansetron/maxeran
- Rule out high risk conditions on differential diagnosis (MH, NMS, thyrotoxicosis)

Hx: Detailed hx to reveal concomitant use of psychotropic meds, new meds, neuroleptics (need to r/o NMS). Symptoms: confusion, agitation, convulsion, coma, mydriasis (miosis in NMS), shivering, flushing, hyperthermia, muscle rigidity, myoclonus, hyperreflexia, autonomic instability, GI symptoms (rare in NMS); rarely rhabdo.

PE: Vitals (orthostatic, temperature) volume status, autonomic instability, CNS changes, muscle tone, reflexes, myoclonus, respiratory compromise/failure

Investigations: Goal to narrow DDx - CBC, lytes, Creatinine, CK, Coags, pan-culture, tox screen, ECG, +/- CXR, AXR to r/o secretory tumours.

Optimization: Psych and ICU consult, delay elective surgery, discontinue serotonergic meds, activatedcharcoal if recent ingestion

Room Setup: Standard CAS + A-line, CVP. Avoid meperidine, dextromethorphan, tramadol, fentanyl, ondansetron, maxeran. Have vasopressors, vasodilators available. Cyproheptadine for severe symptoms – 12mg NG load then 2mg q2h until symptoms resolve

Supportive Care: ABCs, intubation if appropriate; antipyretics, cooling, sedation, paralysis for hyperthermia; benzos for myoclonus, rigidity & agitation, consider phenytoin; NdMBs if benzos ineffective for rigidity; B-blockers (propranolol, esmolol) for 5-HT antagonism, HTN – sedation +/- SNP, HTN– volume +/- NE, phenyl, epi;

Post-operative: Likely ICU setting.

Syndrome of In Appropriate Anti- Diuretic Hormone (SIADH)

Hyponatremia, elevated urine osmolality, excessive urine sodium excretion, and decreased serum osmolality

1. Etiology or Co-existing disease
   a. Tumor – lung, pancreas, prostate, lymphoma
   b. CNS – trauma, SAH, tumor, infection
   c. Pulmonary (infection, CF), Drugs (opiates oxytocin, chlorpropamide, vincristine),Pain, idiopathic, iatrogenic
2. Hyponatremia and volume status – potential for volume overload
   a. cerebral edema, seizures, coma
3. Complications associated with treatment
   a. central pontine myelinolysis from overly rapid correction
   b. DI from 394 demeclocycline
4. DDx of hyponatremia
   a. Hypovolemic – CSWS, Diuretics, Addison 's, nephritis, RTA, Metabolic Alkalosis, vomiting, diarrhea, burns, pancreatitis, trauma
   b. Euvolemic – adrenal insufficiency, hypothyroidism, Drugs, SIADH
   c. Hypervolemic – ARF, CRF, nephrotic syndrome, CHF, cirrhosis

Anesthetic Goals/Conflicts:

- Maintain hemodynamic stability, fluid and electrolyte balance
- Correct underlying reversible aetiologies (infection, tumour, medications, iatrogenic)
- Avoid overcorrection or overly rapid correction resulting in CPM

Hx: surgical history (Neurological Symptoms), symptoms of hyponatremia/cerebral edema (lethargy, weakness, confusion, altered reflexes, Seizures, coma), urinary frequency & amount.

PE: vitals, Volume status (possible overload), Respiratory for edema, Neuro – areflexia, decreased LOC, pseudobulbar palsy, asterixis, muscle weakness

Investigations: Lytes, BUN, creatinine, and glucose. Look for low osmolality (<280 mOsm/kg), elevated Urinary Na (>20 mmol/L) & Osmolarity >100 mOsm/L; CXR for edema, CT head – edema, hemorrhage

Optimization: Correct symptomatic hyponatremia until asymptomatic, usually 120mmol/L, rate of 1- 2mEq/L/ Hour (3% NaCl 1-2ml/kg/hr); asymptomatic 0.5mEq/L/Hr; with true volume depletion, serum Na will increase. ~ 1mEq/L per liter of 0.9% NaCl infused – once ADH is turned off, serumNa may rapidly correct, may need DDAVP to slow correction; Increase in Serum Na = (infuscate [Na] – serum Na) / (TBW+1), Na deficit = TBW x (140- [Na]); eliminate precipitating cause, **free water restriction is mainstay of SIADH treatment (500-1000ml/d),** Demeclocycline (300- 600mg/d) to induce reversible nephrogenic DI, sufficient to decrease TBW by 0.5-1.0 L/day

Anesthetic Options: All feasible – assess Neurologic status

Room Setup: CAS + 5 lead, Art line for serum Na levels, CVP for volume, foley

Intraoperative Management: Avoid drugs known to lower seizure threshold, avoid hypotonic fluids, minimize stress response – ADH secretion, avoid drugs that induce ADH release – morphine, barbiturates, Beta agonists

Post-operative: Monitor urine output, serum Na, Fluid restriction 500-1000 mL/d, differentiate SIADH from cerebral salt wasting in the neurosurgical population (CSWS is associated with volume depletion, SIADH is EU/ hypervolemic)

Complications: Central pontine myelinolysis – S/S = quadriplegia, seizures, coma, and death; RFinclude ETOH, liver Dz, malnutrition, hypokalemia, burns, premenopausal women, severe chronic hyponatremia, onset may be delayed 1-2 days after correction

Sickle Cell Disease

1. Chronic hemolytic anemia
    a. chronic transfusion (Hct>30%), **difficult Cross match**, risk of hemolytic transfusionreactions from allo-immunization
2. Multisystem disease with end-organ dysfunction
    a. CNS - **Stroke**
    b. Pulmonary - acute chest syndrome, recurrent pneumonia, possible **RLD** from pulmonary infarction - **pHTN** and RVF
    c. CVS - LVH from chronic anemia
    d. Other – **CRF**, Splenic infarct (may be asplenia and immunocompromised), Iron overload
3. Potential for peri-operative exacerbations of vaso-occlusive crises
    a. acute pain crisis, acute chest syndrome
4. Chronic pain and opioid tolerance

Anesthetic Goals/Conflicts:

- Pre-operative optimization (consult hematology, consider hydroxyurea (increase [HbF]),consider prophylactic blood transfusion)
- Avoid precipitants of crisis
    - Hypoxia; Hypovolemia, Hyper viscosity, dehydration, Acidosis, Hypothermia, Infection, stasis, EtOH.
    - Ensure good perioperative pain control.

Hx: Exacerbations/Triggers (hospitalizations, frequency); extent of **end-organ damage** (primarily pain, CVA, CHF, pHTN, RVF, RLD, hypoxemia, bronchospasm, CRF, priapism, cholelithiasis, liver infarcts, hemolytic or aplastic anemia, splenic infarcts, hemosiderosis, chronic infection); **predictors of post-**

operative complications - Increase. age, complications (lung disease), hospitalization, abnormal CXR, African haplotype, pregnancy, infection, type of Sx (Chole=D&C=C/S or Hyster > Abd Sx > myringotomy >Hip Surgeries

PE: Vitals with RA SaO_2; wheeze, crackles; Vol status, LVF, pHTN/RVF; neuro deficits;

Investigations: CBC, Lytes, Ur, Cr, Coags, Hb electrophoresis, CXR +/-ABG, ECG +/- ECHO, +/- CT head

Optimization: Heme Consult; Hydroxyurea (increase. HbF); Euvolemia; Blood Tests for high-risk procedures (Hg>100); Avoid respiratory depressants; Cancel elective (acute crisis); Delay urgent (tooptimize Hb > 100

Anesthetic Options: GA; RA ok; TEA beneficial for pain management; Tourniquet use Ok

Room Setup: CAS + 5 lead; T probe; Invasive monitoring

Intraoperative Management: Standard; Follow above mentioned Goals

Complications:

vaso-occlusive crisis - PAIN (ppt by cold, dehydration, stress, menses, EtOH, OSA; pain is typical feature, associated with fever, swelling, N&V; Rx: Tylenol, NSAIDS, PCA opioids, hydration, temperature management); Acute

chest syndrome (2‘to vaso-occlusion, infraction, pneumonia; new lobar infiltrate, fever, increase. WOB,chest pain 2-3 days postop; Rx: as per pneumonia: pulmonary toilet, mobilization, analgesia, incentive spirometry, physio, Ventolin, steroids, Abx, Blood Tx);

Aplastic crisis;

Splenic Sequestration (rapid RBC trapping & fall of Hct, and hypovolemia/shock, LUQ pain; Rx: volume and PRBC, delayed splenectomy); RUQ Syndrome (hepatic ischemia, fever, jaundice, liver failure; Rx: fluids, analgesic, Blood Tx)

Cholecystectomy – most common procedure, high risk, laparoscopy is OK

Obstetrics – increase. risk of SA, prematurity, previa, abruption, PP infection: increase. pain crisis in 3rd. tri – noeffect on UBF/fetus, Maternal mortality ~1%, Fetal mortality as high as 20%, keep Hg > 80 for Vaginal delivery & 100 for C/S.

Spinal Stenosis

1. Geriatric patients (potential for multiple co-morbid illnesses and altered pharmacologyand physiology)
2. Chronic pain with potential concomitant behavioural and psychiatric limitations and drug tolerance
3. Need for multimodal approach for pain management
4. Surgical consideration for spine surgery
    a. Prone position
    b. Blood loss and conservation
    c. Fluid shift
    d. Post-operative pain
    e. Potential neurological monitoring
5. Lack of good evidence around standards for diagnostic, pharmacological and surgical modalities

Anesthetic Goals:

- Careful surgical candidates' selection
- Optimize co-morbid illness
- Obtain thorough history and physical and exclude other potential DDx
    - Ao aneurysm, vascular claudication, PMR, herniated disc, osteoporosis
    - **Key distinguishing feature is intermittent neurogenic claudication**
        - Induced by standing or walking with erect posture
- Document pre-operative neurological deficits
- Multimodal pain management – activity modification, passive ROM, PT, gabapentin,NSAIDs, opioids, epidural steroids, surgical decompression.

Epidural Steroid Injections

Indications:

- May help some patients with back and leg pain (first line is still ice, NSAIDs, rest → exercise)
- Reserved for patients with **symptoms of radiculopathy**
- Pain that **persists more than 4-6 weeks, sciatica and spinal stenosis**
- Epidural steroid injection should be reserved for patients with **symptoms of radiculopathy** (disc herniation or spinal stenosis with evidence of nerve root impingement)
- Radicular symptoms may be secondary to nerve root inflammation and edema, release of arachidonic acid metabolites, neuropeptides such as substance P, VIP, and CGRP released from the nucleus pulposus through the annulus.

Contraindications:

- Ongoing use of anticoagulant medications, local infection, discitis
- Prominent motor deficit or paresis suggestive of severe root or cauda equine compression (bowel & bladder dysfunction)
- Failure of previous injections
- Imaging studies demonstrating severe spinal stenosis

Technique:

- Epidural steroid injections have been traditionally given through either a caudal or interlaminar route; transforaminal route effective if experienced
- Volume used varies: 5-10ml recommended at the lumbar level, 3-6mls at C-spine.
- Fluoroscopy is recommended in the following:
  - post-laminectomy patients, obese patients, cervical epidural steroid injections, patients who don 't respond to the first injection.
- Incorrect needle placement occurs in 20-38% of caudal and 30% of translaminar injections
- The transforaminal approach is especially beneficial in post-laminectomy patients where the drug may not reach the level of pathology due to scarring from previous surgery.
- Injectate - Lidocaine 20-30mg
  - Triamcinolone most common (40-80mg), or methyl prednisolone 80mg
    - Methylprednisolone is not recommended in cervical transforaminal injections because it precipitates and the precipitant may be unintentionally injected into the vertebral artery.
  - Chase with 2cc NS – avoid seeding the tract with steroid
- Repeat every 2-3 weeks for total of 3 injections

Complications:

- PDPH (1-5%), hematoma, increased radicular symptoms (1%), Infection, unintentional subarachnoid injection, intraneural injection

Outcomes:

- Few well controlled studies but reasonable alternative to risks/costs of surgery
- Most reliable studies suggest that injections provide significant benefits to some patients with primarily radicular symptoms but the benefit is of limited duration (2-3months)
- Transforaminal injections seem to have predictive value in deciding whether a patient might benefit from surgery.

Medications for Status Epilepticus

Generic name	Loading dose	Maintenanc edose	Half-life	Therapeutic range (for status)
Lorazepam	0.1 mg/kg at2 mg/ min	Repeat initially to max of 0.3 mg/kg; then dose q 2–3Hours	8–25 Hours	0.2–0.5 μg/ml
Diazepam	0.15 mg/kg at5 mg/ min	Not typically usedas maintenance therapy	28–54 Hours	0.2–0.8 μg/ml
Phenytoin	20 mg/kg at 50 mg/min (max of 30 mg/kg)	1.5 mg/kg tid	24	20–25 μg/ml
Fosphenytoin	20 mg/kg at 50 mg/kg (max of30 mg/kg) [a]	1.5 mg/kg tid[a] butnot neededif venous access is safe	24	20–25 μg/ml
Phenobarbital	20 mg/kg at 50–75 mg/min(max of 30 mg/kg)	2–4 mg/kg qd	90 hours (70Hours in	30–50 μg/ml
Midazolam	0.2 mg/kg	0.75– 10 μg/kg/min	3 Hours	
Propofol	1–2 mg/kg	2–15 mg/kg/Hour	2 Hours	(2.4–4 μg/ml) b
Valproate	20–40 mg/kg	4–8 mg/kg tid	15 Hours	(70–150 μg/ml)
Pentobarbital	10–15 mg/kg	0.5–1 mg/kg/Hour	10–20 Hours	(10–20 μg/ml) b
Thiopental	100–200 mg	3–5 mg/kg/Hour	12–36 Hours	(15–50 μg/ml) b

Stellate Ganglion Block

Indications:

- Sympathetically mediated pain (CRPS, PHN, phantom limb, HSV, reimplantation pain)
- Circulatory insufficiency – post-embolectomy vasospasm, Raynaud 's, Scleroderma
- Long QT syndrome

Contraindications:

- General: Infection, Coagulopathy, lack of consent, allergy, lack of resuscitation equipment or skill
- Specific: Contra-lateral recurrent nerve injury, severe lung disease (FEV1 < 1L)

Equipment:

- Routine monitors, trained assistant, resuscitation equipment, 1.5-increaseh 25-gauge needle

Technique:

- Place patient 's head midline with neck slightly extended. Skin is prepped with antiseptic andthe skin injected with local. The C6 transverse process is palpated and the carotid is retractedlaterally. Needle is inserted to bone (1-2cm), withdraw slightly and inject 0.5-1 cc of local injected as test dose. The needle is advanced to bone again, retracted slightly again and thenfurther local to a total of 8-10 cc is injected (use Marcaine 0.25% without epi)

Successful Block:

- Horner 's, ipsilateral nasal congestion & conjunctiva flushing, vasodilated and warm extremity

Complications:

- Direct trauma: pneumo, esophageal perforation, carotid or IJ puncture; Local anesthetic effects: inadvertent epidural, brachial plexus, intrathecal, intravenous or vertebral artery injection with associated seizures, bradycardia, RLN (60%) or phrenic nerve paralysis

Systemic Lupus Erythematosus

1. Potential **difficult airway**
    - Deforming arthritis, Cricoarytenoid arthritis, RLN palsy
2. Systemic Complications of SLE
    - CNS - seizure, stroke, mood, organic disease, transverse myelitis
    - Cardiac – **Myocarditis** (conduction disease, CHF), **Pericarditis** (effusions), non-infectious **Endocarditis** (AI, MR), Accelerated **CAD**, HTN/pHTN
    - Respiratory – **RLD (ILD,** pleuritis, effusions), **pHTN/RVF**, infection, pulmonary hemorrhage
    - Hematologic - hypercoagulable (APA), anemia, thrombocytopenia, abnormal bleeding
    - Other – CRF, Nephritic, Nephrotic, vasculitis, arthritis, immobility
3. Complications related to medical management
    - **Steroids** (coshing's, hyperglycemia, adrenal suppression), Immunosuppressants / antimalarials, NSAIDs, **Anticoagulants**, ASA
4. Potential for exacerbation of SLE with surgery, stress, infection and pregnancy
5. SLE and Pregnancy:
    - Increased risk of pre-term, IUGR, PIH, possible contraindications to neuraxial, risk of neonatal lupus and Anti-Ro mediated congenital heart block

Anesthetic Goals/Conflicts:

- Potentially challenging airway and myocardial dysfunction
- Coagulation defects / thromboembolism and neuraxial techniques
- Avoid drugs that exacerbate Lupus – Procainamide, Phenytoin, Hydralazine, Penicillin, Isoniazid, Enalapril, Captopril, Clonidine

Hx: Investigate for end-organ dysfunction as above, in particular renal failure, cardio-respiratory involvement, previous endocarditis (consider prophylaxis), arthritis, thrombo-embolic complications and medical therapy.

PE: Detailed airway exam, Neck & TMJ ROM, laryngeal function, hoarseness, detailed cardiorespiratory exam for effusions, tamponade (rare), valvular pathology, CHF, Document pre-existing neuropathies

Investigations: CBC (anemia, thrombocytopenia), E7 (renal dysfunction), ECG (conduction Disease,LVH, pHTN); Coags, X-match, Anti-phospholipid Ag/ Lupus Anticoagulant/Anticardiolipin, +/- factor assay if prolonged PTT, LFTs (hepatitis); CXR (CHF, effusions, infiltrates); PFTs (restrictive), Echocardiography (LV/RV dysfunction, valvular dysfunction)

Optimization: Heme/Rheum/Obs consults; Stress Dose Steroids; SBE prophylaxis

Options: Neuraxial may be contraindicated (thrombocytopenia, prolonged PTT – not a contraindication ifd/t Anti-Phospholipid Antibody, is a contraindication if d/t factor deficiency)

Room Setup: Based on end-organ dysfunction; Consider TEA if appropriate with lung disease; Consider smaller ETT if cricoarytenoid arthritis

Intraoperative Management: Depends on underlying organ dysfunction; Safe and controlled management of potentially difficult airway; Consider potential for myocardial dysfunction oninduction; If on cyclophosphamide prolonged response to suxamethonium and mivacurium due to inhibition of plasma cholinesterase; If renal insufficiency present, avoid renally excreted drugs and renal toxins

Emergence: Fully reversed, awake, may require prolonged ventilation if severe respiratory dysfunction

Post-operative: Beware of post-operative stridor (steroids), thromboembolic events, CHF & arrhythmias, renal insufficiency, adrenal insufficiency, coagulopathy and hemorrhage, seizures, CNS dysfunction, fulminant hepatitis

Tachycardia: Emergency

Most important question is **sinus tachycardia** or not?

Sinus Tachycardia

DDx

1. Hypoxia / hypercarbia
2. Drugs
   - Administration → chronotropes, cocaine, MAOI, stimulants
   - Withdrawal → opioid, BDZ, EtOH, clonidine, β-blocker
3. Pain or light anesthesia – surgical or non-surgical (full bladder, tourniquet)
4. Shock → hypovolemia, PTX, pericardial, sepsis, anaphylaxis, anemia
5. Endocrine
   - Hypoglycemia
   - Hyperthyroidism
   - MH / NMS
   - Pheochromocytoma

Emergency Management

1. Inform surgeon, Scan monitors: rate, rhythm, BP, $EtCO_2$, SaO_2
2. Hand ventilates with 100% O_2
3. Examine patient
   - Assess pulse
   - Auscultate both lungs and examine trachea
   - Examine peripherally and forehead for evidence of anaphylaxis
4. Develop DDx and treat as per ACLS protocol

Non-Sinus Tachycardia DDx

1. SVT: Regular
2. A-fib: Irregular
3. MAT
4. VT / VF

Non-Sinus Tachycardia Emergency Management

1. Determine rhythm and treat as per ACLS
2. Reason for arrhythmia
   - Pre-existing
   - Ischemia → rate, ACS
   - Electrolyte abnormalities

Tamponade

1. Emergency Situation with potential for cardiovascular collapse on induction
2. Pathophysiologic changes
    a. Impaired diastolic filling
    b. Fixed stroke volume
    c. Rate dependent CO
    d. Maximal sympathetic stimulation
3. Aetiologies / co-existing diseases
    a. Blood: post-cardiac Sx, post-MI, aortic dissection, trauma
    b. Other: infectious, malignant, radiation, SLE, uremia, autoimmune

Anesthetic Goals/Conflicts:

- If hemodynamically significant, **drain pericardium prior to anesthesia / PPV**
- **Avoid increase in intrathoracic pressure**
    - o Maintain spontaneous ventilation, avoid coughing & straining
- Cardiovascular: ***fast, full and tight***
    - o Preload: FULL
    - o Contractility: maintain
    - o Rate: maintain / possibly increase
    - o Rhythm: strict NSR
    - o Afterload: maintain
    - o MVO2: monitor for ischemia
- ***These patients are maximally sympathetically stimulated***
    - *o You need to replace the sympathetic drive removed by your anesthetic*

Hx: Determine underlying etiology (dissection, free wall dissection, trauma, post sx, malignancy, autoimmune (SLE/RA/Scleroderma), infectious, radiation). Hx of dyspnea, fatigue, CHF, hypotension, tachycardia.

PE: Vitals: **hemodynamically unstable?** ↓BP ↑HR, signs of CHF. Distant heart sounds, pulsus paradoxus (↓SBP > 10mmHg with inspiration), narrow pulse pressure, possible friction rub. JVD (NoteKussumaul 's sign increase in JVP during inspiration (opposite of normal) occurs with constrictive pericarditis, not withtamponade!) AI if aortic dissection. CVP: Elevated CVP. PAC- diastolic press equalization ~15-20mmHg, corresponding to pericardial pressure

Investigations: CBC/Lytes/Cr (ATN due to shock), INR/PTT, CXR (enlarged cardiac silhouette). ECG:Electrical alternans, low voltage, ST-T elevation, tachycardia. ECHO: visualize effusion, chamber compression, cardiac output, septal shift, chamber volumes.

Optimization: Large bore IV access, volume resuscitation, pericardial drain, epinephrine infusion, atropine for pericardial manipulation. If unable to drain prior to induction, have patient prepped and surgeon in the room.

Anesthetic Options: Local for pericardial drain/window maintains SV, however can lead to coughing,straining. GA: controlled airway, allows sternotomy/thoracotomy, however risk of CVS collapse on induction/PPV. Early cardioversion for arrhythmias.

Room Setup: 5lead, invasive lines, TEE/PAC, drugs: Epi/NE, pericardiocentesis drain, chest prepped.

Intraoperative Management: fluid / PC Drain then GA for definitive Rx. / LA, opioid, small amount ofamnestic, +- paralysis / Consider spontaneous breathing induction, can supplement with airway topicalization but do not delay if unstable. Small TV, increase. RR, observe HD goals.

Post-operative: HDU, observe for recurrence of tamponade. Consider PCA or T Epidural for sternotomy of post-operative pain. Complications: Post-tamponade pulmonary edema: due to increase RV CO, NTG, diuretics

TCA Overdose

Mechanism of action: Stimulation of catecholamine release and block reuptake, Central and peripheral anticholinergic agents, inhibit Na and K channels in brain and heart, Direct alpha blocking.

1. Multisystem effects: Coma, convulsive, cardiac arrythmias and acidosis
    a. CNS: depression, possible seizures (persists ~ 24-48 hrs)
        i. ACh side effects: Dry mouth, constipation, urinary retention, vision
    b. CVS: Postural hypotension, Dose related prolonged QT and QRS widening (>100msec)
        i. Risk of ventricular arrhythmias with QT > 0.16 - serial ECGs (persists for 10 days)

2. Medical Management
    a. Gi decontamination - risk of aspiration
    b. Seizures – Diazepam, Sodium bicarbonate (reduce free fraction), Phenytoin
    c. Dysrhythmias – Alkalization, Lidocaine, Phenytoin (avoid class 1a, amiodarone)
    d. Heart block - Isoproterenol
    e. Hypotension – Volume, Sodium bicarbonate, Sympathomimetics, Inotropes

Anesthetic Goals/Conflicts:

- Usual HCO_3^- is 1-2 MEQ/kg to keep QRS < 100 msecs goal pH 7.5-7.55
- ECG – Abnormal QRS, prolonged QRS, abnormal size and ration of R and S waves in AVR
- R/O hypoglycemia, CO intoxication, bHCG on lab, monitored setting.

Temperature: Emergency

DDx hyperthermia

1. Physiologic (e.g., sepsis)
2. Drugs
    - MH / NMS
    - Pheochromocytoma
    - Hyperthyroidism
    - Serotonergic syndrome
    - Anticholinergic syndrome
    - Transfusion reaction
    - Stimulants: cocaine, amphetamines
3. Endocrine: Hyperthyroidism
4. Exogenous
    - Warming blankets, heating pads

DDx hypothermia

1. Increased heat loss
    - Environmental Exposure
    - Drugs → vasodilation
        - Alcohol
        - Toxins
        - Sepsis
    - Iatrogenic: CPB, CRRT, Cold infusions
2. Decreased heat production
    - Endocrine
        - Hypopituitarism

- Hypoadrenalism
    - Hypothyroid
    - Hypoglycemia
  - Malnutrition
  - Extremes of age
  - Impaired shivering (anesthesia)
3. Impaired regulation: central vs peripheral
4. Other
   - sepsis
   - pancreatitis

Tetralogy of Fallot

1. Complex congenital heart disease characterized by VSD, RVOT obstruction, overriding Ao, RVH
2. Both fixed and dynamic RVOT obstruction
   - Fixed RVOT obstruction – variable R to L shunt & pulmonary blood flow
   - Dynamic RVOT obstruction (infundibular spasm) – increase. R to L shunting & hypoxia
3. Associated abnormalities and conditions
   - paradoxical embolus – avoid air bubbles in lines
   - Thrombophilia 2'to polycythemia
   - 25% have another congenital abnormality
     - Tracheoesophageal fistula and Trisomy 21
4. SBE prophylaxis

Anesthetic Goals / Conflicts

- Hemodynamic Goals
  - Full preload – Stiff RV, stent open RVOT
  - Dec. Contractility to reduce dynamic RVOT obstruction
  - Maintain afterload to minimize R – L shunt and promote pulmonary blood flow
  - Avoid increase. PVR – hypoxia, acidosis, aggressive PPV/PEEP
- Tet -spell – sudden hypoxia / acidosis 2'to infundibular spasm or dec. SVR – increase. R to L shunt
  - 100% O2 +/- gental PPV, fluid bolus, sedation (dec. SNS), knee chest position (Increase. SVR & preload), phenylephrine 1-2ug/kg, propranolol 10-20 ug/kg (dec. infundibular spasm)

Thoracic Aneurysm

1. Emergency Case: full stomach, HD unstable patient
2. Potential for OLV
3. Potential for massive blood loss, fluid shifts, transfusion and hypothermia
4. Intraoperative hemodynamic changes with potential for ischemia - heart, brain, kidneys, and spinal cord
   a. Special monitoring for SC ischemia (SSEP, MEP) and techniques to optimize SC perfusion
   b. Post-operative organ dysfunction: MI, ARF, SC ischemia
5. Co-morbidities: CAD / DM / Chronic kidney disease / HTN / Smoking/Advanced age
6. Post-operative pain

Anesthetic Goals/Conflicts:

- maintain stable hemodynamics throughout peri-operative period
- maintain favourable myocardial oxygen supply / demand relationship
- watch for evidence of peri-operative organ dysfunction (SC, kidneys)
- peri-operative pain control

Hx: Co-morbidities: active cardiac conditions (AHA guidelines), acute vs chronic dissection, symptoms

PE: Evidence of HF, LV and RV dysfunction, AR, cardiac tamponade (JVD, distant HS, HTN, pulsus paradoxus), carotid bruit, neurologic exam

Investigations: CBC, PTT, INR, X-match, lytes, BUN, EKG, TTE, Consider PFT/CXR, invasive cardiac testing according to AHA, CT/CTA of Aneurysm - review for location, level of cross clamp

Optimization: correct anemia (maintain Hb>9.0 g/dL), avoid tachycardia, optimize volume status, continue beta-blockers, hold ACEI/ARB, hold anticoagulants/antiplatelet agents and bridge, ifnecessary, Consider: cardiology, nephrology consultation

Anesthetic Options: GA +/- OLV, PCA vs epidural for post-operative analgesia

Room Setup: CAS (5 lead EKG), IV prox 'l to XC, pre-induction A-line, CVP, +/- TEE/PAC/DLETT+FOB, fluid warmer, cell saver, blood, SC monitoring (SSEP, MEP)

Intraoperative Management:

Induction Titrated (vs. aspiration) if emergency surgery, patient prepped and surgeon in room prior to induction,

Maintenance: volatiles readily titratable, consider effect of epidural on hemodynamics - Prior to cross clamp: avoid over-resuscitation, heparin and mannitol, Cross clamp →

Hypertension (increase afterload), NTG and nitroprusside ready, Removal of cross clamp → **Hypotension,** volume resuscitation prior, dec anesthetic, prepare for **metabolic acidosis** with reperfusion - hyperventilate, HCO3, staged release of cross clamp will help minimize effects and ifunable to control hypotension, surgeon may have to re-apply cross clamp (be ready for rebound hypertension)

Post-operative: Switch DLT to SLT, to CSICU intubated, gradual slow emergence.

Thoracoscopic Surgery

1) Underlying etiology
    - Malignancy – 4 M 's
    - IPF or COPD
    - Pleural disease
    - Pericardial disease
2) Requires OLV with good lung deflation (unable to CPAP operative lung)
3) CO2 insufflation of the thorax and its potential complications
    - dec. pre-load, increase. LV afterload, potential for CO_2 embolism, risk of sudden cardiovascular collapse

Anesthetic Goals:

- Guided by underlying etiology and comorbidities
- Maintain adequate oxygenation
- Post-operative Pain Control
- Multimodal, TEA, paravertebral catheters

Hx and PE and Investigations:

- Determine severity and complications of underlying disease
- Screen and assess comorbidities
- Assess ease of intubation and OLV technique
- Assess ability to tolerate OLV
    - Side of Surgery (right side has 10% more blood flow than left) / Poor PaO2 on Two Lung Ventilation
      / Pre-operative FEV1 (inverse correlation) / Supine position

- Contraindications:
    - o Extensive pleural adhesions, Extensive inflammatory process, Previous pleural fusion, Unresectable lesion, Coagulation defect, Inability to tolerate one-lung ventilation, Severe COPD, Dependence on mechanical ventilation with high peak pulmonary pressures, Hemodynamic instability, Hypovolemic shock, Cardiogenic shock, Ongoing cardiac ischemia, post-acute MI

Optimization: Standard for Thoracic and OLV

Room Setup: Standard

Management: GA usually preferred but TEA is possible with local and intercostal nerve blocks Induction dictated by comorbid illnesses; Maintenance as per usual OLV cases.

Post-operative: multimodal pain management

Complications: Related to DLETT/OLV; Cardiac: HD instability, arrhythmias; Conversion to Open (25%); Persistent Air leak > 5 days (5%); -Down Lungll syndrome (increase secretions, atelectasis, re-expansion pulmonary edema, pneumonia); Bleeding, infection etc.

Acute Spinal Cord Injury

1. **Emergency Trauma with C/T/L-spine injury**
    - Full stomach, Hemorrhage & hemodynamic instability, Intoxication, Additional injuries (CHI with increase. ICP in 25%), Hypothermia
2. **Potentially difficult airway**
3. **Prevention of secondary spinal cord injury** (SCI) from hypoxemia or hypotension
    - Goal MAP > 80-85, Volume resuscitates, HD support (Dopamine, pressors)
4. Specific considerations of acute spine injury
    - C-spine precautions and airway protection - High aspiration risk (loss of cough ability (T2-L1))
    - Respiratory insufficiency History / injury above T7
        - o Intercostal paralysis (T1-T11), Diaphragmatic paralysis (C3-C5), Pulmonary edema
    - Severe ANS abnormalities
        - o Potential for neurogenic shock (hypotension & bradycardia (vasovagal))
        - o Thermoregulation loss & poikilothermic
    - Hyperkalemia History / Succinyl from 24 hours to 6 months post-injury

Anesthetic Goals/Conflicts:

1. Prevent Secondary SCI
    - Full spinal precautions – imaging can be delayed until after more urgent management
    - Safe airway management, Avoid hypoxia and hypotension
2. DDx: Neurogenic vs hypovolemic shock: lose ability to ↑ HR in response to hypovolemia
3. Conflict: SCI, Difficult AW, CHI (↑ICP) vs Uncooperative patient; RSI vs. Aspiration Risk

Spinal shock (1-3 weeks) = flaccidity and areflexia (has nothing to do History / HD stability)
Neurogenic shock = sympathectomy History / PNS dominance; Vasodilation– hypotension responsive to pressors; Bradycardia and loss of baroreceptor reflex arc to hypotension (responsive to atropine)
ATLS approach: 1'(ABCDE) then 2'survey (AMPLE + head to toe exam)

Hx: AMPLE; Old charts; MOI; Associated injuries; Intoxication; Resus History; Comorbid Disease

PE: Vitals (HR, BP); C-spine precautions; Monitor; Large IVs; ABCDE; Respiratory function; Neuro exam
Canadian C-Spine: GCS 15 and stable – Age <65, Normal neuro exam, no dangerous mechanism (fall >3ft; MVC >100km/hr, roll-over, ejection, ATV, bicycle; axial load) – low-risk factors present (simple rear-end, sitting position, ambulatory, delayed neck pain, absent midline pain – active rotation OK – No x-ray

Investigations: CBC; Coags; E7; Cx Match; ABG (respiratory insufficiency), vital capacity – 15mls/kg; Tox screen; CXR; C-spine (C1-T1, boney alignment, cartilage spaces, soft tissue – 10mm at atlas, 4mm C2-C4, 15mm below C4, AbN if >5mm increase); CT Head/Spine; FAST; ECG

Optimization: ATLS; Oxygen/Vent/Volume; maintain MAP> 80mmHg; Asp prophylaxis; Anti-sialagogue (AFOI); Steroids – methylprednisolone 30mg/kg within 8hrs (controversial)

Anesthetic Options: Usually GA for emergency fixation or decompression

Room Setup: CAS + 5lead, temperature, A-line, CVC (Chronotropes, pressers); Foley; Warming; ER drugs; Cell saver; prone patient.

Intraoperative Management: AFOI if possible (assess CNS); RSI + Inline stabilization +/- Cricoid if uncooperative; Watch for ↑ICP (conflict); Avoid SUX >24H; Maintain SCPP; Prone position (most dangerous time); protective vent strategy if ALI; possible SSEP / MEP monitoring

Emergence: Keep intubated vs extubation for neuro assessment; Be wary of aw swelling;

Post-operative: HDU/ICU

Total Spinal

1. Emergency requiring prompt diagnosis and simultaneous management
    a. discontinue local anaesthetics
2. Supportive management – including sedation
    a. Airway – consider intubation and ventilation
        i. Consider PPV may further reduce preload!
    b. Hemodynamic sequelae (complete sympathectomy)
        i. severe hypotension, bradycardia, cardiac arrest
3. Consideration in pregnancy - Above PLUS
    a. FHR monitoring
    b. left uterine displacement
    c. leg elevation +/- reverse Trendelenburg if hyperbaric LA used

Anesthetic Goals/Conflicts:

- Support airway with intubation and ventilation
- Support circulation with fluid, vasopressors and atropine
- Avoid awareness with sedation and counsel patient once situation resolves

Intraoperative Management:

1. Call a code
2. Stop injection of LA
3. Support airway, consider intubation
4. Support BP with fluids/inotropes: atropine if brady, ephedrine, move quickly to epinephrine
5. Ensure adequate sedation
6. If obstetric patient, ensure adequate fetal monitoring and support uterine perfusion pressure
7. Inform obstetrician
8. Discuss what happened with patient once spinal resolves

Risk factors for un-expected cardiac arrest following spinal: Male, ASA 1, use of beta blockers, resting HR < 60, Age < 50, prolonged PR interval.? related to high vagal tone

Paradoxical Bezhold Jarsisch reflex

- Mechanoreceptors in the heart (LV>>Atria) / afferent c-fibers / efferent vagus
- Activation with nociception → reflex hypotension, bradycardia, coronary artery dilatation
- The paradox - receptors in the wall of the underfilled LV may erroneously STIMULATE - results in paradoxical bradycardia and decreased contractility adding to the sudden arterial hypotension

-Reversell Bainbridge

- stretch receptors located in the right atrial wall and the Cavo atrial junction → ↑ right-sided filling pressure → vagal afferent signals to the cardiovascular center in the medulla → inhibit parasympathetic activity → increased heart rate
- The changes in heart rate are dependent on the underlying heart rate before stimulation.

Stereotactic Surgery

Stage I: localisation of nucleus/seizure foci/tumour. Stage II: implantation of stimulator. Stage III: tunnelling

1. Avoidance of sedatives (burr hole under local anaesthetic)
2. Uncontrolled airway at risk of obstruction with challenging access (key for frame immediately available)
3. Coexisting Disease
    a. Parkinson 's - aspiration risk, autonomic instability, increased perioperative complications, management of medications – held pre-operative, avoidance of beta-blockers as this would decrease tremor, avoid antidopaminergic medications
    b. Seizures – hold anti-epileptics
    c. Tumor, Chronic pain, Depression, neurodegenerative disease (dystonia, MS),
4. Complications
    a. intra-cerebral hematoma, Sz,
    b. hypertension, bradycardia, arrhythmia
    c. Sitting Position - VAE, postural hypotension

Anesthetic Goals/Conflicts:

1) Awake, comfortable and cooperative patient
2) Stable hemodynamics (avoid HTN, hydralazine)
3) Avoid sedatives as it alters electrophysiologic footprint required for nucleus localization

Hx: standard anaesthetic history and physical with additional attention to the etiologic considerations, and their medications (e.g., anti-Parkinson/seizure medications), history of coagulopathy, antiplatelet medications, herbal, co-existing diseases, hypertension

PE: standard physical with special attention to etiological factors requiring surgery

Investigations: CBC, coags, lytes, Group & Screen. CT scan. ECG

Optimization: anti-parkinsonian medications held prior to DBS; avoid anti-dopaminergic meds

Anesthetic Options: Stage II: monitored anaesthesia care if DBS – must avoid all agents which decrease tremor (end-point of stimulation) as the patient must be very cooperative. Stage III: GETA

Room Setup: standard CAS monitors + 5 lead EKG, emergency resuscitation drugs and airway equipment. Antihypertensives and anticonvulsants available

Intraoperative Management: MAC for stage II and GETA for Stage III. Monitor for complications: haemorrhage, VAE, seizures, cardiac dysrhythmias – especially bradycardia (stimulation of deep structures near the hypothalamus)

Post-operative: minimal pain post-operative.

Tracheal Resections

1) Difficult airway with the potential for obstruction and disruption with induction and PPV
   a. Delineation of anatomy (CT/spirometry/ECHO)
2) Maintenance of oxygenation and ventilation in the setting of an open airway
   a. Standard orotracheal intubation / Insertion of a tube into the opened trachea distal toarea of resection / HFJV through stenotic area / HFPPV / CPB
3) Priority on maintaining postoperative integrity of the tracheal anastomosis
   a. Immediate extubation
4) Etiology and complications of disease:
   a. 4M 's of cancer (mass, metabolic, metastases, medication)
   b. Potential for anterior mediastinal mass and superior vena cava syndrome
   c. Pulmonary sepsis
5) Severe co-existing pulmonary disease is a contraindication to surgery

Anesthetic Goals/Conflicts:

- *Pre-operative assessment to determine*
  - *the nature, location, and extent of trachea to be resected*
  - *presence of pre-existing disease (specifically cardiopulmonary reserve)*
- *Attain Anesthesia without causing airway obstruction*
- *Planned approach with surgical team to securing airway distal to obstruction/ventilation*
- *Avoid post-operative ventilation for risk of disrupting tracheal anastomosis*

Hx: Dyspnea, dynamic symptoms, associated co-morbidities (pulmonary), type of lesion (vascular/tumour), functional capacity, degree of obstruction, contraindications to HFJV (peds, COPD, Bullae)

PE: Dynamic airway obstruction, stridor/wheeze, vascular compression, evidence of heart failure, COPD, Rt heart failure, pHTN (Loud S2, RV heave, elevated JVP)

Investigations: CBC / Lytes / Coag / ABG / ECG / CXR / **CT** / bronchoscopy / spirometry with flowvolume

Optimization: Consider pre-operative chemo/irradiation/ airway stent; with severe obstruction consider high FiO_2, increase. humidity, steroids, racemic epi, Heliox; minimize pre-operative sedation; avoid anti - sialagogues (inspissation's)

Room Setup: Arterial Line (Lt – no compression), SaO_2 on Rt, various ETT tubes (armoured, MLT), FOB, HFJV catheters, Surgeon with rigid bronchoscope, ETT to intubate in the field; Heliox; +/-CVP

Intraoperative Management: Close communication between surgeon and anesthesiologist. SV with high FiO_2, AFOI vs. SVGA, SLT (endobronchial intubation) vs. DLT, secure distal to lesion, bilateral ETT tubes, or OLV, or ligatures around PA 's to decrease blood flow to non-ventilated lung; if unable to secure distal - HFJV or HFPPV SLT: HJV through small bore ETT tubes or catheters and surgeon works Aron small catheter >> Must have enough room for gas egress!! Unable to suction debits with this method. Or you can use HFPPV (TV 50- 250ml) through small catheter at rates of 150/min (minimal movement, and contamination of lungs). HFFPV of one lung is usually sufficient! Finally, >> CPB >> risk of heparinization and intrapulmonary hemorrhage precludes it's use!

Post-operative: Keep head in flexion to decrease tension on suture line. Early extubation desired, but make sure ETT is not near the suture line. Avoid vigorous chest physio

Complications: Trach disruption, RLN injury, airway edema. Massive hemoptysis (usually fatal)

Tracheoesophageal Fistula

1. Possible difficult intubation & BMV with gastric distension with increased risk of aspiration
2. Possible respiratory distress secondary to aspiration – acute and chronic
3. Co-existing congenital anomalies
    a. VATER/VACTERL including CHD
4. Neonatal/prematurity considerations
    a. altered airway anatomy, cardiac, respiratory, metabolic, and physiologic changes
    b. complications of prematurity – revision to fetal circulation
5. Post-operative intensive care and pain management

Anesthetic Goals / Conflicts

1. Secure the airway distal to the fistula while avoiding PPV (RSI vs. SV)
    a. risks of intubating the fistula, inability to PPV, gastric aspiration
2. Protect the lungs from aspiration pre-operatively
3. Identify coexisting anomalies, specifically CHD
4. Diagnose and treat hypoxemia intraoperatively
5. Prevent post-operative pain and complications

Hx & Px: OB hx, PCA/GA, premature, Growth, congenital anomalies (**V**ertebral, **A**nal atresia, **C**HD, **TE**F, **R**adial/renal dysplasia, **L**imb anomalies), CHF (WOB, failure to thrive, heave, murmurs), Shunting(Cyanosis, clubbing), Vitals including pre/post ductal SaO2

Inv: CBC, electrolytes, +/- ABG, CXR (pulmonary blood flow, heart shape) +/- ECHO if signs of CHD

Optimization: Prevent aspiration (NPO, HOB elevated, consider G-tube pre-operative) treat aspiration (Abx, physio delay case to optimize), Peds cardio consult to r/o CHD, pouch tube / suction

Room Setup: Multiple cuffed/uncuffed ETT, ENT with rigid bronchoscope, FOB, fogarty balloon catheter, warming blanket / lights

Monitors: CAS, temperature, Aline, pre & post ductal SaO_2, precordial stethoscope (L Ax to Dx endobronchial intubation)

Management: Suction oral pharynx, pouch +/- gastric tube, avoid PPV (gastric distension – impaired/impossible ventilation, aspiration, impaired venous return), RSI (intentional endobronchial intubation and withdrawal, FOB to confirm) vs. SV (Sevoflurane vs. TIVA), topicalize airway , rigid bronchoscopy to delineate anatomy, +/- fogarty balloon to occlude fistula, ETT distal to lesion; Maintenance with TIVA/Sevoflurane + opioid, titrated FiO_2 to maintain preductal $SaO_2 > 90\%$, NdMB, minimize PIP (reduce gastric distension), avoid hypothermia/hypoglycemia

Emergence/Disposition: likely postop ventilation (pre-existing pulmonary complications, tracheomalacia, tracheal wall defect), extubation if term, healthy, otherwise normal, warm, reversed, stable infant, protect anastomosis (neck flexion, avoid reintubation, avoid gastric suctioning below level of repair, post-operative pain – epidural/caudal

Complications: Hypoxemia (mispositioned ETT – (endobronchial, fistula), gastric distension and hypoventilation, surgical retraction, aspiration pneumonitis, cardiac shunting etc.) Hypotension (surgical retraction, gastric distension, hemorrhage, CHF), Post-operative (GERD, aspiration, leak, esophageal stricture, tracheomalacia, pneumoTx

Tracheostomy

1. Emergency case as dictated by the etiology
    a. Trauma - facial smash, penetrating neck injury
    b. Upper airway obstruction
    c. ICU patient with prolonged OETT
2. Shared airway
    a. Potential for catastrophic loss of airway
        i. Possible difficult airway
    b. Potential for airway fire
3. Co-existing disease states
    a. Critically ill - MOD
    b. Trauma – CHI, C-Spine injury, occult injuries
    c. Chronic Tracheostomy – RLD, chronic aspiration, pHTN, Sz, developmental delay, neuromuscular disorders

Anesthetic Goals/Conflicts:

1. Maintain airway patency
    a. Back-up airway plan
2. Good communication with surgical team
3. Support/Optimize underlying disease state
4. high O_2 (desaturation) vs. low FiO2 (protect against airway fire)

Hx: Indication, airway patency (stridor, dyspnea, wheeze), Respiratory reserve, Co-morbidities and implications, Chronic Trach – indication (aspiration, developmental delay, neuromuscular weakness) type of trach tube (size, cuffed, single cannula, custom), recent trach change, need forchronic ventilation, vent settings, comorbid disease (RLD, pHTN)

PE: vitals, airway patency/swelling, easy of intubation/re-intubation, Grade of original intubation, ventsettings, FiO2, neck circ., cardiopulmonary exam – wheezes, crackles, loud P2, RV heave

Investigations: CBC, coags, ABG, G+S, PFTs, CXR, ECHO / CT scan dictated by history & physical

Optimization: GA vs Awake, perform procedure in OR if possible, NPO/NG to suction, optimize FiO2 & vent. settings, optimize co-morbidities, change trach to cuffed (1/2 size smaller), patient position (shoulder roll)

Room Setup: Difficult airway cart, Cook catheter, ± Jet ventilator, +/- Art. Line

Intraoperative Management: awake with local infiltration, caution with FiO_2

Post-operative: HDU observation initially, humidified O_2, caution suctioning of secretions, sterile precautions, cuff pressure 15-20 mm Hg, stoma/track not fully established for 5 days = higherrisk, Laryngoscope and small ETT at the bedside

Complications: loss of airway – false lumen, hemorrhage, loss of surgical plane; airway fire; Stoma – infection, hemorrhage, granuloma; Tracheo-innominate fistula – hemorrhage 7 days post-operative; laryngeal injury; tracheal stenosis

Transsphenoidal Surgery

1. Mass effects
    a. Neurologic impairment (bitemporal hemianopsia)
    b. Raised ICP (rare, but possible if causes obstructive hydrocephalus)
2. Neurohormonal effects / Endocrinopathies
    a. Non-functional adenomas
    b. Endocrine deficiencies 2° mass – Panhypopituitarism
        i. (G, L, F, T, A, P) -Go Look For The Adenoma Pleasell
    c. Hypersecretory tumors - 60% (prolactin > GH > ACTH, TSH rare)
        i. Cushing 's, acromegaly
3. Surgical Issues / Complications
    a. Head up positioning-Poor pt & airway access, bleeding (throat pack), VAE risk
    b. Neurologic injury- optic nerve or chiasm, cranial nerves III, IV, V, VI
    c. Potential for massive, difficult to access hemorrhage - cavernous sinus involvement
    d. Post-operative endocrine dysfunction (DI 40%), CSF leak/meningitis risk
    e. Crisp emergence-min coughing, N/V

Anesthetic Goals/Conflicts:

- Optimize perioperative endocrine function (stress dose steroids), consult endocrinology
- Assess and manage any increase. ICP, avoiding aggravating factors
- Controlled emergence (minimizing bucking / coughing / vomiting to decrease the risk of bleeding and CSF leak
  Monitor for postoperative complications e.g.: DI (40%)

Hx & Px: signs of ICP (a.m. headache, N/V), mass effects (VF defects – bitemporal hemianopsia), &pituitary deficiency (most non-functional with Sx of
Hyposecretion in the order (Go Look for The Adenoma Please)

Hypersecretory prevalence (Please Get Active Tumors). Prolactin - galactorrhea, amenorrhea, dec libido/ impotence; GH - Acromegaly; ACTH - Cushing 's Dz; Endo/neurosurgeon consults

Inv: CBC, Lytes, Glucose, BUN, Cr, Group & Screen, (look for anemia, ↓/↑glycemia, electrolyte abnormalities, ↓Na 2° to hypocortisolemia, DI, SIADH, renal insufficiency), Ca – r/o ↑Ca (MEN type I), TSH, T4, ACTH, cortisol level, insulin-like growth factor-1, testosterone, LH, PRL, βHCG –for women with amenorrhea prior to surgery. CT (tumor: Sella turcica or suprasellar, mass effects, ICP) Stage I: microadenoma (<1 cm) no Sella expansion Stage II-IV: macroadenoma (>1 cm) may extend beyond Sella

Optimization: Endocrine consult, hydrocortisone 50-100 mg pre-induction & historically q6-8h until weaned postop (consider Dex), antibiotic prophylaxis against meningitis, PONV prophylaxis

Anesthetic Options: GETA and NMB for microsurgery

Room Setup: CAS monitors + 5lead, A-line, Large bore IV, Foley to monitor DI (40%), throat pack, VAE risk (precordial Doppler, atrial CVC/Bunegin), +/- Lumbar drain (↑ surgical exposure/↓CSF leak)

Intraoperative Management: FOB if acromegaly or Cushing 's (difficult ventilation / intubation); oral RAE ETT (smaller if acromegaly). Balanced technique, TIVA if VEPs monitored (or MAC < 0.8, but VEPs sensitive to volatile), no nitrous oxide (pneumocephalus, VAE), NMB ensures patient still. Crisp emergence for neuro assessment. No bucking/coughing/vomiting), remove throat pack & suction carefully +/- laryngoscopy

Complications: Intraoperative – VAE, massive hemorrhage – venous vs. arterial, CN damage, thrombosis & CVA; Post-operative – DI (40%), SIADH (usually delayed), Adrenal insufficiency(CV collapse – steroid coverage), Bleeding (increase. ICP, brainstem compression, CN dysfunction), CSF leak (risk of meningitis, consider lumbar drain), hypothalamic injury, cerebral ischemia, Stroke

Transtracheal Jet Ventilation

Considerations:

1. Typically, emergency situation with potential hypoxia/hypercarbia
2. Generally difficult airway with potential for abnormal airway anatomy
3. Potential complications: pneumothorax, decreased cardiac output, ALI, subcutaneous emphysema with loss of airway
4. Need for subsequent definitive management

Big take home points:

Temporizing maneuver only

Need to ensure adequate exhalation of gas (**place oral/nasal airway and maintain jawthrust**) Monitor closely for changes in hemodynamics, signs of barotrauma

Contraindications:

Complete upper airway obstruction

Chronic pulmonary disease (particularly bullous lung disease)

Severe CAD or other cardiac conditions which might result in an exaggerated drop in cardiac outputSevere obesity

Complications: Catheter kinking, local hemorrhage, subcutaneous/mediastinal emphysema, esophageal injury,
pneumothorax

Where it fits in difficult airway algorithm:

If unable to BVM and unable to ventilate with LMA then this is a temporizing maneuver while further airway tools, surgical equipment and surgeon are mobilized.

How to do it:

- Extend neck (roll under neck)
- Identify cricothyroid membrane
- Add 15° bend to distal 2.5 cm of 12-16'IV catheter
- Attach 20 cc syringe (± fluid)
- 12-16'IV catheter inserted 30° caudad off the perpendicular throughcricothyroid membrane
- Once in trachea remove needle thread 14'catheter to hub
- Reconfirm position by aspirating air
- Connect to oxygen source (commercial jet ventilator, E cylinder, anesthesia machine.
- Ventilate with 1:1 IE ratio if using E cylinder, titrate to chest movement if using commercial jet ventilator

Trauma

1) C-Spine/TBI
2) Aspiration risk
3) Potential for multisystem injury (and occult injuries)
4) Hypovolemia
5) Hypothermia
6) Potential toxic ingestion

Anesthetic Goals/Conflicts:

- ATLS resuscitation
    - ABCDE, Monitors, IV access, Volume resuscitation – look for end points SBP > 100, HR <100, UO > 0.5ml/kg/hr, decreasing lactate, reverse acidosis
- Normal INR, PTT, maintain platelets > 50, normal serum Ca
- Temperature > 35
- Aspiration risk vs C-spine injury
- RSI in hypovolemic patient
- C-spine injury in uncooperative/combative patient (airway management)

Hx: AMPLE, mech of injury (high energy? E.g., ejection, ped struck, motorcycle, >100 km/hour, fatality at scene…)

Px: Rapid primary assessment. Vitals + temperature, airway patency, trachea (midline), ensure c-spine stabilization, JVP, flail segment obvious, AE bilateral/adequate (i.e., quickly rule out airway obstruction, flail chest, massive hemo, open pneumo, tension pneumo), adequacy of peripheral perfusion, quality of heart sounds (tamponade). Then secondary survey looking for pulmonary contusion, simple pneumo, tracheobronchial injury, aortic disruption, esophageal injury (traversingmediastinal injury), myocardial contusion. Ensure appropriate lines and adjuncts being used (e.g., foley etc....). Assess for evidence of occult bleeding (abdominal, femurs...), long bone fractures and assess measures to control hemorrhage. Eventually log roll looking for hidden injuries including Thoracolumbar spine.

Investigations: C-spine, Trauma labs (CBC, Coags, ABG, Lytes, Bun, Cr, Tox Screen, crossmatch, Calcium (if transfusing), CXR (although many of above injuries should not wait for CXR), C-spinefilms (plain film +/- CT), CT chest/Abd/head… depending on site of trauma, Angio or Echo depending on clinical findings

Optimization: See goals above. Aspiration prophylaxis.

Room setup: CAS + 5. Art line, CVP (minor trauma may not require), foley, SCDs, fluid warmer +/- rapid infuser, warming blanket, TEE only for special circumstances (e.g., significant myocardial contusion or aortic dissection). Severe hypothermia may require active rewarming (veno-veno) and correction of metabolic/hematologic status prior to surgical management.

Anesthetic options: Regional requires euvolemia and correction of coagulation and metabolic status. As result, a GA is generally indicated.

Intraoperative management: Anticipate exaggerated response to induction. Intraoperatively, goals are unchanged. Aggressive prevention/treatment of hypothermia, acidosis, hypovolemia… Watch for fat emboli, particularly in patient with significant pulmonary injury.

Postoperative disposition: High dependency unit.

Traumatic Brain injury & Increased ICP

1. Etiology of increase ICP
   - mass, edema, hemorrhage
2. Monitor & manage increase ICP
   - risk of cerebral ischemia and herniation
3. Prevention of secondary brain injury
4. Complications
   - Seizures, neurogenic pulmonary edema, myocardial dysfunction, DIC, DI, SIADH
5. Considerations of trauma
   - Emergency, Aspiration risk, HD instability, C-spine precautions, life-threatening injuries – overt & occult, intoxication/uncooperative

Anesthetic Goals/Conflicts:

- Conflicts
  - awake intubation (difficult airway, C-spine) vs. increase ICP
  - HD unstable (abruption, hemorrhage) vs. increase. ICP
  - Non-neurosurgical procedure with coexisting increase. ICP
- Prevent secondary brain injury
  - avoid hypoxia, hypercarbia, hyperglycemia, hyperthermia
  - maintain CPP (60 mmHg), Hgb
  - elevated HOB
- Avoid abrupt increase in BP and ICP

Hx: AMPLE, Etiology of injury/increase. ICP (trauma = ATLS), Stable or unstable, current ICPmanagement, symptoms, identify occult injuries

PE: If trauma, primary & secondary survey, C-Spine precautions, **GCS**, pupils, basal skull #, Cushing 's response (HTN, brady), irregular breathing, focal neurologic signs

Inv: CBC, G&S, lytes, urea, Cr, serum osmolality, INR, PTT, ABG to assess $ETCO_2$ gradient

Imaging: CXR, C-spine film, +/-pelvic X-ray, CT head (+/- C-spine), FAST U/S (CT) if unstable

Optimization: Secure airway, mild hyperventilation → $PaCO_2$ 30 – 35 mmHg, promote venous drainage (elevated HOB, head in neutral position), diuresis: mannitol 0.5-1 g/kg, furosemide 0.25-0.5 mg/kg, consider hypertonic saline: 5 cc/kg 3%, or 2 cc/kg 7.5%, secondary prevention(normothermia, normoglycemia, normocapnia, sodium), ensure adequate resuscitation, large bore IV access, blood products, surgical decompression/EVD

Anesthetic Options: GA

Room Setup: CAS (5 lead EKG), A-line, CVP, temperature, foley, ICP monitoring, CSF drain, vasoactive agents, ICP agents (mannitol, Lasix), BIS monitor for assessment of function (SR ratio)

Intraoperative Management: Secure airway (RSI vs. awake vs. primary surgical) c-spine precautions, cricoid is controversial, avoid ketamine and N_2O. Suxamethonium. TIVA (prop/remi) preferred over inhalational agents. IV/ tracheal lidocaine. Maintain CPP 60mmHg (MAP ~ 90mmHg), don 'tdelay for monitoring

Post-operative: may keep intubated and ventilated to ICU, or smooth rapid emergence for neuroassessment. Monitor and manage DI/SIADH

Complications: increase. ICP/herniation (diuretics, coma, NdMB, craniectomy), DIC, SIADH/DI, myocardial dysfunction, Seizures, ARDS, ICU prophylaxis (ulcer, DVT)

TURP & TURP Syndrome

2. Coexisting disease common in this population
    - IHD, ARF (post-renal), elderly
3. Considerations of intraoperative complications
    - TURP syndrome (2%)
        - Fluid overload & pulmonary edema; electrolyte abnormalities; hyperglycinemia, hyperammonemia
    - Concealed hemorrhage (avg. 2-4 cc/min, but 2.5% require PRBCs)
    - Dysrhythmias (1%)
    - Hypothermia
    - Bladder perforation – 1%
    - Septicemia (usually gram negative)
    - DIC (rare complication associated with prostate cancer)
4. Positioning: Lithotomy → Nerve Injury; Trendelenburg → CVS/Pulmonary effects

Anesthetic Goals/Conflicts:

- Optimization of co-existing diseases
- Prevention or early recognition of TURP syndrome
- Attention to blood loss and appropriate replacement
- Conflict: preference for neuraxial technique to monitor CNS symptoms vscontraindications to neuraxial

Hx: Headache, N/V, agitation, visual changes, dLOC are signs of TURP syndrome. Pre-operative hx: AMPLE with focus on comorbidities and discussion re:neuraxial anesthesia

PE: Standard pre-anesthetic physical: vitals, CVS (JVP, Arrhythmia), Mental status, respiratory, back.

Investigations: Lytes (hyponatremia, hyperkalemia), CBC (hemolytic anemia), ABG, Creatinine,coags, Serum osmolality, ammonium, T&S, ECG, +/- echo,

Optimization: As indicated by pre-operative assessment, blood available if prostate >40g, Prostaticstenting with laser treatment is an alternative

Anesthetic Options: GA (respiratory support, contraindication to regional), Regional (SAB to T9-10 has advantage of detecting CNS changes, pain with bladder perforation – suprapubic (extraperitoneal) or upper abdominal (intraperitoneal)pain

Room Setup: Emergency drugs, CAS + 5-lead, temperature probe, CVP, A-line if severe co-existing disease

Intraoperative Management: Regional: T9-10, Lithotomy position →physiologic changes, nerve palsies.
TURP Syndrome: hypertension, bradycardia and mental status changes are classic triad.
Respiratory: pulmonary edema, elevated JVP; CVS: arrhythmias, hypotension later; CNS: pupillary reflex sluggish or absent with glycine toxicity but intact with cerebral edema.
Prevention: appropriate irrigation agent, minimize resection time, hemostasis, avoid high irrigating pressures (limit bag height to 30-40cm, frequent drainage), avoid hypotonic IV fluids, check lytes in Pts with CRF, metabolic abnormalities (hyponatremia).
Treatment: Early recognize, inform surgeon, ABC Approach. Consider invasive monitoring, Investigations (Lytes, BUN, Cr, glucose, CBC, ABG, ECG) Treat Hyponatremia, diuresis with furosemide, hypertonic saline (1-2ml/kg/hour do not correct >1.5mEq/L/Hour). Sz – midazolam, STP, Propofol, consider phenytoin 10-20mg/kg load;

Post-operative: for severe cases: ICU, q1h blood work

Special: Problems in PAR include: post-operative delirium, hypotension, respiratory distress. Need toconsider these patients 'comorbidities. (See seminar)

Twins

1. Parturient
   a. Exaggerated physiologic changes of pregnancy
2. Increased risk for maternal/fetal complications
   a. preterm labour; uterine atony and PPH, PIH; fetal distress (especially in 2Nd neonate), fetal abnormalities (T-T transfusion), malpresentation and cord prolapsed
3. Management for twin delivery:
   a. monitoring of 2 fetuses; resus equips for 2 neonates; possible need for C/S or forceps

Anesthetic Goals/Conflicts:

1. Early labour epidural
2. Maintain adequate maternal and uteroplacental hemodynamics

Hx: Standard anaesthetic history, previous obstetrical hx and any problems with current pregnancy, current gestation; Fetal history: number, recent US, position, lung maturity etc.

PE: good airway exam, Vitals, cardiopulmonary exam

Investigations: CBC, diff, coags, review U/S report(s)

Optimization: labour epidural in place early

Room Setup: standard, monitoring for multiple fetuses

Intraoperative Management: Method of delivery depends on presentation of fetuses; Indication for C-section if: Twin A presentation is breech or shoulder, twin-twin transfusion, discordant growth, congenital abnormalities.
Higher risk for emergent C/S; Management as for any OB patient with monitoring for 2 and LUD is especially important; Large IV for risk of PPH; Epidural better than spinal if long C-section is predicted.

Post-operative: Increased risk for PPH.

Special: Multiple gestation puts mom and babies at increased risk for just about every possible complication of pregnancy. For the list, see the seminar.

Vasculitis

Classified as large, medium and small vessel.

1. Multisystem disease with end-organ dysfunction:
    - CNS: encephalopathy, vision
    - Lung: Pulmonary hemorrhage, cavitation
    - CVS: Aortitis, ischemia from arterial stenosis (claudication, cerebral, RAS, CHF)
    - Kidney: renal failure
2. Medications:
    - Immunosuppressive drugs and end organ damage
    - Steroids and need for stress dosing

Anesthetic Goals/Conflicts:

- Diagnosis by angiography/biopsy
- Consider short course of steroids, immunosuppressants or cytotoxic agents for symptomatic dx

Failure to Wean DDx

1. CNS: Pain / Anxiety
2. Respiratory Mechanics
3. Lung Parenchymal or AW obstruction
4. Primary Cardiac
5. Neuromuscular weakness

Anesthetic Goals/Conflicts:

- Treat pain and anxiety
- R/O Cardiac etiology: Systolic or Diastolic dysfunction
- R/O Neuromuscular weakness: Adequate nutrition, Electrolytes, Phosphate, assess diaphragmfunction.
- R/O lung parenchymal issues: ABG, CXR
- R/O other factors impairing respiratory mechanics i.e. Abd Compartment Syndrome.

Wegner's Granulomatosis

1. Potential difficult aorway
   a. Laryngeal stenosis, friable bleeding tissue (gentle, small ETT)
2. Multisystem granulomatous disease:
   a. CNS: cerebral aneurysm 's, peripheral neuropathy
   b. CVS: Cardiac valve destruction, abn conduction, myocardial ischemia
   c. Respiratory: Sinusitis, laryngeal stenosis, epiglottic destruction, VQ mismatch, pneumonia, hemoptysis, bronchial destruction
   d. Renal: Hematuria, Azotemia, progressive renal failure
3. Possible contraindication to arterial line due to peripheral arteritis
4. Consideration for medical therapy and immunosuppressants:
   a. Cyclophosphamide (decreases plasma cholinesterase) = mainstay of treatment

Anesthetic Goals/Conflicts:

- Careful airway management
- Document neurologic deficits prior to regional techniques

Wide Complex Tachycardia

- Anesthetic emergency with the need to simultaneously diagnose and treat using ACLS treatment algorithm.
- Consider the multiple aetiologies
- Consider cardiology consult if applicable

Anesthetic Goals/Conflicts:

- Get early help, call a code
- Notify surgeon and nursing staff, IV, O2 monitor….
- Stable vs Unstable: meds and maneuvers vs. immediate synchronized cardioversion
- Cycle monitors with differential diagnosis in mind

WPW

1. Potential for acute SVT, VF, sudden cardiac death and hemodynamic compromise or collapse
    a. ACLS, Defibrillation, Adenosine (if no atrial fib or flutter), Global antiarrhythmics (amiodarone, procainamide)
2. Avoid sympathetic stimulation/tachycardia-anxiety, hypovolemia, ketamine
3. Atrial fibrillation and/or atrial flutter
    a. Avoid AV nodal blockers – adenosine, BB, CCB, digoxin
4. Comorbidities
    a. Epstein's anomaly

Anesthetic Goals/Conflicts:

- Identify patients with WPW
- Avoid increased SNS activity, a fib/flutter and AV nodal blocking drigs (BB, CCB, Dig)
    - enhanced anterograde conduction through the accessory pathways
- Be prepared to treat tachydysrhythmias with cardioversion, or drugs – amiodarone, procainamide infusion (10 mg/kg at 20 mg/min)

Hx: AMPLE, syncope, palpitations, FMHx sudden death, previous arrhythmias / treatments

Investigations: lytes Mg, ECG: delta wave, short PR, widened QRS (antegrade conduction)

Optimization: continue antiarrhythmic agents (maintain NSR) unless EP studies, anxiolytics pre-operative

Room Setup: procainamide, amiodarone, anxiolysis, Crash cart, defib pads,

Intraoperative Management: avoid ketamine and pancuronium; avoid volatiles if ablation procedures – increase. accessory pathway refractory time; caution with atropine, glycopyrrolate (tachycardia), ensure adequate analgesia; Cardiac monitored bed post-operative

Special:

- only a worry when the accessory pathway conducts Atrium → Ventricle AND when the patient goes into AFIB or A-Flutter
    - risk that the rapid atrial rate can be conducted into the ventricle and result in hemodynamic collapse from VFIB/Flutter
    - AV node maximal conduction rate = ~ 220 – Pt 's age
    - Accessory pathway maximal conduction rate = NO MAXIMUM
- ECG – very rapid, wide complex tachy (resembling V-tach) with irregular ventricular complexes
- In this situation, **you should avoid AV nodal blocking drugs** (adenosine, BB, CCB, Dig) asthis may result in the impulses being transmitted down the accessory pathway

Safe to use global antiarrhythmics or cardioversion - Amiodarone (adult dose 150 mg bolus, Peds 5mg/kgover 20 min), Procainamide (may get transient increase conduction through AV node before blocking down) (adult dose is 10mg/kg IV over 15min, peds 15mg/kg)

Wrist Block and Hand Block (Never use Epi!)

Indications: For surgery on hands and fingers, no specific contraindications: contraindication to brachial plexus blockade: rescue of incomplete brachial plexus block

Complications: Minimal, hematoma/infection/nerve injury possible, wrist tourniquet well tolerated Duration Lido 2% ~ 2-5hrs, Bupivacaine 0.5% 5-15 hrs. Use 4-6 ml per nerve! Onset10-15mins

Median Nerve: Located bw flexor carpi radialis and Palmaris longus. At the level of the wrist, the motorbranch has already left posteriorly, therefore can 't use nerve stims! Inject at the level of the ulnar styloid process at a depth of 1.5 cm (fascial pop) bw the two tendons. (3-4ml).

Ulnar Nerve: Lies bw ulnar artery and flexi carpi ulnaris. Volar approach: at the level of the styloid, inject3 mls bw ulnar artery and FCU tendon. For ulnar approach: Introduce from the ulnar side of the tendon approx. 5- 10mm past tendon, inject 3-5ml. Can elicit paresthesia's or use N. Stim (only one!) Can also inject 2-3mls above tendon which blocks cutaneous branches which branch off 5cm above styloid.

Radial Nerve: Sensory block only, field block at the anatomic snuff box made by extensor pollicuslongus and EP brevis. Inject using 2 injections in an -X‖ shape. 4-6ml.

Digital Nerve Blocks: For surgery on fingers, 2-3 ml per side, do not use epinephrine!

The main digital nerves are derived from median and ulnar nerves, accompanied by digital vessels and run on the ventrolateral aspect of the finger. Small dorsal digital nerves run on the dorsolateral aspect of the finger and supply innervations to the back of the fingers as far as the proximal joint. (4 small nerves atthe base of each corner)

Technique: 25G 1.5‖ A 23- to 25-gauge needle is inserted at the medial and lateral aspects of the baseof the selected digit. A total of 2–3 mL of local anesthetic without epinephrine is injected on eachside near the periosteum.

Complications: Nerve injury is primary complication
Therefore, avoid epinephrine

References:

1. http://www.ncepod.org.uk/reports.htm. Abdominal Aortic Aneurysm: A service in need of surgery? Published in 2005 by the National Confidential Enquiry into Patient Outcome and Death.
2. Hirsch AT, Haskal ZJ, Hertzer NR et al. ACC/AHA 2005 Practice Guidelines for the management of patients with peripheral arterial disease. Circulation 2006;113(11):e463-654
3. Berkowitz ID, Raja SN, Bender KS, et al. Dwarfs: pathophysiology and anesthetic implications. Anesthesiology. 1990;73(4):739-759.
4. Cevik B, Colakoglu S. Anesthetic management of achondroplastic dwarf undergoing cesarean section—a case report.Middle East J Anaesthesiol. 2010:20(6):907-910.
5. Jain A, Jain K, Makkar JK, et al. Anaesthetic management of an achondroplastic dwarf undergoing radical nephrectomy—a case report.South Afr J Anaesth Analg. 2010;16(2):77-79.
6. Krishnan BS, Eipe N, Korula G. Anaesthetic management of a patient with achondroplasia. Paediatr Anaesth. 2003;13(6):547-549.
7. Mayhew JF, Katz J, Miner M, et al. Anaesthesia for the achondroplastic dwarf.Can Anaesth Soc J. 1986;33(2):216-221.
8. Oppitz F, Speulda E. Anesthesia recommendations for patients suffering from achondroplasia.orpha.net/data/patho/Pro/en/ Achondroplasia_EN.pdf. Accessed June 30, 2015.
9. Mitra S, Dey N, Gomber KK. Emergency cesarean section in a patient with achondroplasia: an anesthetic dilemma.J Anesth Clin Pharmacol. 2007;23(3):315-318.
10. Tetzlaff J, Benedetto P. Skin and bone disorders. In: Fleisher L, ed.Anesthesia and Uncommon Diseases, 6th Edition. Philadelphia, PA: Saunders; 2012.
11. R.A. Leslie, E.K. Johnson, G. Thomas, and A.P.L. Goodwin, (2011). Anaesthesia for craniotomy. Dr Podcast Scripts for the Final FRCA (pp. 242 – 248). Cambridge University Press, New York, USA.
12. G. Edward Morgan, Maged. S Mikhail, and Michael J. Murray. (2006, 2002). Anesthesia for Neurosurgery. Clinical Anesthesiology Fourth edition (pp. 631 – 647). New York, Chicago, San Francisco, Lisbon, London, Madrid, Mexico City, M i l a n New Delhi, San Juan, Seoul, Sydney, and Toronto: Lange Medical Books/ McC
13. J. B ... linical Ana ... : Can
14. http: ... al-sign
15. Add ... sease and othe ... omms/ publ ... Scholar
16. Alpć ... -Lamy sync ... d Oral Patl ... .06.023. [Pul
17. Arn ... patients with ... ediatr. 200 ... ef] [Google Sch
18. Arn ... patients with mucopolysaccharidosis I: findings from the MPS I Registry. J Pediatr Surg. 2012;47:477–484. doi: 10.1016/j.jpedsurg.2011.09.042. [PubMed] [CrossRef]

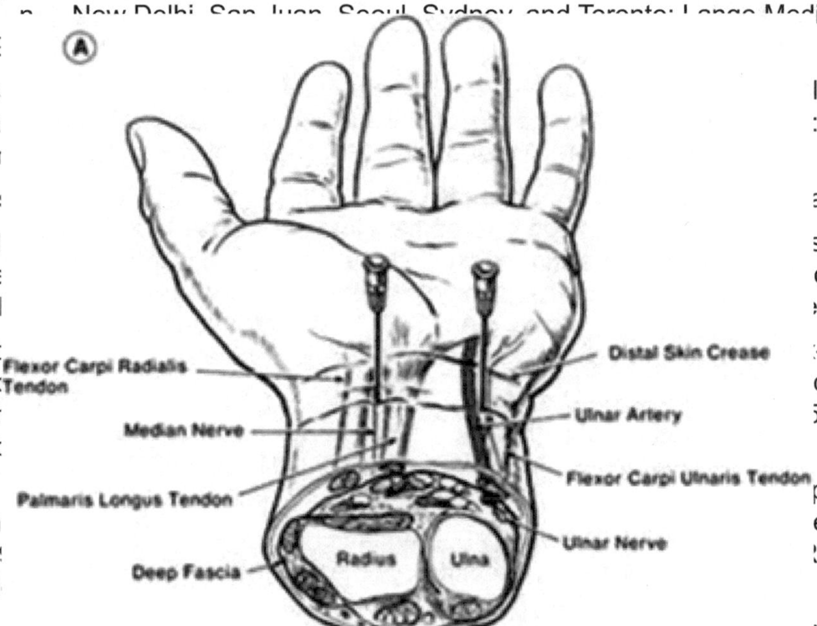

[Google Scholar]

19. Belani KG, Krivit W, Carpenter BLM, et al. Children with mucopolysaccharidosis: perioperative care, morbidity, mortality, and new findings. J Pediatr Surg. 1993;28:403–408. doi: 10.1016/0022-3468(93)90240-L. [PubMed] [CrossRef] [Google Scholar]

20. Bonow RO, Carabello BA, Chatterjee K, et al. 2008 focused update incorporated into the ACC/AHA 2006 guidelines for the management of patients with valvular heart disease: a report of the American College of Cardiology/American Heart Association Task Force on Practice Guidelines (Writing Committee to Revise the 1998 Guidelines for the Management of Patients With Valvular Heart Disease): endorsed by the Society of Cardiovascular Anesthesiologists, Society for Cardiovascular Angiography and Interventions, and Society of Thoracic Surgeons. Circulation. 2008;118:e523–e661. doi: 10.1161/CIRCULATIONAHA.108.190748. [PubMed] [CrossRef] [Google Scholar]

21. Braunlin EA, Hunter DW, Krivit W, et al. Evaluation of coronary artery disease in the Hurler syndrome by angiography. Am J Cardiol. 1992;69:1487–1489. doi: 10.1016/0002-9149(92)90908-H. [PubMed] [CrossRef] [Google Scholar]

22. Braunlin EA, Harmatz PR, Scarpa M, et al. Cardiac disease in patients with mucopolysaccharidosis: presentation, diagnosis and management. J Inherit Metab Dis. 2011;34:1183–1197. doi: 10.1007/s10545-011-9359-8.[PMC free article] [PubMed] [CrossRef] [Google Scholar]

23. Buhain WJ, Rammohan G, Berger HW. Pulmonary function in Morquio's disease: a study of two siblings. Chest. 1975;68:41–45. doi: 10.1378/chest.68.1.41. [PubMed] [CrossRef] [Google Scholar]

24. Dangel JH. Cardiovascular changes in children with mucopolysaccharide storage diseases and related disorders - clinical and echocardiographic findings in 64 patients. Eur J Pediatr. 1998;157:534–538. doi: 10.1007/s004310050872.[PubMed] [CrossRef] [Google Scholar]

25. Dilber E, Celiker A, Karagöz T, Kalkanoglu HS. Permanent transfemoral pacemaker implantation in a child with Maroteaux Lamy syndrome. Pacing Clin Electrophysiol. 2002;25:1784–1785. doi: 10.1046/j.1460-9592.2002.01784.x.[PubMed] [CrossRef] [Google Scholar]

26. Fesslová V, Corti P, Sersale G, et al. The natural course and the impact of therapies of cardiac involvement in the mucopolysaccharidoses. Cardiol Young. 2009;19:170–178. doi: 10.1017/S1047951109003576. [PubMed] [CrossRef] [Google Scholar]

27. Fleisher LA, Beckman JA, Brown KA, et al. 2009 ACCF/AHA focused update on perioperative beta blockade incorporated into the ACC/AHA 2007 guidelines on perioperative cardiovascular evaluation and care for noncardiac surgery: a report of the American College of Cardiology Foundation/American Heart Association Task Force on Practice Guidelines. J Am Coll Cardiol. 2009;54:e13–e118. doi: 10.1016/j.jacc.2009.07.010.[PubMed] [CrossRef] [Google Scholar]

28. Frawley G, Fuenzalida D, Donath S, Yaplito-Lee J, Peters H (2012) A retrospective audit of anesthetic techniques and complications in children with mucopolysaccharidoses. Pediatr Anesth. doi:10.1111/j.1460-9592.2012.03825.x [PubMed]

29. Giugliani R, Harmatz P, Wraith JE. Management guidelines for mucopolysaccharidosis VI. Pediatrics. 2007;120:405–418. doi: 10.1542/peds.2006-2184. [PubMed] [CrossRef] [Google Scholar]

30. Hirth A, Berg A, Greve G. Successful treatment of severe heart failure in an infant with Hurler syndrome. J Inherit Metab Dis. 2007;30:820. doi: 10.1007/s10545-007-0613-z.[PubMed] [CrossRef] [Google Scholar]

31. Hishitani T, Wakita S, Isoda T, Katori T, Ishizawa A, Okada R. Sudden death in Hunter syndrome caused by complete atrioventricular block. J Pediatr. 2000;136:268–269. doi: 10.1016/S0022-3476(00)70117-X. [PubMed] [CrossRef] [Google Scholar]

32. Ingelmo PM, Parini R, Grimaldi M, et al. Multidetector computed tomography (MDCT) for preoperative airway assessment in children with mucopolysaccharidoses. Minerva Anestesiol. 2011;77:774–780. [PubMed] [Google Scholar]

33. Jeong HS, Cho DY, Ahn KM, Jin DK. Complications of tracheotomy in patients with mucopolysaccharidoses type II (Hunter syndrome) Int J Pediatr Otorhinolaryngol. 2006;70:1765–1769. doi: 10.1016/j.ijporl.2006.05.021.[PubMed] [CrossRef] [Google Scholar]

34. John A, Fagondes S, Schwartz I, et al. Sleep abnormalities in untreated patients with mucopolysaccharidosis type VI. Am J Med Genet A. 2011;155A:1546–1551. [PubMed] [Google Scholar]

35. Kamin W. Diagnosis and management of respiratory involvement in Hunter syndrome. Acta Paediatr Suppl. 2008;97:57–60. doi: 10.1111/j.1651-2227.2008.00650.x.[PubMed] [CrossRef] [Google Scholar]

36. Kimball TR. Pediatric stress echocardiography. Pediatr Cardiol. 2002;23:347–357. doi: 10.1007/s00246-001-0198-5.[PubMed] [CrossRef] [Google Scholar]

37. Kirkpatrick K, Ellwood J, Walker RWM. Mucopolysaccharidosis type I (Hurler syndrome) and anesthesia: the impact of bone marrow transplantation, enzyme replacement therapy, and fiberoptic intubation on airway management. Paediatr Anaesth. 2012;22:745–751. doi: 10.1111/j.1460-9592.2012.03897.x. [PubMed] [CrossRef] [Google Scholar]

38. Kurdi MS, Deshpande SS. Mucopolysaccharidoses—an adventurous anaesthetic encounter. Indian J Anaesth. 2008;52:453– 458. [Google Scholar]

39. Leal GN, de Paula AC, Leone C, Kim CA. Echocardiographic study of paediatric patients with mucopolysaccharidosis. Cardiol Young. 2010;20:254–261. doi: 10.1017/S104795110999062X. [PubMed] [CrossRef] [Google Scholar]

40. Leighton SEJ, Papsin B, Vellodi A, Dinwiddie R, Lane R. Disordered breathing during sleep in patients with mucopolysaccharidoses. Int J Pediatr Otorhinolaryngol. 2001;58:127–138. doi: 10.1016/S0165-5876(01)00417-7.[PubMed] [CrossRef] [Google Scholar]

41. Linstedt U, Maier C, Joehnk H, Stephani U. Threatening spinal cord compression during anesthesia in a child with mucopolysaccharidosis VI. Anesthesiology. 1994;80:227–229. doi: 10.1097/00000542-199401000-00034. [PubMed] [CrossRef] [Google Scholar]

42. Martins AM, Dualibi AP, Norato D, et al. Guidelines for the management of mucopolysaccharidosis type I. J Pediatr. 2009;155:S32– S46. doi: 10.1016/j.jpeds.2009.07.005.[PubMed] [CrossRef] [Google Scholar]

43. McLaughlin AM, Farooq M, Donnelly MB, Foley K. Anaesthetic considerations of adults with Morquio's syndrome—a case report. BMC Anesthesiol. 2010;10:2. doi: 10.1186/1471-2253-10-2. [PMC free article] [PubMed] [CrossRef] [Google Scholar]

44. Mendelsohn NJ, Harmatz P, Bodamer O, et al. Importance of surgical history in diagnosing mucopolysaccharidosis type II (Hunter syndrome): data from the Hunter Outcome Survey. Genet Med. 2010;12:816–822. doi: 10.1097/GIM.0b013e3181f6e74d. [PubMed] [CrossRef] [Google Scholar]

45. Miller G, Partridge A. Mucopolysaccharidosis type VI presenting in infancy with endocardial fibroelastosis and heart failure. Pediatr Cardiol. 1983;4:61–62. doi:

10.1007/BF02281012. [PubMed] [CrossRef] [Google Scholar]

46. Misumi I, Chikazawa S, Ishitsu T, et al. Atrioventricular block and diastolic dysfunction in a patient with Sanfilippo C. Intern Med. 2010;49:2313–2316. doi: 10.2169/internalmedicine.49.4210. [PubMed] [CrossRef] [Google Scholar]

47. Mohan UR, Hay AA, Cleary MA, Wraith JE, Patel RG. Cardiovascular changes in children with mucopolysaccharide disorders. Acta Paediatr. 2002;91:799–804. doi: 10.1111/j.1651-2227.2002.tb03330.x. [PubMed] [CrossRef] [Google Scholar]

48. Moores C, Rogers JG, McKenzie IM, Brown TCK. Anaesthesia for children with mucopolysaccharidoses. Anaesth Intensive Care. 1996;24:459–463. [PubMed] [Google Scholar]

49. Muenzer J. Overview of the mucopolysaccharidoses. Rheumatology (Oxford) 2011;50(Suppl 5):v4–v12. doi: 10.1093/rheumatology/ker394. [PubMed] [CrossRef] [Google Scholar]

50. Muhlebach MS, Wooten W, Muenzer J. Respiratory manifestations in mucopolysaccharidoses. Paediatr Respir Rev. 2011;12:133–138. doi: 10.1016/j.prrv.2010.10.005.[PubMed] [CrossRef] [Google Scholar]

51. Murgu SD, Colt HG. Tracheobronchomalacia and excessive dynamic airway collapse. Respirology. 2006;11:388–406. doi: 10.1111/j.1440-1843.2006.00862.x. [PubMed] [CrossRef] [Google Scholar]

52. Myer CM., III Airway obstruction in Hurler's syndrome–radiographic features. Int J Pediatr Otorhinolaryngol. 1991;22:91–96. doi: 10.1016/0165-5876(91)90101-G. [PubMed] [CrossRef] [Google Scholar]

53. Nagano R, Takizawa S, Hayama N, et al. Three-dimensional CT and histopathological findings of airway malacia in Hunter syndrome. Tokai J Exp Clin Med. 2007;32:59–61.[PubMed] [Google Scholar]

54. Orchard PJ, Milla C, Braunlin E, et al. Pre-transplant risk factors affecting outcome in Hurler syndrome. Bone Marrow Transplant. 2010;45:1239–1246. doi: 10.1038/bmt.2009.319.[PubMed] [CrossRef] [Google Scholar]

55. Pelley CJ, Kwo J, Hess DR. Tracheomalacia in an adult with respiratory failure and Morquio syndrome. Respir Care. 2007;52:278– 282. [PubMed] [Google Scholar]

56. Ransford AO, Crockard HA, Stevens JM, Modaghegh S. Occipito-atlanto-axial fusion in Morquio-Brailsford syndrome. A ten-year experience. J Bone Joint Surg Br. 1996;78:307–313. [PubMed] [Google Scholar]

57. Rovelli AM. The controversial and changing role of haematopoietic cell transplantation for lysosomal storage disorders: an update. Bone Marrow Transplant. 2008;41(Suppl 2):S87–S89. doi: 10.1038/bmt.2008.62.[PubMed] [CrossRef] [Google Scholar]

58. Rowe R, Cohen RA. An evaluation of a virtual reality airway simulator. Anesth Analg. 2002;95:62–66. doi: 10.1097/00000539- 200207000-00011. [PubMed] [CrossRef] [Google Scholar]

59. Semenza GL, Pyeritz RE. Respiratory complications of mucopolysaccharide storage disorders. Medicine (Baltimore) 1988;67:209– 219. [PubMed] [Google Scholar]

60. Shih SL, Lee YJ, Lin SP, Sheu CY, Blickman JG. Airway changes in children with mucopolysaccharidoses. Acta Radiol. 2002;43:40–43. doi: 10.1034/j.1600-0455.2002.430108.x. [PubMed] [CrossRef] [Google Scholar]

61. Simmons MA, Bruce IA, Penney S, Wraith E, Rothera MP. Otorhinolaryngological manifestations of the mucopolysaccharidoses. Int J Pediatr Otorhinolaryngol. 2005;69:589–595. doi: 10.1016/j.ijporl.2005.01.017.[PubMed] [CrossRef] [Google

Scholar]

62. Sims HS, Kempiners JJ. Special airway concerns in patients with mucopolysaccharidoses. Respir Med. 2007;101:1779–1782. doi: 10.1016/j.rmed.2007.02.013. [PubMed] [CrossRef] [Google Scholar]

63. Tandon V, Williamson JB, Cowie RA, Wraith JE. Spinal problems in mucopolysaccharidosis I (Hurler syndrome) J Bone Joint Surg Br. 1996;78:938–944. doi: 10.1302/0301-620X78B6.1279. [PubMed] [CrossRef] [Google Scholar]

64. Theroux MC, Nerker T, Ditro C, Mackenzie WG. Anesthetic care and perioperative complications of children with Morquio syndrome. Paediatr Anaesth. 2012;22:901–907. doi: 10.1111/j.1460-9592.2012.03904.x. [PubMed] [CrossRef] [Google Scholar]

65. Thorne JA, Javadpour M, Hughes DG, et al. Craniovertebral abnormalities in Type VI mucopolysaccharidosis (Maroteaux-Lamy syndrome) Neurosurgery. 2001;48:849–852. [PubMed] [Google Scholar]

66. Valayannopoulos V, Nicely H, Harmatz P, Turbeville S. Mucopolysaccharidosis VI. Orphanet J Rare Dis. 2010;5:5. doi: 10.1186/1750- 1172-5-5. [PMC free article] [PubMed] [CrossRef] [Google Scholar]

67. Van den Broek L, Backx APCM, Coolen H, et al. Fatal coronary artery disease in an infant with severe mucopolysaccharidosis type I. Pediatrics. 2011;127:e1343–e1346. doi: 10.1542/peds.2009-2047. [PubMed] [CrossRef] [Google Scholar]

68. Walker RWM, Darowski M, Morris P, Wraith JE. Anaesthesia and mucopolysaccharidoses. A review of airway problems in children. Anaesthesia. 1994;49:1078–1084. doi: 10.1111/j.1365-2044.1994.tb04360.x. [PubMed] [CrossRef] [Google Scholar]

69. Walker RWM, Allen DL, Rothera MR. A fibreoptic intubation technique for children with mucopolysaccharidoses using the laryngeal mask airway. Paediatr Anaesth. 1997;7:421–426. doi: 10.1046/j.1460-9592.1997.d01-102.x. [PubMed] [CrossRef] [Google Scholar]

70. Walker PP, Rose E, Williams JG. Upper airways abnormalities and tracheal problems in Morquio's disease. Thorax. 2003;58:458–459. doi: 10.1136/thorax.58.5.458.[PMC free article] [PubMed] [CrossRef] [Google Scholar]

71. Walker RWM, Colovic V, Robinson DN, Dearlove OR. Postobstructive pulmonary oedema during anaesthesia in children with mucopolysaccharidoses. Paediatr Anaesth. 2003;13:441–447. doi: 10.1046/j.1460-9592.2003.00969.x.[PubMed] [CrossRef] [Google Scholar]

72. Wippermann CF, Beck M, Schranz D, Huth R, Michel-Behnke I, Jüngst BK. Mitral and aortic regurgitation in 84 patients with mucopolysaccharidoses. Eur J Pediatr. 1995;154:98–101. doi: 10.1007/BF01991908. [PubMed] [CrossRef] [Google Scholar]

73. Wold SM, Derkay CS, Darrow DH, Proud V. Role of the pediatric otolaryngologist in diagnosis and management of children with mucopolysaccharidoses. Int J Pediatr Otorhinolaryngol. 2010;74:27–31. doi: 10.1016/j.ijporl.2009.09.042. [PubMed] [CrossRef] [Google Scholar]

74. Wraith JE, Beck M, Giugliani R, Clarke J, Martin R, Muenzer J. Initial report from the Hunter Outcome Survey. Genet Med. 2008;10:508–516. doi: 10.1097/GIM.0b013e31817701e6. [PubMed] [CrossRef] [Google Scholar]

75. Kumar V, Abbas AK, Fausto N. Robbins and Cotran Pathologic Basis of Disease. 7th ed. St. Louis, Mo: WB Saunders; 2005. [Google Scholar]

76. 2. Tallgren M, Höckerstedt K, Isoniemi H, Orko R, Lindgren L. Intraoperative death in cardiac amyloidosis with increased QT dispersion in the electrocardiogram. Anesth Analg. 1995;80:1233–5. [PubMed] [Google Scholar]

77. 3. Kotani N, Hashimoto H, Muraoka M, Kabara S, Okawa H, Matsuki A. Fatal perioperative myocardial infarction in four patients with cardiac amyloidosis. Anesthesiology. 2000;92:8735.[PubMed] [Google Scholar]

78. 4. Wang MM, Pollard JB. Postoperative ventricular fibrillation and undiagnosed primary amyloidosis. Anesthesiology. 2000;92:871– 2.[PubMed] [Google Scholar]

79. 5. Weingarten TN, Hall BA, Richardson BF, Hofer RE, Sprung J. Periorbital ecchymoses during general anaesthesia in a patient with primary amyloidosis: A harbinger for bleeding? Anesth Analg. 2007;105:1561–3. [PubMed] [Google Scholar]

80. 6. Campos JH. A reaction to tape after tracheal extubation in a patient with systemic amyloidosis. J Clin Anesth. 1999;11:126– 8.[PubMed] [Google Scholar]

81. 7. Sucker C, Hetzel GR, Grabensee B, Stockschlaeder M, Scharf RE. Amyloidosis and bleeding: Pathophysiology, diagnosis, and therapy. Am J Kidney Dis. 2006;47:947–55. [PubMed] [Google Scholar]

82. 8. Blum A, Sohar E. The diagnosis of amyloidosis. Ancillary procedures. Lancet. 1962;1:721–4. [PubMed] [Google Scholar]

83. Stoelting's Anesthesia and Co-Existing Disease, Chapter 11, pg 262-263

84. https://www.openanesthesia.org/als-anesthetic-concerns/

85. Hepner DL, Castells MC. Latex allergy: An update. Anesth Analg 2003; 96:1219-29.

86. Katz JK, Holzman RS, Brown RH et al. Natural rubber latex allergy: considerations for anesthesiologists. http://www.asahq.org/publicationsAndServices/latexallergy.pdf

87. Walker I, Howard R. Latex allergy – perioperative management clinical guideline.

88. http://www.ich.ucl.ac.uk/clinical_information/clinical_guidelines/cmg_guideline_000 17

89. Rees S. Anaesthesia Tutorial of the week. Anaphylaxis. http://www.anaesthesiauk. com/article.aspx?articleid=100741

90. The Association of Anaesthetists of Great Britain and Ireland (2003) Suspected anaphylactic reactions associated with Anaesthesia. www.aagbi.org
6. Brown R, Schauble J, Hamilton R. Prevalence of latex allergy among anesthesiologists: Identification of sensitized but asymptomatic individuals. Anesthesiology. 1998; 89:287-89.

91. https://www.frca.co.uk/Documents/178%20Ankle%20block%20Landmark%20 and%20Ultrasound%20techniques%20LR.pdf

92. H Wulf Epidural anaesthesia and spinal haematoma. Can J Anaesth: 1996, 43(12);1260-71

93. K Robins, S Saravanan, E J Watkins Ankylosing spondylitis and epidural haematoma. Anaesthesia: 2005, 60(6);624-5

94. Y K Batra, A Sharma, S Rajeev Total spinal anaesthesia following epidural test dose in an ankylosing spondylitic patient with anticipated difficult airway undergoing total hip replacement. Eur J Anaesthesiol: 2006, 23(10);897-8

95. M Steffek, R Owczuk, M Szlyk-Augustyn, M Lasinska-Kowara, M Wujtewicz Total spinal anaesthesia as a complication of local anaesthetic test-dose administration through an epidural catheter. Acta Anaesthesiol Scand: 2004, 48(9);1211-3

96. Mayo Clinic. Anorexia nervosa. Diseases & Conditions February 20, 2018.

97. National Institute of Mental Health. Eating Disorders. Bethesda, MD: National Institutes of Health; November 2017.

98. Kulshrestha A, Bajwa S. Nutritional and eating disorders: Clinical impact and considerations during anesthesia procedures. Journal of Medical Nutrition and

Nutraceuticals. 2012;1(2):77–82.

99. Seller CA, Ravalia A. Anaesthetic implications of anorexia nervosa. Anaesthesia. 2003;58(5):437–443.

100. Hirose K, Hirose M, Tanaka K, Kawahito S, Tamaki T, Oshita S. Perioperative management of severe anorexia nervosa. British Journal of Anaesthesia. 2014;112(2):246–254.

101. Mehanna HM, Moledina J, Travis J. Refeeding syndrome: What it is, and how to prevent and treat it. British Medical Journal. 2008;336(7659):1495–1498.

102. Poulida S, Hadzilia S, Stamatakis E, Valsamidis D. Ambulatory anesthesia in a patient with anorexia nervosa: 2AP1– 11. European Journal of Anaesthesiology. 2012;29:33.

103. R.A. Leslie, E.K. Johnson, G. Thomas, and A.P.L. Goodwin, (2011). Valvular defects. Dr Podcast Scripts for the Final FRCA (pp. 3441). Cambridge University Press, New York, USA.

104. G. Edward Morgan, Maged. S Mikhail, and Michael J. Murray. (2006, 2002). Anesthesia for Patients with Cardiovascular Disease. Clinical Anesthesiology Fourth edition (pp. 441 – 490). New York, Chicago, San Francisco, Lisbon, London, Madrid, Mexico City, Milan, New Delhi, San Juan, Seoul, Sydney, and Toronto: Lange Medical Books/McGraw-Hill - Medical Publishing Division.

105. J. Barker, S. Maguire, S. Mills et al., (2009). Valvular heart disease. The Clinical Anaesthesia Viva Book Second edition. (pp. 262263). New York, USA: Cambridge University Press.

106. Mandell LA, Niederman MS. Aspiration Pneumonia. N Engl J Med. 2019 Feb 14;380(7):651-663. [PubMed]

107. Kudo H, Ide H, Nakabayashi M, Goto T, Wakakuri A, Iwata N, Kuroki Y. [The effectiveness of the complete lateral position method in elderly patients with severe dysphagia]. Nihon Ronen Igakkai Zasshi. 2019;56(1):59-66. [PubMed]

108. Cicala G, Barbieri MA, Spina E, de Leon J. A comprehensive review of swallowing difficulties and dysphagia associated with antipsychotics in adults. Expert Rev Clin Pharmacol. 2019 Mar;12(3):219-234. [PubMed]

109. Neill S, Dean N. Aspiration pneumonia and pneumonitis: a spectrum of infectious/noninfectious diseases affecting the lung. Curr Opin Infect Dis. 2019 Apr;32(2):152-157. [PubMed]

110. Bowerman TJ, Zhang J, Waite LM. Antibacterial treatment of aspiration pneumonia in older people: a systematic review. Clin Interv Aging. 2018;13:2201-2213. [PMC free article] [PubMed]

111. Marin S, Serra-Prat M, Ortega O, Clavé P. Cost of oropharyngeal dysphagia after stroke: protocol for a systematic review. BMJ Open. 2018 Dec 14;8(12):e022775. [PMC free article] [PubMed]

112. Liu C, Cao Y, Lin J, Ng L, Needleman I, Walsh T, Li C. Oral care measures for preventing nursing home-acquired pneumonia. Cochrane Database Syst Rev. 2018 Sep 27;9:CD012416. [PMC free article] [PubMed]

113. Barrett Mørk FC, Gade C, Thielsen M, Frederiksen MS, Arpi M, Johannesen J, Jimenez-Solem E, Holst H. Poor compliance with antimicrobial guidelines for childhood pneumonia. Dan Med J. 2018 Nov;65(11) [PubMed]

114. Jam R, Mesquida J, Hernández Ó, Sandalinas I, Turégano C, Carrillo E, Pedragosa R, Valls J, Parera A, Ateca B, Salamero M, Jane R, Oliva JC, Delgado-Hito P. Nursing workload and compliance with non-pharmacological measures to prevent ventilator-associated pneumonia: a multicentre study. Nurs Crit Care. 2018

Nov;23(6):291-298. [PubMed]Kazachkov M, PalmaChopra A, Condos R, Efrati O, Fitzgerald K, Fridman D, Goldenberg RM, Goldhaber A, Kaufman DA, Kothare SV, Levine J, Levy J, Lubinsky AS, Maayan C, Moy LC, Rivera PJ, Rodriguez AJ, Sokol G, Sloane MF, Tan T, Kaufmann H. Respiratory care in familial dysautonomia: Systematic review and expert consensus recommendations. Respir Med. 2018 Aug;141:37-46. [PMC free article]

115. R.A. Leslie, E.K. Johnson, G. Thomas, and A.P.L. Goodwin, (2011). Chronic obstructive pulmonary disease and asthma. Dr Podcast Scripts for the Final FRCA (pp. 156 – 162). Cambridge University Press, New York, USA.

116. G. Edward Morgan, Maged. S Mikhail, and Michael J. Murray. (2006, 2002). Anesthesia for Patients with Respiratory Disease. Clinical Anesthesiology Fourth edition (pp. 571 – 585). New York, Chicago, San Francisco, Lisbon, London, Madrid, Mexico City, Milan, New Delhi, San Juan, Seoul, Sydney, and Toronto: Lange Medical Books/McGraw-Hill - Medical Publishing Division.

117. https://sfai.se/wp-content/uploads/2018/06/Full-Guideline-Regional-2018.pdf

118. Handoll H, and Koscielniak-Nielsen ZJ, Single, Double, or Multiple Injection Techniques for Axillary Brachial Plexus Block for Hand, Wrist, or Forearm Surgery; Anesth Analg 2006; 103(1):248

119. Neal JM, Hebel JR, Gerancher JC, Hogan QH, Brachiual Plexus Anesthesia: Essentials of our current understanding, Regional Anesthesia and Pain Medicine, 2002; 27(4); 402–428

120. Nicholls B, Conn D, Roberts A, Abbott Pocket Guide to Practical Peripheral Nerve Blockade. July 2006 D.L. Brown, Atlas of Regional Anaesthesia, 3rd edition, 2005, Saunders

121. Statement by the Honorary Secretary of the Conference of Medical Royal Colleges and their Faculties in the UK on 11 Oct 1976; Diagnosis of Brain Death. British Medical Journal 1976; 2:1187-1188

122. Department of Health; A Code of Practice for the Diagnosis of Brain Stem Death. HMSO, London 1998.

123. https://www.frca.co.uk/Documents/115%20Brainstem%20death.pdf

124. Fayez A Mahmoud, Intraoperative Hypotension. (381-383). Pass Way Key Concepts for The European Diploma of Anesthesia And Intensive Care Part II 1st edition; Jeddah 2020.

125. 1. Kazan R, Bracco D, Hemmerling TM. Reduced cerebral oxygen saturation measured by absolute cerebral oximetry during thoracic surgery correlates with postoperative complications. Br J Anaesth. 2009;103:811–6. [PubMed] [Google Scholar]

126. 2. Karzai W, Schwarzkopf K. Hypoxemia during one-lung ventilation: Prediction, prevention, and treatment. Anesthesiology. 2009;110:1402–11. [PubMed] [Google Scholar]

127. 3. Sutton CJ, Naguib A, Puri S, Sprenker CJ, Camporesi EM. One-lung ventilation in infants and small children: Blood gas values. J Anesth. 2012;26:670–4. [PubMed] [Google Scholar]

128. 4. Remolina C, Khan AU, Santiago TV, Edelman NH. Positional hypoxemia in unilateral lung disease. N Engl J Med. 1981;304:523–5. [PubMed] [Google Scholar]

129. 5. Addington WW, Kettel LJ, Cugell DW. Alkalosis due to mechanical hyperventilation in patients with chronic hypercapnia. Am Rev Respir Dis. 1966;93:736–41. [PubMed] [Google Scholar]

130. J. Barker, S. Maguire, S. Mills et al., (2009). Burns. The Clinical Anaesthesia Viva

Book Second edition. (pp. 62 – 66). New York, USA: Cambridge University Press.

131. 1. Atkinson JC, Frank MM. Oral manifestations and dental management of patients with hereditary angioedema. J Oral Pathol Med 20:139–142, 1991. [PubMed] [Google Scholar]

132. 2. Moellman JJ, Bernstein JA. Diagnosis and management of hereditary angioedema: An emergency medicine perspective. J Emerg Med 43:391–400, 2012. [PubMed] [Google Scholar]

133. 3. Bygum A, Andersen KE, Mikkelsen CS. Self-administration of intravenous C1-inhibitor therapy for hereditary angioedema and associated quality of life benefits. Eur J Dermatol 19:147–151, 2009. [PubMed] [Google Scholar]

134. 4. Bernstein JA, Coleman S, Bonnin AJ. Successful C1 inhibitor short-term prophylaxis during redo mitral valve replacement in a patient with hereditary angioedema. J Cardiothorac Surg 5:86, 2010. [PMC free article] [PubMed] [Google Scholar]

135. 5. Levy JH, Freiberger DJ, Roback J. Hereditary angioedema: Current and emerging treatment options. Anesth Analg 110:1271–1280, 2010. [PubMed] [Google Scholar]

136. 6. Hermans C. Successful management with C1-inhibitor concentrate of hereditary angioedema attacks during two successive pregnancies: A case report. Arch Gynecol Obstet 276:271–276, 2007. [PubMed] [Google Scholar]

137. Yentis S, May A, Alhotra S. Analgesia, anaesthesia and pregnancy. A Practical Guide. Cambridge University Press. 2007

138. Levy DM. Emergency Caesarean Section: Best Practice. Anaesthesia. 2006; 61: 786-791 Confidential Enquiry into Maternal and Child Health http://www.cemach.org.uk/

139. Royal College of Obstetricians and Gynaecologists' Clinical Effectiveness Support Unit. The National Sentinel Caesarean Section Audit Report. London RCOG, 2001 http://www.rcog.org.uk/resources/public/pdf/nscs_audit.pdf

140. NICE guidelines for caesarean section

141. http://www.nice.org.uk/guidance/index.jsp?action=download&o=29331

142. Fayez A Mahmoud, Carcinoid Syndrome. (3). Pass Way Key Concepts for The European Diploma of Anesthesia And Intensive Care Part II 1st edition; Jeddah 2020.

143. R.A. Leslie, E.K. Johnson, G. Thomas, and A.P.L. Goodwin, (2011). Pre-operative assessment and management of patients with cardiac disease. Dr Podcast Scripts for the Final FRCA (pp. 7 – 13). Cambridge University Press, New York, USA.

144. G. Edward Morgan, Maged. S Mikhail, and Michael J. Murray. (2006, 2002). Anesthesia for Patients with Cardiovascular Disease. Clinical Anesthesiology Fourth edition (pp. 441 – 490). New York, Chicago, San Francisco, Lisbon, London, Madrid, Mexico City, Milan, New Delhi, San Juan, Seoul, Sydney, and Toronto: Lange Medical Books/McGraw-Hill - Medical Publishing Division.

145. https://en.wikipedia.org/wiki/Revised_Cardiac_Risk_Index

146. https://www.ncbi.nlm.nih.gov/pmc/articles/PMC5066735/

147. http://unos.org/data/ (Accessed on September 28, 2018).

148. Guidance from the International Society of Heart and Lung Transplantation regarding the SARS CoV-2 pandemic. https://is hlt.org/ishlt/media/documents/SARS-CoV-2_-Guidance-for-Cardiothoracic-Transplant-and-VAD-centers.pdf (Accessed on J une 02, 2020).

149. Loupy A, Aubert O, Reese PP, et al. Organ procurement and transplantation during the COVID-19 pandemic. Lancet 2020; 395:e95.

150. Bottiger BA, Nicoara A, Snyder LD, et al. Frailty in the End-Stage Lung Disease or Heart Failure Patient: Implications for the Perioperative Transplant Clinician. J Cardiothorac Vasc Anesth 2019; 33:1382.

151. Russo MJ, Chen JM, Sorabella RA, et al. The effect of ischemic time on survival after heart transplantation varies by donor age: an analysis of the United Network for Organ Sharing database. J Thorac Cardiovasc Surg 2007; 133:554.

152. Crossley GH, Poole JE, Rozner MA, et al. The Heart Rhythm Society (HRS)/ American Society of Anesthesiologists (ASA) Expert Consensus Statement on the perioperative management of patients with implantable defibrillators, pacemakers and arrhythmia monitors: facilities and patient management this document was developed as a joint project with the American Society of Anesthesiologists (ASA), and in collaboration with the American Heart Association (AHA), and the Society of Thoracic Surgeons (STS). Heart Rhythm 2011; 8:1114.

153. Vincent JL, De Backer D. Circulatory shock. N Engl J Med 2013; 369:1726.

154. De Backer D, Biston P, Devriendt J, et al. Comparison of dopamine and norepinephrine in the treatment of shock. N Engl J Med 2010; 362:779.

155. Kheng CP, Rahman NH. The use of end-tidal carbon dioxide monitoring in patients with hypotension in the emergency department. Int J Emerg Med 2012; 5:31.

156. Jones AE, Craddock PA, Tayal VS, Kline JA. Diagnostic accuracy of left ventricular function for identifying sepsis among emergency department patients with nontraumatic symptomatic undifferentiated hypotension. Shock 2005; 24:513.

157. Singer M, Deutschman CS, Seymour CW, et al. The Third International Consensus Definitions for Sepsis and Septic Shock (Sepsis-3). JAMA 2016; 315:801.

158. Shankar-Hari M, Phillips GS, Levy ML, et al. Developing a New Definition and Assessing New Clinical Criteria for Septic Shock: For the Third International Consensus Definitions for Sepsis and Septic Shock (Sepsis-3). JAMA 2016; 315:775.

159. Adrie C, Laurent I, Monchi M, et al. Postresuscitation disease after cardiac arrest: a sepsis-like syndrome? Curr Opin Crit Care 2004; 10:208.

160. Smulders YM. Pathophysiology and treatment of haemodynamic instability in acute pulmonary embolism: the pivotal role of pulmonary vasoconstriction. Cardiovasc Res 2000; 48:23.

161. Barber AE, Shires GT. Cell damage after shock. New Horiz 1996; 4:161. 10- Cannon JW. Hemorrhagic Shock. N Engl J Med 2018; 378:370.

162. Angus DC, van der Poll T. Severe sepsis and septic shock. N Engl J Med 2013; 369:840.

163. Hinshaw LB. Sepsis/septic shock: participation of the microcirculation: an abbreviated review. Crit Care Med 1996; 24:1072.

164. GarciKakihana Y, Ito T, Nakahara M, et al. Sepsis-induced myocardial dysfunction: pathophysiology and management. J Intensive Care 2016; 4:22.Shoemaker WC. Temporal physiologic patterns of shock and circulatory dysfunction based on early descriptions by invasive and noninvasive monitoring. New Horiz 1996; 4:300.Chien S. Role of the sympathetic nervous system in hemorrhage. Physiol Rev 1967; 47:214.

165. Tuchschmidt JA, Mecher CE. Predictors of outcome from critical illness. Shock and cardiopulmonary resuscitation. Crit Care Clin 1994; 10:179.

166. Casey LC, Balk RA, Bone RC. Plasma cytokine and endotoxin levels correlate with

survival in patients with the sepsis syndrome. Ann Intern Med 1993; 119:771.

167. Levy MM, Fink MP, Marshall JC, et al. 2001 SCCM/ESICM/ACCP/ATS/SIS International Sepsis Definitions Conference. Crit Care Med 2003; 31:1250.

168. a-Alvarez M, Marik P, Bellomo R. Sepsis-associated hyperlactatemia. Crit Care 2014; 18:503.

169. [1] Stevenson LW, Perloff JK. The Dilated cardiomyopathy: clinical aspects. Cardiol Clin. 1988;6:187– 218. [PubMed] [Google Scholar]

170. [2] Stoelting RK, Dierdorf SF. Anaesthesia and Coexisting Disease.(3rd ed) New York: Churchill Livingstone; 1993. Cardiomyopathy. In: Stoelting RK (Ed) pp. 97–102. [Google Scholar]

171. [3] Molhoek SG, Bax JJ, Erven RV. Effectiveness of resynchronization therapy in patients with end stage heart failure. Am J Cardiol. 2002;90:379–83. [PubMed] [Google Scholar]

172. [4] Schechter WS, Kim C, Martinez M. Anesthetic induction in a child with end-stage cardiomyopathy. Can J Anaesth. 1995;42:404–08. [PubMed] [Google Scholar]

173. [5] Sharma R, Francis DP, Pitt B. Hemoglobin perdicts survival in patients with chronic heart failure: a sub study of the ELITE II trial. Eur Heart J. 2004;25(12):1021–28. [PubMed] [Google Scholar]

174. Patelis N, Diakomi M, Maskanakis A, Maltezos K, Schizas D, Papaioannou M. General versus local anesthesia for carotid endarterectomy: Special considerations. Saudi J Anaesth 2018;12:612-7.

175. Kavaklı AS, Ayoğlu RU, Öztürk NK, et al. Simultaneous Bilateral Carotid Endarterectomy under Cervical Plexus Blockade. Turk J Anaesthesiol Reanim 2015;43:367-70.

176. Zdrehuş C. Anaesthesia for carotid endarterectomy - general or loco- regional? Rom J Anaesth Intensive Care 2015;22:17-24.

177. Kfoury E, Dort J, Trickey A, et al. Carotid endarterectomy under local and/ or regional anesthesia has less risk of myocardial infarction compared to general anesthesia: An analysis of national surgical quality improvement program database. Vascular 2015;23:113-9.

178. Guay J. Regional anesthesia for carotid surgery. Curr Opin Anaesthesiol 2008; 21:638-44.

179. Radak D, de Waard D, Halliday A, Neskovic M, Tanaskovic S. Carotid endarterectomy has significantly lower risk in the last two decades: should the guidelines now be updated? J Cardiovasc Surg 2018;59:586-99.

180. Licker M. Regional or general anaesthesia for carotid endarterectomy: Does it matter? Eur J Anaesthesiol 2016;33:241-43.

181. Pasin L, Nardelli P, Landoni G, et al. Examination of regional anesthesia for carotid endarterectomy. J Vasc Surg 2015;62:631-4.e1 [http://dx.doi. org/10.1016/j. jvs.2015.03.074].

182. Ciccozzi A, Angeletti C, Guetti C, et al. Regional anaesthesia techniques for carotid surgery: the state of art. J Ultrasound 2014;17:175- 83.

183. Handoll H, and Koscielniak-Nielsen ZJ, Single, Double, or Multiple Injection Techniques for Axillary Brachial Plexus Block for Hand, Wrist, or Forearm Surgery; Anesth Analg 2006; 103(1):248

184. Neal JM, Hebel JR, Gerancher JC, Hogan QH, Brachiual Plexus Anesthesia: Essentials of our current understanding, Regional Anesthesia and Pain Medicine, 2002; 27(4); 402–428

185. Nicholls B, Conn D, Roberts A, Abbott Pocket Guide to Practical Peripheral Nerve Blockade. July 2006 D.L. Brown, Atlas of Regional rd Anaesthesia, 3 edition, 2005, Saunders

186. R.A. Leslie, E.K. Johnson, G. Thomas, and A.P.L. Goodwin, (2011). Chronic obstructive pulmonary disease and asthma. Dr Podcast Scripts for the Final FRCA (pp. 156 – 162). Cambridge University Press, New York, USA.

187. G. Edward Morgan, Maged. S Mikhail, and Michael J. Murray. (2006, 2002). Anesthesia for Patients with Respiratory Disease. Clinical Anesthesiology Fourth edition (pp. 571 – 585). New York, Chicago, San Francisco, Lisbon, London, Madrid, Mexico City, Milan, New Delhi, San Juan, Seoul, Sydney, and Toronto: Lange Medical Books/McGraw-Hill - Medical Publishing Division.

188. Bothwick E, Ferguson A. Perioperative acute kidney Injury: risk factors, recognition, management and outcomes.Clinical review. BMJ. 2010; 340:c3365

189. Stewart J et al. Adding insult to injury. National Confidential Enquiry into Patient Outcome and Death; 2009. www.ncepod.org

190. http://www.renal.org/Clinical/GuidelinesSection/AcuteKidneyInjury.aspx

191. Mehta RL, Kellum JA, Shah SV, Molitoris BA, Ronco C, Warnock DG, Levin A et al. Acute Kidney Injury Network: report of an initiative to improve outcomes in acute injury. Critical Care 2007; 11:R31doi:10.1186/cc5713

192. Smith T, Pinnock C, Lin T. Fundamentals of anaesthesia, 3 ed. Cambridge University Press; 2009

193. Atherton AC. Physiology: Renal blood flow, glomerular filtration and plasma clearance. Anaesthesia and Intensive Care Medicine 2009; 10:271-275

194. Bihoric A et al Long term risk of mortality and AKI during hospitalisation after major surgery Ann Surg 2009;240:851-8

195. Abelha FJ et al Outcome and quality of life of patients with AKI after major surgery Nefrologica 2009;29:404- 14

196. https://www.drugabuse.gov/publications/research-reports/cocaine/what-are-effects-maternal-cocaine-use

197. National Institute on Drug Abuse. (2016). Cocaine research report: What are the effects of maternal cocaine use?

198. United States Department of Justice, Drug Enforcement Administration. (2017). Drugs of Abuse.

199. National Institute on Drug Abuse. (2016). Cocaine research report: What is Cocaine?

200. Center for Integrated Healthcare. (2013). Cocaine.

201. Lambert, B. L., & Bauer, C. R. (2012). Developmental and behavioral consequences of prenatal cocaine exposure: a review. Journal of Perinatology: Official Journal of the California Perinatal Association, 32(11), 819–828.

202. J. Barker, S. Maguire, S. Mills et al., (2009). Carbon monoxide poisoning. The Clinical Anaesthesia Viva Book Second edition. (pp. 66 – 67). New York, USA: Cambridge University Press.

203. 203. Wilson, Peter R.; Stanton-Hicks, Michael; Bruehl, Stephen; Harden, R. Norman (2007-05-01). “Proposed New Diagnostic Criteria for Complex Regional Pain Syndrome”. Pain Medicine. 8 (4): 326–331. doi:10.1111/j.1526-4637.2006.00169.x. ISSN 1526-2375. PMID 17610454.

204. ^ Schwartzman RJ, Erwin KL, Alexander GM (May 2009). “The natural history of complex regional pain syndrome”. The Clinical Journal of Pain. 25 (4): 273–80.

doi:10.1097/AJP.0b013e31818ecea5. PMID 19590474. S2CID 10909080.

205. ^ Proposed new diagnostic criteria for complex regional pain syndrome. Harden RN, Bruehl S, Stanton-Hicks M, Wilson PR. Pain Med. 2007 May-Jun;8(4):326-31.

206. ^ Jump up to: a b Marinus J, Moseley GL, Birklein F, et al. (July 2011). “Clinical features and pathophysiology of complex regional pain syndrome”. Lancet Neurology. 10 (7): 637–48. doi:10.1016/S1474-4422(11)70106- 5. PMC 5511749. PMID 21683929.

207. ^ Jump up to: a b c “Complex regional pain syndrome - Symptoms and causes”. Mayo Clinic.

208. ^ Jump up to: a b Bruehl, Stephen; Harden, R. Norman; Galer, Bradley S.; Saltz, Samuel; Backonja, Miroslav; Stanton- Hicks, Michael (January 2002). “Complex regional pain syndrome: are there distinct subtypes and sequential stages of the syndrome?”. Pain. 95 (1–2): 119–124. doi:10.1016/s0304-3959(01)00387-6. ISSN 0304- 3959. PMID 11790474. S2CID 20773804.

209. ^ “Complex regional pain syndrome”. nhs.uk. 2017-10-19.

210. Conn JW. Primary aldosteronism, a new clinical syndrome. J Lab Clin Med 1955; 45: 3–17

211. Winship SM, Winstanley JHR, Hunter JM. Anaesthesia for Conn’s syndrome. Anaesthesia 1999; 54: 564–74

212. Aprahamian C, Thompson BM, Finger WA, Darin JC. Experimental cervical spine injury model: Evaluation of airway management and splinting techniques. Ann Emerg Med. 1984;13:584–587. [PubMed] [Google Scholar]

213. Bednar DA. Efficacy of orthotic immobilization of the unstable subaxial cervical spine of the elderly patient: Investigation in a cadaver model. Can J Anaesth. 2004;47:251–256. [PMC free article] [PubMed] [Google Scholar]

214. Bess RS, Lenke LG. Blood loss minimization and blood salvage techniques for complex spinal surgery. Neurosurg Clin N Am. 2006;17:227–234. [PubMed] [Google Scholar]

215. Bilello JF, Davis JW, Cunningham MA, Groom TF, Lemaster D, Sue LP. Cervical spinal cord injury and the need for cardiovascular intervention. Arch Surg. 2003;138:1127–1129.[PubMed] [Google Scholar]

216. Brimacombe J, Keller C, Künzel KH, Gaber O, Boehler M, Pühringer F. Cervical spine motion during airway management: a cinefluoroscopic study of the posteriorly destabilized third cervical vertebrae in human cadavers. Anesth Analg. 2000;91:1724–1728. [PubMed] [Google Scholar]

217. Sofer S, Dagan R.Harefuah. 1991 Oct;121(7-8):232-5.PMID: 1783311 Hebrew.

218. Berry FA.Otolaryngol Clin North Am. 1981 Aug;14(3):533-56.PMID: 7029411 Review. No abstract available.

219. 11. Delibasi T, Ustun I, Aydin Y, Berker D, Erol HK, Gul K, et al. Early severe pre-eclamptic findings in a patient with Cushing’s syndrome. Gynecol Endocrinol. 2006;22:710–2. [PubMed] [Google Scholar]

220. 12. Park SY, Rhee Y, Youn JC, Park YN, Lee S, Kim DM, et al. Ectopic Cushing’s syndrome due to concurrent corticotropin-releasing hormone (CRH) and adrenocorticotropic hormone (ACTH) secreted by malignant gastrinoma. Exp Clin Endocrinol Diabetes. 2007;115:13–6. [PubMed] [Google Scholar]

221. 13. Esfahani AF, Chavoshi M, Noorani MH, Saghari M, Eftekhari M, Beiki D, et al. Successful application of technetium- 99m-labeled octreotide acetate scintigraphy in the detection of ectopic adrenocorticotropin-producing bronchial carcinoid lung tumor: A case report. J Med Case Reports. 2010;4:323. [PMC free article][PubMed]

[Google Scholar]

222. Aptiz C, Webb G, Redington A. Tetralogy of Fallot. Lancet 2009 374: 1462-71

223. Singh V. Tetralogy of Fallot: surgical perspective, treatment and management. E-Medicine the http://emedicine.medscape.com/article/904652 (accessed 8 April 2011)

224. 1. Richmond S. Newborn Life Support. Resuscitation Council (UK) http://www.resus.org.uk/pages/nls.pdf (accessed 15th November 2005)

225. 2. Wall S, Lee AC , Niermeyer S et al. Neonatal resuscitation in low-resource settings: what, who and how to overcome challenges to scale up? International Journal of Obstetrics 2009 107:S47-S64

226. 3. Woods DL Newborn Care Manual. Perinatal Education Programme. International Association of Maternal and Neonatal Health. http://www.gfmer.ch/PEP/NCM_Home.htm (accessed 15th November 2009).

227. Deighan M, Ash S, McMorrow R.Int J Obstet Anesth. 2014 Feb;23(1):75-9. doi: 10.1016/j.ijoa.2013.10.006. Epub 2013 Oct 31.PMID: 24361190

228. Karlet MC.AANA J. 2000 Apr;68(2):141-8.PMID: 10876461 Review.

229. Nolan SJ, Thornton J, Murray CS, Dwyer T.Cochrane Database Syst Rev. 2015 Oct 9;(10):CD008649. doi: 10.1002/14651858.CD008649.pub2.PMID: 26451533 Updated. Review.

230. https://pubmed.ncbi.nlm.nih.gov/17019190/

231. 231. 3. Hill MD, Brooks W, Mackey A, et al; for CREST Investigators. Stroke after carotid stenting and endarterectomy in the

232. Carotid Revascularization Endarterectomy Versus Stenting Trial (CREST). Circulation. 2012;126(25):3054– 3061. https://doi.org/10.1161/CIRCULATIONAHA.112.120030[PMC free article] [PubMed] [Google Scholar]

233. 232. 4. Taylor WAS, Thomas NWM, Wellings JA, Bell BA. Timing of postoperative intracranial hematoma development and implications for the best use of neurosurgical intensive care. J Neurosurg.1995;82(1):48– 50. https://doi.org/10.3171/jns.1995.82.1.0048[PubMed] [Google Scholar]https://www.ncbi.nlm.nih.gov/pmc/articles/PMC6338181/

234. Nair-Collins M, Northrup J, Olcese J. Hypothalamic-Pituitary Function in Brain Death: A Review. J Intensive Care Med. 2014 Mar 31. [Epub ahead of print] PubMed PMID: 24692211.

235. https://www.openanesthesia.org/diabetes-insipidus-dx/

236. Sonksen P, Sonksen J. Insulin: understanding its action in health and disease. Br J Anaesth 2000, 85: 69-79 McAnulty GR, Robertshaw HJ, Hall GM. Anaesthetic management of patients with diabetes mellitus. Br J Anaesth 2000, 85: 80-90 French G. Clinical management of diabetes mellitus during anaesthesia and surgery. Update in Anaesthesia 2000, 11: Article 13

237. https://www.frca.co.uk/article.aspx?articleid=100704

238. Haematology: Basic Principles and Practice (6 ed.). Elsevier Saunders. 2012. ISBN 978-1437729283.

239. ^ Clark, Michael; Kumar, Parveen J. (1998). Clinical Medicine: A Textbook for Medical Students and Doctors (4 ed.). Philadelphia: W.B. Saunders. ISBN 0-7020-2458-9.

240. ^ "Disseminated Intravascular Coagulation". The Lecturio Medical Concept Library. Retrieved 12 July 2021.

241. https://en.wikipedia.org/wiki/Disseminated_intravascular_coagulation

242. 1. Practice guidelines for the management of the difficult airway: A report by the American Society of Anesthesiologists Task Force on Management of the Difficult Airway. Anesthesiology 1993; 78: 597.

243. https://journals.lww.com/anesthesia-analgesia/fulltext/2003/04000/the_difficult_airway_algorithm_of_the_american.64.aspx

244. https://www.frca.co.uk/Documents/139%20Anaesthesia%20for%20children%20with%20down's%20syndrome.pdf

245. https://en.wikipedia.org/wiki/Drowning

246. https://www.cincinnatichildrens.org/health/e/ecmo

247. https://en.wikipedia.org/wiki/Eisenmenger%27s_syndrome

248. American Society of Anesthesiologists. Standards for Basic Anesthetic Monitoring. www.asahq.org/Search.aspx?q=standar ds+basic+anesthetic+monitoring (Accessed on March 29, 2016).

249. https://www.asahq.org/standards-and-guidelines (Accessed on May 21, 2019).

250. Radman T, Lisanby SH. New directions in the rational design of electrical and magnetic seizure therapies: individualized Low Amplitude Seizure Therapy (iLAST) and Magnetic Seizure Therapy (MST). Int Rev Psychiatry 2017; 29:63.

251. https://www.uptodate.com/contents/anesthesia-for-electroconvulsive-therapy

252. Kerri. M. Robertson., David. A. Lubarsky., Sudharma. Ranasinghe., (2006). PEDIATRIC ANESTHESIA. Anesthesiology BOARD REVIEW Second Edition. (pp. 301 – 311). New York, Chicago, San Francisco, Lisbon, London, Madrid, Mexico City, Milan, New Delhi, San Juan, Seoul, Sydney, and Toronto: Lange Medical Books/McGraw-Hill - Medical Publishing Division.

253. https://www.nejm.org/doi/full/10.1056/NEJMicm1009990

254. https://www.mayoclinic.org/diseases-conditions/malignant-hyperthermia/symptoms-causes/syc-20353750

255. Capdevila X, Biboulet P, Bouregba M, Barthelet Y, Rubenovitch J, d'Athis F. Comparison of the Three-in-One and Fascia Iliaca Compartment Blocks in Adults: Clinical and Radiographic Analysis. Anesth Analg1998; 86:1039-44

256. Lang SA, Yip RW, Chang PC. The femoral 3-in-1 block revisited. J Clin Anesth 1993; 5:292-296

257. Ridgway S, Herrick M. Perioperative nerve dysfunction and peripheral nerve blockade. Contin Educ Anaesth Crit Care Pain (2006) 6 (2): 71-74.

258. Murray JM, Derbyshire S, Shields MO. Lower limb blocks. Anaesthesia, 2010; 65 (Suppl. 1): 57-66 femoral nerve blockade.

259. https://www.frca.co.uk/Documents/249%20Femoral%20Nerve%20Block-%20Landmark%20approach.pdf

260. Figueireido S, Tsatsaris V, Mignon A.Ann Fr Anesth Reanim. 2007 Jul-Aug;26(7-8):699-704. doi: 10.1016/j.annfar.2007.05.006. Epub 2007 Jun 14.PMID: 17572043 Review. French.

261. Levy DM.Anaesthesia. 2006 Aug;61(8):786-91. doi: 10.1111/j.1365-2044.2006.04711.x.PMID: 16867092 Review.

262. https://pubmed.ncbi.nlm.nih.gov/8076233/

263. https://heart.bmj.com/content/91/6/839

264. https://www.ncbi.nlm.nih.gov/books/NBK531480/

265. https://pubmed.ncbi.nlm.nih.gov/19506473/

266. https://www.orpha.net/data/patho/Ans/en/Glucose-6-phosphate-dehydrogenase-deficiency.pdf

267. https://www.frca.co.uk/Documents/238%20Guillain%20Barre%20Syndrome.pdf

268. Maron BJ: Hypertrophic cardiomyopathy: A systematic review. JAMA 2002; 287:1308–20

269. Maron BJ, McKenna WJ, Danielson GK, Kappenberger LJ, Kuhn HJ, Seidman CE, Shah PM, Spencer WH, Spirito P, Ten Cate FJ, Wigle ED: ACC/ESC clinical expert consensus document on hypertrophic cardiomyopathy: A report of the American College of Cardiology Task Force on Clinical Expert Consensus Documents and the European Society of Cardiology Committee for Practice Guidelines (Committee to Develop an Expert Consensus Document on Hypertrophic Cardiomyopathy). J Am Coll Cardiol 2003; 42:1687–713

270. Maron BJ, Casey SA, Poliac LC, Gohman TE, Almquist AK, Aeppli DM: Clinical course of hypertrophic cardiomyopathy in a regional United States cohort. JAMA 1999; 281:650–5

271. Klues HG, Schiffers A, Maron BJ: Phenotypic spectrum and patterns of left ventricular hypertrophy in hypertrophic cardiomyopathy: morphologic observations and significance as assessed by two-dimensional echocardiography in 600 patients. J Am Coll Cardiol 1995; 26:1699–708

272. J Pharm Bioallied Sci. (2013) The potential anesthetic threats, challenges and intensive care considerations in patients with HIV infection. doi: 10.4103/0975-7406.106554. Retrieved from https://www.ncbi.nlm.nih.gov/pmc/articles/PMC3612332/

273. Ann Ib Postgrad Med. 2009 Jun; 7(1): 31–35. Retrieved from https://www.ncbi.nlm.nih.gov/pmc/articles/PMC4111002/

274. G. Edward Morgan, Maged. S Mikhail, and Michael J. Murray. (2006, 2002). Management of Patient with Fluid & Electrolyte Disturbances. Clinical Anesthesiology Fourth edition (pp. 662 – 690). New York, Chicago, San Francisco, Lisbon, London, Madrid, Mexico City, Milan, New Delhi, San Juan, Seoul, Sydney, and Toronto: Lange Medical Books/McGraw-Hill - Medical Publishing Division.

275. R. Mihai and J. R. Farndon. Parathyroid disease and calcium metabolism. British Journal of Anaesthesia (2000);85:29-43

276. Hannah Blanshard. Oxford handbook of Anaesthesia. Oxford University Press, UK, 2006;162

277. Anna Batchelor. Oxford handbook of Anaesthesia. Oxford University Press, UK, 2006;558

278. Review of Medical Physiology,:Hormonal control of calcium metabolism and physiology of bone; Ganong . 22nd Edition, Chapter 21;USA ; 2005,382-395

279. Russell T Wall.398-402. Stoelting's Anesthesia and Co-existing disease, fifth edition, Churchill Livingstone, Philadelphia, 2008; 398- 402.

280. Michael F. Roizen and Nader M. Enany. Diseases of the endocrine system, Chapter 13, Anesthesia and uncommon disease; Edition: 5,USA, 2005;413-420

281. https://www.frca.co.uk/Documents/142%20Anaesthesia%20&%20the%20parathyroid%20gland.pdf

282. R.A. Leslie, E.K. Johnson, G. Thomas, and A.P.L. Goodwin, (2011). Hypertension. Dr Podcast Scripts for the Final FRCA(pp. 19 – 22). Cambridge University Press, New York, USA.

283. G. Edward Morgan, Maged. S Mikhail, and Michael J. Murray. (2006, 2002). Anesthesia for Patients with Cardiovascular Disease. Clinical Anesthesiology Fourth edition (pp. 441 – 490). New York, Chicago, San Francisco, Lisbon, London, Madrid, Mexico City, Milan, New Delhi, San Juan, Seoul, Sydney, and Toronto: Lange Medical Books/McGraw-Hill - Medical Publishing Division.

284. J. Barker, S. Maguire, S. Mills et al., (2009). Hypertension and ischaemic heart disease. The Clinical Anaesthesia Viva Book Second edition. (pp. 114 – 118). New York, USA: Cambridge University Press.

285. The measurement of adult blood pressure and management of hypertension before elective surgery: Joint Guidelines from the Association of Anaesthetists of Great Britain and Ireland and the British Hypertension Society. 2016 Mar;71(3):326-37. doi: 10.1111/anae.13348. Epub 2016 Jan 17. Retrieved from: https://www.ncbi.nlm.nih.gov/pubmed/26776052

286. https://www.frca.co.uk/Documents/162%20Anaesthesia%20for%20thyroid%20surgery.pdf

287. http://blog.vetbloom.com/anesthesia-analgesia/perioperative-hypoxemia/

288. https://www.anesthesiaconsiderations.com/increased-airway-pressure

289. https://www.aana.com/docs/default-source/practice-aana-com-web-documents-(all)/professional-practice-manual/informed- consent-for-anesthesia-care.pdf?sfvrsn=8a0049b1_8

290. Bier A: Uber einen neun weg local anaesthesia an den gliedmassen zuerzeugen. Arch Klin Chir 1908;86:1007–1016.

291. Bier A: On a new method of local anesthesia. Muench Med Wschir 1909; 56:589.

292. Bier A: Concerning venous anesthesia. Berl Klin Wschr 1909;46: 477–489.

293. Bier A: On local anesthesia with special reference to vein anesthesia. Edinburgh Med J 19105:103–123.

294. Morrison J: Intravenous local anesthesia. Br J Surg 1930–1931;18:641–647.

295. Herreros L: Regional anesthesia by the intravenous route. Anesthesiology 1946;7:558–560.

296. https://www.nysora.com/techniques/intravenous-regional-anesthesia/intravenous-regional-block-upper-lower-extremity-surgery/

297. https://pubmed.ncbi.nlm.nih.gov/15062198/

298. https://academic.oup.com/bja/article/115/5/676/230337

299. Paediatric cardiology: an introduction. Archer N, Burch M. Chapman Hall Medical. Philadelphia 1998

300. https://www.frca.co.uk/Documents/Recognising%20Cardiac%20Disease%20in%20Children%20final.pdf

301. https://www.chop.edu/conditions-diseases/laryngeal-trauma
302. G. Edward Morgan, Maged. S Mikhail, and Michael J. Murray. (2006, 2002). Anesthesia for Otorhinolaryngologic Surgery. Clinical Anesthesiology Fourth edition (pp. 837 – 848). New York, Chicago, San Francisco, Lisbon, London, Madrid, Mexico City, Milan, New Delhi, San Juan, Seoul, Sydney, and Toronto: Lange Medical Books/McGraw-Hill - Medical Publishing Division.
303. https://www.healthline.com/health/lithium-toxicity
304. G. Edward Morgan, Maged. S Mikhail, and Michael J. Murray. (2006, 2002). Anesthesia for patients with liver Disease. Clinical Anesthesiology Fourth edition (pp. 789 – 802). New York, Chicago, San Francisco, Lisbon, London, Madrid, Mexico City, Milan, New Delhi, San Juan, Seoul, Sydney, and Toronto: Lange Medical Books/McGraw-Hill - Medical Publishing Division.
305. Trotter, JF. 'Practical Management of acute liver failure in the intensive care unit'. Curr Opin Crit Care 2009, 15:163-167 3- Auzinger G, Wendon J. 'Intensive care management of acute liver failure'. Curr Opin Crit Care 2008, 14:179-188
306. Bhatia V, Singh R, Acharya SK. 'Predictive value of arterial ammonia for complications and outcome in acute liver failure'. Gut 2006, 55(1):98-104
307. Gunning KEJ. "Acute Liver Failure'. Anaesthesia UK – accessed 05/10/2011 5. O'Grady JG, Schalm SW, Williams R. 'Acute liver failure: redefining the syndromes'. Lancet 1993; 342:273-5
308. Hirschfiled GM, Gibbs P, Griffiths WJH. 'Adult liver transplantation; what non-specialists need to know'. BMJ 2009, 338:b1670.
309. R.A. Leslie, E.K. Johnson, G. Thomas, and A.P.L. Goodwin, (2011). Local anaesthetic toxicity. Dr Podcast Scripts for the Final FRCA (pp. 453 – 460). Cambridge University Press, New York, USA.
310. J. Barker, S. Maguire, S. Mills et al., (2009). IVRA for Dupuytrens contracture and LA toxicity. The Clinical Anaesthesia Viva Book Second edition. (pp. 136 – 139). New York, USA: Cambridge University Press.
311. https://www.nhlbi.nih.gov/health-topics/long-qt-syndrome
312. Norgren L, Hiatt WR, Dormandy JA, et al. TASC II Working Group. Inter-society consensus for the management of peripheral arterial disease (TASC II). J Vasc Surg 2007; 45 Suppl: S5-67. [PubMed] [Google Scholar]
313. Howard DP, Banerjee A, Fairhead JF, et al. Population-based study of incidence, risk factors, outcome, and prognosis of ischemic peripheral arterial events: implications for prevention. Circulation2015; 132: 1805-15. [PMC free article] [PubMed] [Google Scholar]
314. Creager MA, Kaufman JA, Conte MS. Clinical practice. Acute limb ischemia. N Engl J Med 2012; 366: 2198-206. [PubMed] [Google Scholar]
315. Ascher E. Haimovici's Vascular Surgery, 5th ed. Oxford: Blackwell, 2014.
316. R.A. Leslie, E.K. Johnson, G. Thomas, and A.P.L. Goodwin, (2011). One-lung ventilation. Dr Podcast Scripts for the Final FRCA (pp. 199 – 203). Cambridge University Press, New York, USA.
317. G. Edward Morgan, Maged. S Mikhail, and Michael J. Murray. (2006, 2002). Anesthesia for Thoracic Surgery. Clinical Anesthesiology Fourth edition (pp.

585 – 614). New York, Chicago, San Francisco, Lisbon, London, Madrid, Mexico City, Milan, New Delhi, San Juan, Seoul, Sydney, and Toronto: Lange Medical Books/McGraw-Hill - Medical Publishing Division.

318. J. Barker, S. Maguire, S. Mills et al., (2009). Pneumonectomy. The Clinical Anaesthesia Viva Book Second edition. (pp.194 – 196). New York, USA: Cambridge University Press.

319. https://www.uptodate.com/contents/lung-transplantation-anesthetic-management

320. https://www.orphananesthesia.eu/en/rare-diseases/published-guidelines/marfan-syndrome/978-marfan-syndrome-2/file.html

321. R.A. Leslie, E.K. Johnson, G. Thomas, and A.P.L. Goodwin, (2011). Blood groups. Dr Podcast Scripts for the Final FRCA(pp. 104 – 109). Cambridge University Press, New York, USA.

322. G. Edward Morgan, Maged. S Mikhail, and Michael J. Murray. (2006, 2002). Fluid Management & Transfusion. Clinical Anesthesiology Fourth edition (pp. 690 – 708). New York, Chicago, San Francisco, Lisbon, London, Madrid, Mexico City, Milan, New Delhi, San Juan, Seoul, Sydney, and Toronto: Lange Medical Books/McGraw-Hill - Medical Publishing Division.

323. J. Barker, S. Maguire, S. Mills et al., (2009). Massive blood transfusion. The Clinical Anaesthesia Viva Book Second edition. (pp. 157 – 160). New York, USA: Cambridge University Press.

324. https://www.omnicalculator.com/health/blood-loss

325. https://academic.oup.com/bjaed/article/7/1/6/509175

326. https://en.wikipedia.org/wiki/Metabolic_acidosis

327. Ferrari LR, Zurakowski D, Solari J, Rahbar R. Laryngeal cleft repair: the anesthetic perspective. Paediatr Anaesth. 2013 Apr;23(4):334-41.[PubMed]

328. Allen E, Fingeret A. StatPearls [Internet]. StatPearls Publishing; Treasure Island (FL): Jul 27, 2020. Anatomy, Head and Neck, Thyroid. [PubMed]

329. Ferlito A. The natural history of early vocal cord cancer. Acta Otolaryngol. 1995 Mar;115(2):345-7. [PubMed]

330. Schleicher A, Groeben H. Anesthetic considerations for tracheobronchial surgery. J Thorac Dis. 2020 Oct;12(10):6138- 6142. [PMC free article] [PubMed]

331. https://www.ncbi.nlm.nih.gov/books/NBK572099/

332. R.A. Leslie, E.K. Johnson, G. Thomas, and A.P.L. Goodwin, (2011). Valvular defects. Dr Podcast Scripts for the Final FRCA (pp. 34 - 41). Cambridge University Press, New York, USA.

333. G. Edward Morgan, Maged. S Mikhail, and Michael J. Murray. (2006, 2002). Anesthesia for Patients with Cardiovascular Disease. Clinical Anesthesiology Fourth edition (pp. 441 – 490). New York, Chicago, San Francisco, Lisbon, London, Madrid, Mexico City, Milan, New Delhi, San Juan, Seoul, Sydney, and Toronto: Lange Medical Books/McGraw-Hill - Medical Publishing Division.

334. J. Barker, S. Maguire, S. Mills et al., (2009). Valvular heart disease. The Clinical Anaesthesia Viva Book Second edition. (pp. 262 - 263). New York,

USA: Cambridge University Press.

335. https://rarediseases.info.nih.gov/diseases/7065/mucopolysaccharidosis

336. G. Edward Morgan, Maged. S Mikhail, and Michael J. Murray. (2006, 2002). Anesthesia for Patients with Neurologic & Psychiatric Disease. Clinical Anesthesiology Fourth edition (pp. 647 – 662). New York, Chicago, San Francisco, Lisbon, London, Madrid, Mexico City, Milan, New Delhi, San Juan, Seoul, Sydney, and Toronto: Lange Medical Books/McGraw- Hill - Medical Publishing Division.

337. https://en.wikipedia.org/wiki/Multiple_sclerosis#Epidemiology

338. https://takeonduchenne.eu/what-are-neuromuscular-disorders/?gclid=Cj0KCQiAw9qOBhC-ARIsAG- rdn4mklc2H_zQDZjjNoalvPCO04S8LMacyFdr6z6FtfrBKEOouG4c-0laAiKbEALw_wcB

339. R.A. Leslie, E.K. Johnson, G. Thomas, and A.P.L. Goodwin, (2011). Myasthenia and muscle disease. Dr Podcast Scripts for the Final FRCA (pp. 147 – 152). Cambridge University Press, New York, USA.

340. G. Edward Morgan, Maged. S Mikhail, and Michael J. Murray. (2006, 2002). Anesthesia for Patients with Neurologic & Psychiatric Disease. Clinical Anesthesiology Fourth edition (pp. 647 – 662). New York, Chicago, San Francisco, Lisbon, London, Madrid, Mexico City, Milan, New Delhi, San Juan, Seoul, Sydney, and Toronto: Lange Medical Books/McGraw- Hill - Medical Publishing Division.

341. J. Barker, S. Maguire, S. Mills et al., (2009). Myasthenia gravis. The Clinical Anaesthesia Viva Book Second edition. (pp. 163 – 166). New York, USA: Cambridge University Press.

342. https://www.myotonic.org/sites/default/files/MDF_LongForm_ AnesGuidelines_01C.pdf

343. https://www.bjaed.org/article/S1743-1816(17)30181-6/fulltext#relatedArticles

344. https://www.frca.co.uk/article.aspx?articleid=100728

345. 2. Mulvihill JJ, Parry DM, Sherman JL, Pikus A, Kaiser-Kupfer MI, Eldridge R. NIH conference. Neurofibromatosis 1 (Recklinghausen disease) and neurofibromatosis 2 (bilateral acoustic neurofibromatosis) Ann Intern Med. 1990 Jul 1;113(1):39–52. An update. [PubMed] [Google Scholar]

346. 3. Nussbaum R, McInnes R, Willard HF. Thompson & Thompson Genetics in Medicine. Philadelphia, PA: W.B. Saunders; 2007;119-120:292–293. [Google Scholar]

347. 4. Cawthon RM, O'Connell P, Buchberg AM, et al. Identification and characterization of transcripts from the neurofibromatosis 1 region: the sequence and genomic structure of EVI2 and mapping of other transcripts. Genomics. 1990 Aug;7(4):555–565. [PubMed] [Google Scholar]

348. https://www.ncbi.nlm.nih.gov/pmc/articles/PMC3726098/

349. Anaesthetic considerations for non-obstetric surgery during pregnancy Reitman et al.British Journal of AnaesthesiaDecember 2011

350. J. Barker, S. Maguire, S. Mills et al., (2009). Bariatric surgery and drugs for obesity. The Clinical Anaesthesia Viva Book Second edition. (pp. 52 – 56). New York, USA: Cambridge University Press.

351. https://www.frca.co.uk/article.aspx?articleid=100758

352. R.A. Leslie, E.K. Johnson, G. Thomas, and A.P.L. Goodwin, (2011). Obstructive sleep apnoea. Dr Podcast Scripts for the Final FRCA (pp. 229 – 232). Cambridge University Press, New York, USA.

353. J. Barker, S. Maguire, S. Mills et al., (2009). Obstructive sleep apnoea. The Clinical Anaesthesia Viva Book Second edition.(pp. 172 – 175). New York, USA: Cambridge University Press.

354. https://accessmedicine.mhmedical.com/content.aspx?bookid=564&sectionid=42800568

355. R.A. Leslie, E.K. Johnson, G. Thomas, and A.P.L. Goodwin, (2011). Pacemakers and implantable cardioverter devices. Dr Podcast Scripts for the Final FRCA (pp. 41 – 47). Cambridge University Press, New York, USA.

356. J. Barker, S. Maguire, S. Mills et al., (2009). Pacemakers. The Clinical Anaesthesia Viva Book Second edition. (pp. 175 – 178). New York, USA: Cambridge University Press.

357. - R.A. Leslie, E.K. Johnson, G. Thomas, and A.P.L. Goodwin, (2011). Pain. Dr Podcast Scripts for the Final FRCA (pp. 460 – 479). Cambridge University Press, New York, USA.

358. Miguel R. Interventional treatment of cancer pain: the fourth step in the World Health Organization analgesic ladder? Cancer Control. 2000;7:149–56. [PubMed] [Google Scholar]

359. Miljanich GP. Ziconotide: neuronal calcium channel blocker for treating severe chronic pain. Curr Med Chem. 2004;11:3029–40. [PubMed] [Google Scholar]

360. Miljanich GP, Ramachandran J. Antagonists of neuronal calcium channels: structure, function, and therapeutic implications. Annu Rev Pharmacol Toxicol. 1995;35:707–34.[PubMed] [Google Scholar]

361. Mohammed I, Hussain A. Intrathecal baclofen withdrawal syndrome- a life-threatening complication of baclofen pump: Acase report. BMC Clin Pharmacol. 2004;4:1–5.[PMC free article] [PubMed] [Google Scholar]

362. Morales E, Mucksavage JJ. Cyclooxygenase-2 inhibitor-associated acute renal failure: case report with rofecoxib and review of the literature. Pharmacotherapy. 2002;22:1317–21.[PubMed] [Google Scholar]

363. 1. Kelly PJ. Pallidotomy in Parkinson's disease. Neurosurgery. 1995;36:1154–7. [PubMed] [Google Scholar]

364. 2. DeLong MR, Juncos JL. Parkinson's Disease and Other Movement Disorders. In: Kasper DL, Fauci AS, Longo DL, Braunwald E, Hauser SL, Jameson JL, editors. Harrison's Principles of Internal Medicine. 17th ed. New York: McGraw-Hill Medical Publishers; 2008. pp. 2406–17. [Google Scholar]

365. 1. Lonnqvist P-A, Morton NS. Postoperative analgesia in infants and children. Br J Anaesth 2005; 95: 59 – 68
2. Berde CB, Sethna NF. Analgesics for the Treatment of Pain in Children. N Engl J Med 2002; 347: 1094 – 1103
3. Howard RF, Lloyd-Thomas A. Pain management in children. In: Sumner E and Hatch DJ eds. Paediatric Anaesthesia. London, U.K. Arnold. 1999.

366. - Kerri. M. Robertson., David. A. Lubarsky., Sudharma. Ranasinghe., (2006). EENT SURGERY. Anesthesiology BOARD REVIEW Second Edition. (pp. 109 – 113). New York, Chicago, San Francisco, Lisbon, London, Madrid, Mexico City, Milan, New Delhi, San Juan, Seoul, Sydney, and Toronto: Lange Medical Books/McGraw-Hill - Medical Publishing Division.

367. https://www.frca.co.uk/Documents/151%20case%20study%20for%20 Phaeochromocytoma,%20perioperative%20management.pdf

368. Xavier Capdevila, MD, PhD, Philippe Macaire, MD, Christophe Dadure, MD, Olivier Choquet, MD, Philippe Biboulet, MD, Yves Ryckwaert, MD et al. Continuous Psoas Compartment Block for Postoperative Analgesia After Total Hip Arthroplasty: New Landmarks, Technical Guidelines,andClinicalEvaluation. ANESTHANALG2002;94;1606–13

369. S. T. Touray, M. A. de Leeuw, W. W. A. Zuurmond and R. S. G. M. Perez. Psoas compartment block for lower extremity surgery: a meta-analysis. British Journal of Anaesthesia; 2008; 101 (6): 750–60

370. Auroy Y, Benhamou D, Bargues L, Ecoffey C, Bruno Falissard B, Mercier F, Bouaziz H , Samii K. Major Complications of Regional Anesthesia in France. Anesthesiology 2002; 97:1274–80

371. The Abbott pocket guide to practical peripheral nerve blockade. Nicholls, Conn and Roberts.

372. R. A. Leslie, E. K. Johnson, and A. P. L. Goodwin, (2011). Anaesthesia for MRI scanning. Dr Podcast Scripts for the Final FRCA (pp. 264– 268). Cambridge University Press, United Kingdom.

373. Keith. G. Allman, Iain. H. Wilson, and Aidan. O'Donnell. (2011). Anaesthesia for CT, MRI, and Interventional Radiology. OXFORD HANDBOOK OF ANAESTHESIA (pp. 715 – 725). New York: Oxford University Press Inc.,

374. R.A. Leslie, E.K. Johnson, G. Thomas, and A.P.L. Goodwin, (2011). Anaesthesia for craniotomy. Dr Podcast Scripts for the Final FRCA (pp. 242 – 248). Cambridge University Press, New York, USA.

375. G. Edward Morgan, Maged. S Mikhail, and Michael J. Murray. (2006, 2002). Anesthesia for Neurosurgery. Clinical Anesthesiology Fourth edition (pp. 631 – 647). New York, Chicago, San Francisco, Lisbon, London, Madrid, Mexico City, Milan, New Delhi, San Juan, Seoul, Sydney, and Toronto: Lange Medical Books/McGraw-Hill - Medical Publishing Division.

376. J. Barker, S. Maguire, S. Mills et al., (2009). Intracranial pressure. The Clinical Anaesthesia Viva Book Second edition. (pp. 129 – 131). New York, USA: Cambridge University Press.

377. https://www.slideshare.net/JohnDUrbanoRRT/capnography-the-other-vital-sign

378. https://www.frca.co.uk/article.aspx?articleid=100463

379. Bayley G, Walker I. Special considerations in the premature and ex-premature infant. Anaesthesia and Intensive Care Medicine 12(3): 91-94

380. Santin RL, Porat R. Apnea of prematurity. Available at www.emedicine.com/ped/topic1157.htm Walther-Larsen S, Rasmussen LS. The former preterm infant and risk of post-operative apnoea:

381. recommendations for management. Acta Anaesthesiol Scand 2006; 50: 888-93 APA Consensus Guideline on Perioperative Fluid Management in Children v 1.1 September 2007

382. https://www.bjanaesthesia.org/article/S0007-0912(21)00014-3/fulltext#relatedArticles

383. R. A. Leslie, E. K. Johnson, and A. P. L. Goodwin, (2011). Pyloric stenosis. Dr Podcast Scripts for the Final FRCA (pp. 337– 341). Cambridge University Press, United Kingdom.

384. Backman H, Eriksson B, Hedman L, et al. Restrictive spirometric pattern in the general adult population: Methods of defining the condition and consequences on prevalence. Respir Med 2016; 120:116.

385. Koul PA, Hakim NA, Malik SA, et al. Prevalence of chronic airflow limitation in Kashmir, North India: results from the BOLD study. Int J Tuberc Lung Dis 2016; 20:1399.

386. Hedenstierna G, Rothen HU. Respiratory function during anesthesia: effects on gas exchange. Compr Physiol 2012; 2:69.

387. R.A. Leslie, E.K. Johnson, G. Thomas, and A.P.L. Goodwin, (2011). Bone, joint and connective tissue. Dr Podcast Scripts for the Final FRCA (pp. 1 – 7). Cambridge University Press, New York, USA.

388. J. Barker, S. Maguire, S. Mills et al., (2009). Rheumatoid arthritis. The Clinical Anaesthesia Viva Book Second edition. (pp. 217 – 220). New York, USA: Cambridge University Press.

389. 1. Killian G. Ueber directe bronchoscopie. MMW. 1898;27:844–7.[Google Scholar]

390. 2. Clerf LH. Historical aspects of foreign bodies in the air and food passages. South Med J. 1975;68:1449– 54. [PubMed] [Google Scholar]

391. Sandvei MS, Romundstad PR, Müller TB, Vatten L, Vik A. Risk factors for aneurysmal subarachnoid hemorrhage in a prospective population study: the HUNT study in Norway. Stroke. 2009 Jun;40(6):1958–1962. Epub 2009 Feb 19. [PubMed] [Google Scholar]

392. Connolly ES, Jr, Rabinstein AA, Carhuapoma JR, et al. Guidelines for the management of aneurysmal subarachnoid hemorrhage: a guideline for healthcare professionals from the American Heart Association/American Stroke Association. Stroke. 2012 Jun;43(6):1711–1737. Epub 2012 May 3. [PubMed] [Google Scholar]

393. Fontanarosa PB. Recognition of subarachnoid hemorrhage. Ann Emerg Med. 1989 Nov;18(11):1199– 1205. [PubMed] [Google Scholar]

394. https://emedicine.medscape.com/article/2000841-overview

395. https://academic.oup.com/bjaed/article/16/5/173/2389879

396. https://www.ncbi.nlm.nih.gov/books/NBK532983/

397. https://www.nysora.com/regional-anesthesia-for-specific-surgical-procedures/lower-extremity-regional-anesthesia-for- specific-surgical-procedures/foot-and-anckle/ultrasound-guided-sciatic-nerve-block-2/

398. https://www.ncbi.nlm.nih.gov/pmc/articles/PMC5014778/

399. https://www.aana.com/docs/default-source/aana-journal-web-documents-1/scoliosisp277-285.pdf?sfvrsn=812e5ab1_6

400. R.A. Leslie, E.K. Johnson, G. Thomas, and A.P.L. Goodwin, (2011). Epilepsy. Dr Podcast Scripts for the Final FRCA(pp. 279 –282). Cambridge University Press, New York, USA.

401. G. Edward Morgan, Maged. S Mikhail, and Michael J. Murray. (2006, 2002). Anesthesia for Patients with Neurologic & Psychiatric Disease. Clinical Anesthesiology Fourth edition (pp. 647 – 662). New York, Chicago, San Francisco, Lisbon, London, Madrid, Mexico City, Milan, New Delhi, San Juan, Seoul, Sydney, and Toronto: Lange Medical Books/McGraw-Hill - Medical Publishing Division.

402. J. Barker, S. Maguire, S. Mills et al., (2009). Epilepsy. The Clinical Anaesthesia Viva Book Second edition. (pp.100 – 104). New York, USA: Cambridge University Press.

403. Finfer S et al. A comparison of albumin and saline for fluid resuscitation in the intensive care unit. New England Journal of Medicine 2004; 350: 2247-56

404. Hebert PC et al. A multicenter, randomised controlled clinical trial of transfusion requirements in critical care. New England Journal of Medicine 1999; 340: 409-17.

405. Meduri GU. Levels of evidence for the pharmacological effectiveness of prolonged methylprednisolone treatment in unresolving ARDS. Chest 1999; 116: S116-118.

406. Amato MB et al. Effect of protective-ventilation strategy on mortality in the acute respiratory distress syndrome. New England Journal of Medicine 1998; 338: 347-54.

407. ARDS Network. Ventilation with lower tidal volumes as compared with traditional tidal volumes for acute lung injury and the acute respiratory distress syndrome. New England Journal of Medicine 2000; 342: 1301-8

408. Bellomo R et al. Low-dose dopamine in patients with early renal dusfunction: a placebo-controlled randomised trial (ANZICS Clinical Trial Group). Lancet 2000; 356: 2139-43

409. https://www.bjaed.org/article/S2058-5349(19)30153-2/fulltext

410. https://www.anesthesiaconsiderations.com/siadh

411. R.A. Leslie, E.K. Johnson, G. Thomas, and A.P.L. Goodwin, (2011). Anaemia and abnormal haemoglobins. Dr Podcast Scripts for the Final FRCA (pp. 109 – 114). Cambridge University Press, New York, USA.

412. J. Barker, S. Maguire, S. Mills et al., (2009). Sickle cell. The Clinical Anaesthesia Viva Book Second edition.(pp. 224 – 227). New York, USA: Cambridge University Press.

413. https://pubmed.ncbi.nlm.nih.gov/20861423/

414. https://www.spine-health.com/treatment/injections/lumbar-epidural-steroid-injections-low-back-pain-and-sciatica

415. https://www.frca.co.uk/Documents/256%20Stellate%20Ganglion%20Block.pdf

416. Danchenko N, Satia JA, Anthony MS. Epidemiology of sys- temic lupus erythematosus: A comparison of worldwide disease burden. Lupus 2006;15:308–18

417. Masi AT, Kaslow RA. Sex effects in systemic lupus erythemato- sus: A clue to pathogenesis. Arthritis Rheum 1978;21:480–4

418. Gaubitz M. Epidemiology of connective tissue disorders. Rheumatology 2006;45S:iii3–4

419. Kasitanon N, Magder LS, Petri M. Predictors of survival in systemic lupus erythematosus. Med (Baltimore) 2006;85:147–56

420. https://www.dvm360.com/view/anesthetic-monitoring-savvy

421. T. E. Peck, and S. A. Hill, (2014). Central nervous system. Pharmacology for Anaesthesia and Intensive Care. (FOURTH EDITION) (pp. 257 – 270). University of Cambridge, United Kingdom.

422. R. A. Leslie, E. K. Johnson, and A. P. L. Goodwin, (2011). Drugs acting on the central nervous system. Dr Podcast Scripts for the Primary FRCA (pp. 216– 223). Cambridge University Press, United Kingdom.

423. R.A. Leslie, E.K. Johnson, G. Thomas, and A.P.L. Goodwin, (2011). Management of acute spinal cord injury. Dr Podcast Scripts for the Final FRCA (pp. 254 – 258) Cambridge University Press, New York, USA.

424. R.A. Leslie, E.K. Johnson, G. Thomas, and A.P.L. Goodwin, (2011). Late management of patients with spinal cord injury.Dr Podcast Scripts for the Final FRCA (pp. 258 – 264). Cambridge University Press, New York, USA.

425. G. Edward Morgan, Maged. S Mikhail, and Michael J. Murray. (2006, 2002). Anesthesia for the Trauma Patient. Clinical Anesthesiology Fourth edition (pp. 861 – 874). New York, Chicago, San Francisco, Lisbon, London, Madrid, Mexico City, Milan, New Delhi, San Juan, Seoul, Sydney, and Toronto: Lange Medical Books/McGraw-Hill - Medical Publishing Division.

426. J. Barker, S. Maguire, S. Mills et al., (2009). Trauma. The Clinical Anaesthesia Viva Book Second edition. (pp. 248 – 250).New York, USA: Cambridge University Press.

427. https://www.ncbi.nlm.nih.gov/pmc/articles/PMC5874464/

428. https://pubmed.ncbi.nlm.nih.gov/32529139/

429. https://pubmed.ncbi.nlm.nih.gov/23089505/

430. https://anesthesia.ucsf.edu/clinical-resources/tracheoesophageal-fistula-tef

431. Jackson C. Tracheostomy. Laryngoscope 1909; 19: 285-90

432. Terragni P, Antonelli M, Fumagalli R, Faggiano C, Berardino M, Pallavicini FB et al. Early vs late tracheotomy for prevention of pneumonia in mechanically ventilated adult ICU patients: a randomized controlled trial. JAMA. Apr 21 2010;303(15):1483-9

433. Scales D, Thiruchelvam D, Kiss A, Redelmeier DA. The effect of tracheostomy timing during critical illness on long-term survival. Crit Care Med. Sep 2008;36(9):2547-57

434. TRACMAN study. http://www.pslgroup.com/dg/2361ee.htm

435. Ciaglia P, Firsching R, Syniec C. Elective percutaneous dilatational

tracheostomy. A new simple bedside procedure; preliminary report. Chest. Jun 1985; 87: 715-9

436. Byhahn C, Wilke H, Halbig S, Lischke V, Westphal K. Percutaneous tracheostomy: Ciaglia blue rhino versus the basic Ciaglia technique of percutaneous dilational tracheostomy. AnesthAnalg. Oct 2000; 91:882-6

437. Standards for the Care of Adult Patients with Temporary Tracheostomy. Standards and Guidelines. The Intensive Care Society, July 2008

438. Trottier SJ, Hazard PB, Sakabu SA, Levine JH, Troop BR, Thompson JAet al. Posterior tracheal wall perforation during percutaneous dilatational tracheostomy. Chest 1999; 115:1383-9

439. Kost KM. Endoscopic percutaneous dilatational tracheotomy: a prospective evaluation of 500 consecutive cases. Laryngoscope. Oct 2005;115:1-30

440. Cook T, Woodall N, Frerk C. Major Complications of Airway Management in the United Kingdom. National Audit Project 4. The Royal College of Anaesthetists and the Difficult Airway Society. March 2011.

441. https://emedicine.medscape.com/article/1413327-technique

442. 1. Hahn RG et al. Fluid absorption in endoscopic surgery. Br J Anaesth 2006;96:8-20

443. 2. Hahn RG et al. Relations between irrigant absorption rate and hyponatraemia during transurethral resection of the prostate. Acta Anaesthesiol Scand 1988;32:53-60

444. 3. Arieff et al. Endometrial ablation complicated by fatal hyponatraemic encephalopathy. JAMA 1993;270:1230-2

445. 4. Gravenstein D. Transurethral resection of the prostate (TURP) syndrome: a review of the pathophysiology and management. Anaesth Analg 1997;84:438-46

446. 5. O'Donnell AM, Foo ITH. Anaesthesia for transurethral resection of the prostate. Continuing Education in Anaesthesia, Critical Care & Pain 2009;9:92-6

447. 6. Roos NP et al. Mortality and reoperation after open and transurethral resection of the prostate for benign prostatic hyperplasia. NEJM 1989;320:1120-4

448. https://www.frca.co.uk/Documents/155%20Anaesthesia%20for%20 Transurethral%20resection%20of%20the%20prostate%20(TURP). pdf

449. https://pubmed.ncbi.nlm.nih.gov/17881218/

450. https://www.ncbi.nlm.nih.gov/pmc/articles/PMC4024692/

451. . Multz AS, Aldrich TK, Prezant DJ, et al. Maximal inspiratory pressure is not a reliable test of inspiratory muscle strength in mechanically ventilated patients. Am Rev Respir Dis1990;142:529–32.

452. https://thorax.bmj.com/content/57/11/986? cf_chl_jschl_tk =pR9xAAUcjjCGEiXjoGfKFoVhixEl4Onpff2nTS314ZU-1641554023-0-gaNycGzNDVE

453. . Fauci AS, Haynes BF, Ketz P, Wollf SM. Wegener's granulomatosis, Prospective clinical and therapeutic experience with 85 patients for 21

years. Ann Intern Med. 1983;98:76–85.http://dx.doi.org/10.7326/0003-4819-98-1-76. [PubMed] [Google Scholar]

454. Rodrigues CE, Callado MR, Nobre CA, Moura FE, Vieira RM, de Albuquerque LA, et al. Wegener's granulomatosis: prevalence of the initial clinical manifestations-report of six cases and review of the literature. Rev Bras Reumatol. 2010;50:150–64.http://dx.doi.org/10.1590/S0482-50042010000200005. [PubMed] [Google Scholar]

455. https://www.ncbi.nlm.nih.gov/pmc/articles/PMC4894140/

456. https://www.acls.net/aclsalg?gclid=CjwKCAiA5t-OBhByEiwAhR-hm0iKniQl4CYcsb3USdFpfXwFWAkCNEQPSxzAHPpiOjw_Burn2XhqWhoCiAUQAvD_BwE

457. 459. https://www.chelwest.nhs.uk/your-visit/patient-leaflets/surgery-services/nerve-blocks-for-hand-surgery

Made in the USA
Monee, IL
05 November 2026

67808871R00120